Health Visiting

Health Visiting

A Rediscovery

Third Edition

Edited by

Karen A. Luker

FMedSci, PhD, BNurs, SCPHN (HV), NDNCert
QNI Professor of Community Nursing
School of Nursing, Midwifery and Social Work
The University of Manchester
Manchester, UK

Jean Orr

CBE, MSc, BA, HV Cert
Emeritus Professor of Nursing
Queen's University Belfast
Belfast, UK

Gretl A. McHugh

PhD, MSc (Public Health), BNurs (Hons), RN, SCPHN (HV)
Senior Lecturer
School of Nursing, Midwifery and Social Work
The University of Manchester
Manchester, UK

⊛WILEY-BLACKWELL

A John Wiley & Sons, Ltd., Publication

Registered Office
John Wiley & Sons, Ltd, The Atrium, Southern Gate, Chichester, West Sussex, PO19 8SQ, UK

Editorial Offices
9600 Garsington Road, Oxford, OX4 2DQ, UK
The Atrium, Southern Gate, Chichester, West Sussex, PO19 8SQ, UK
111 River Street, Hoboken, NJ 07030-5774, USA

For details of our global editorial offices, for customer services and for information about how to apply for permission to reuse the copyright material in this book please see our website at www.wiley.com/wiley-blackwell.

Library of Congress Cataloging-in-Publication Data
Health visiting : a rediscovery / edited by Karen A. Luker, Jean Orr, Gretl A. McHugh.
- 3rd ed.
    p. ; cm.
  Includes bibliographical references and index.
  ISBN-13: 978-1-4443-3581-1 (pbk. : alk. paper)
  ISBN-10: 1-4443-3581-2
I. Luker, Karen A.   II. Orr, Jean.   III. McHugh, Gretl A.
[DNLM: 1. Community Health Nursing–Great Britain.   2. Evidence-Based
Nursing–Great Britain. WY 106]
LC classification not assigned
  610.73'43–dc23

                                        2011030348

A catalogue record for this book is available from the British Library.

Wiley also publishes its books in a variety of electronic formats. Some content that appears in print may not be available in electronic books.

Set in 9/12.5pt Interstate by SPi Publisher Services, Pondicherry, India
Printed and bound in Malaysia by Vivar Printing Sdn Bhd

1   2012

Contents

List of Contributors   ix

Introduction   1

1 Managing Knowledge in Health Visiting   9
Kate Robinson

Introduction   9
Defining health visiting practice   11
What do health visitors do – and where do they do it?   12
Evidence-based medicine   16
The current landscape of evidence-based practice   22
    Refuting evidence-based practice   22
    So does it work – and if not, why not?   24
    Redefining evidence-based practice   25
Managing knowledge and evidence in practice   27
    Case study 1.1: National policy-making in relation
    to inequalities in health   27
    Case study 1.2: Introducing new technology   28
    Case study 1.3: Creating guidelines in primary care   30
    Case study 1.4: Protocol-based decision-making in nursing   31
    Case study 1.5: Knowledge management in primary care   32
    Lessons from the case studies   33
Communities of practice   35
Reflective practice   37
Clients: what do they know and how do they know it?   40
    Social networking sites   41
The debate   44
Summary   46
References   46
Appendix 1: Activities for Chapter 1   49

2 Health Visiting: Context and Public Health Practice   52
Martin Smith and Maria Horne

Introduction   52
Public health   55
    Defining public   55
    Defining health   56

Defining public health   58
Human rights and public health   62
The principles of health visiting   66
   The search for health needs   66
   The stimulation of an awareness of health needs 67
   The influence on policies affecting health   68
   The facilitation of health enhancing activities 69
Health inequalities   71
Summary   78
References   79
Appendix 2: Activities for Chapter 2   83

3 The Community Dimension   **85**
Rosamund Bryar and Jean Orr

Introduction   85
Defining community   86
Impact of communities on health   89
The role of health visitors with communities   94
Gaining an understanding of the health of your
local community   101
   Windshield survey   102
   Public health walk   102
   Health needs assessment   103
Using health promotion models to support community working   110
Summary   113
References   113
Appendix 3: Activities for Chapter 3   117

4 Approaches to Supporting Families   **120**
Karen I. Chalmers

Introduction   120
Models of intervention in family life   121
   Three models relevant to health visiting practice
   in families with young children   122
   Application of models in practice   125
Policies   126
Evidence for interventions to support families   128
Characteristics of programmes to support families
with young children   129
Early home visiting programmes   130
Current home visiting programmes   132
   Family Nurse Partnership Programme   132
   Flying Start - Wales   136
   Starting Well - Scotland   137
   The Triple - P Programme - Positive Parenting Programme   139

    Sure Start Programmes   140
Working with families   145
    Empirical evidence on relationship development   147
Challenges   149
    Public health agenda   149
    Level of evidence   150
    Adhering to the programme criteria   150
    High needs families   151
    Practice specialisation   151
    Concerns about child safety   152
    Adequate resources   152
Summary   153
References   153
Appendix 4: Activities for Chapter 4   160

5 Safeguarding Children: Debates and Dilemmas for Health Visitors   **163**
Julianne Harlow and Martin Smith

Introduction   163
The key concepts   165
    Defining child   165
    Defining childhood   167
    Defining safeguarding   168
    Defining child abuse   173
    Defining significant harm   179
Incidence and prevalence of child abuse   182
Assessment of vulnerable children   186
    The Framework for the Assessment of Children in Need and Their Families   186
    Common Assessment Framework (CAF)   188
    Graded Care Profile   190
Working together   190
    Confidentiality and information sharing   192
    Supervision   193
Summary   197
References   198
Appendix 5: Activities for Chapter 5   202

6 Evaluating Practice   **205**
Karen A. Luker and Gretl A. McHugh

Introduction   205
Sources of evidence   206
Evaluation - the problem of definition   209
    Conceptualising evaluation   210
The care planning process   214

Actual and potential problems 215
Evaluation and evaluative research 217
Evaluation of healthcare 218
Structure, process and outcome evaluation 219
Additional issues in evaluating the practice of health visiting 227
Record-keeping 231
Problem-orientated recording 232
Summary 235
References 236
Appendix 6: Activities for Chapter 6 239

Bibliography 243
Index 266

List of Contributors

Professor Rosamund Bryar FQNI, PhD, Cert Ed (FE), MPhil, BNurs, RN, SCPHN
(HV), NDNCert, SCM
Professor of Community and Primary Care Nursing
School of Health Sciences
City University London
London, UK

Professor Karen I. Chalmers PhD, MSc(A), BScN, RN
Honorary Professor
School of Nursing, Midwifery and Social Work
The University of Manchester
Manchester, UK

Ms Julianne Harlow MA, BSc(Hons), PGCE, SCPHN-HV(T), RN
Senior Lecturer
Health and Social Care
Faculty of Well-Being and Social Sciences
University of Bolton
Bolton, UK

Dr Maria Horne PhD, MA, BA(Hons), Dip Community Health Studies,
SCPHN (HV), SCM, RN
Health Visiting Lecturer
School of Nursing Midwifery and Social Work
The University of Manchester
Manchester, UK

Professor Karen A. Luker FMedSci, PhD, BNurs, SCPHN (HV), NDNCert.
QNI Professor of Community Nursing
School of Nursing Midwifery and Social Work
The University of Manchester
Manchester, UK

Dr Gretl A. McHugh PhD, MSc (Public Health), BNurs (Hons), RN, SCPHN (HV)
Senior Lecturer
School of Nursing Midwifery and Social Work
The University of Manchester
Manchester, UK

Professor Jean Orr CBE, MSc, BA, HV Cert
Emeritus Professor of Nursing
Queen's University Belfast
Belfast, UK

Professor Kate Robinson PhD, BA, RN, SCPHN (HV)
Professor Emeritus
University of Bedfordshire
Luton, UK

Mr Martin Smith MPH, MFPH, PGCert HEd, FHEA, BA(Hons), DipHV,
SCPHN-HV(T), RN
Specialty Registrar-Public Health
Mersey Deanery School of Public Health
Liverpool, UK

Introduction

Karen A. Luker and Gretl A. McHugh

The University of Manchester
Manchester, UK

Over two decades have passed since the publication in 1992 of the Second Edition of *Health Visiting: Towards Community Health Nursing* and there have been numerous challenges and developments within the National Health Service (NHS), social care and nurse education in the intervening years.

In brief, the role of the nurse has been strengthened both in primary and secondary care by the redrawing of the boundaries between medical and nursing work (for example, nurse prescribing). New careers for nurses have emerged such as, nurse consultants, community matrons, specialist nurses and nonmedical public health specialists. These developments have enabled the nursing profession to have an impact on shaping and developing services for the public.

Skill mix has enabled the refocusing of some roles, for example the building of teams and closer collaborative working among health professionals. Teamwork, with the goal of providing a comprehensive service has been a particular development within the community; with health visiting teams consisting of community staff nurses, nursery nurses, trainee assistant practitioners (TAPs), bilingual support workers and clerical staff.

The health visiting profession is 150 years old in 2012 and the changes and developments in the profession have been immense, and some more welcome than others. A noteworthy change for health visitors was the dissolution of the United Kingdom Central Council for Nursing, Midwifery and Health Visiting (UKCC) (and the four National Boards for England, Northern Ireland, Scotland and Wales) and its replacement in 2002 by the Nursing and Midwifery Council (NMC). The removal of the health visiting profession from statute in 2001 (removing any legal status) and closure of the professional register in 2004

Health Visiting: A Rediscovery, Third Edition. Edited by Karen A. Luker, Jean Orr and Gretl A. McHugh.
© 2012 Blackwell Publishing Ltd. Published 2012 by Blackwell Publishing Ltd.

(ceasing NMC regulation) has been seen as detrimental to the profession and one in which the professional organisation, the Community Practitioners' and Health Visitors' Association (CPHVA), has been lobbying to get reinstated (Unite/CPHVA, 2010). Health visitors considered that with this loss of statute the importance of their work had been overlooked. Health visiting is included as part of the Specialist Community Public Health Nursing (SCPHN) section of the NMC register. The NMC sets standards of education, training and conduct in nursing and midwifery in the UK, including proficiency for SCPHNs to ensure the maintenance of high standards within this specialist area (NMC, 2004) and these standards are currently being reviewed.

During the last ten years the NHS has been continually changing and improving, but when there is a change of the government, there is often a new strategic vision and new challenges for health professionals working in the NHS. The latest NHS plan (DH, 2010a) sets out a number of radical changes in both the organisation and delivery of services for the NHS. The vision is for the commissioning of services to be organised by health professionals closest to the patient and work has begun on the establishment of General Practice (GP) consortia, and this will be the mechanism which supersedes Primary Care Trusts (PCTs) in England to purchase some specialist and secondary care. In addition, there will be an independent NHS Commissioning Board, which will ensure that resources are allocated and accounted for in pursuit of defined health outcomes. The NHS Commissioning Board will tackle inequalities in access to health and lead on quality improvement (DH, 2010a). Organisational changes have been made with the aim of improving the quality of service for patients and similar developments are occurring in Wales, Northern Ireland and Scotland.

Until recently in England, health visitors have been employed by Primary Care Trusts (PCTs) and some now will become employed by the NHS Foundation Hospital Trusts until GP consortia and local authority responsibilities become clearer. It is likely that services for nought to five year olds (including health visiting) will be commissioned by the NHS Commissioning Board which will have some commissioning responsibilities on behalf of Public Health England. Whatever the commissioning arrangements turn out to be the government has pledged to ensure that more disadvantaged families receive intensive support from the health visiting service. In Scotland, health visitors are employed by one of the 14 area NHS boards, usually within Community Health Partnerships (CHPs) of Child, Family and Public Health Services. Following a review of community nurses in Scotland in 2009 there has been resistance to replacing health visitors with a generic community nursing role and this opposition has been successful in keeping the distinctive health visiting/public health role in Scotland. In Wales, the NHS underwent changes in 2009 and established seven Local Health Boards (LHBs) where health visitors are employed. In addition Public Health Wales is a new NHS trust and responsible for delivering a public health services to each of the seven LHBs. Northern Ireland has a combined health and social care structure with five Health and Social Care Trusts where health visitors are employed but its health visiting services are being modernised in line with the rest of the UK.

The government's vision of a patient-centred NHS, with more patient involvement and choice will require nurses/health visitors to work with and to support patients, clients and families with health care decisions. The emphasis is on self-care and on encouraging individuals to be responsible for their own health, a focus which is central to the work of health visitors.

Role of the health visitor

There has always been much debate around the health visitor's role, but over the last decade or more there has been an apparent shift away from the preventive role to one with a focus on child protection and safeguarding children issues. The public health role of the health visitor has never reached its full potential. There is a shortage of health visitors and many areas of the United Kingdom (UK) focus on 'crisis visiting', rather than delivering a broad range of health visiting services. The health visitor has always been seen as the key health professional for the under fives, offering a universal service in line with policy requirements (DH, 2009). There is a renewed recognition that the traditional work of the health visitor is important and the government is investing in training an additional 6000 health visitors to have 4200 new health visitors in place by 2015 (DH, 2011). The title of this Third Edition (*Health Visiting: A Rediscovery*) reflects this initiative.

Health visitors are continuing to be seen as the lead professional for children under five and their families in the delivery of a Universal Child Health Service, in line with the Healthy Child Programme (HCP) (DH, 2009). This HCP sets out the programme of health development reviews, screening, immunisation etc, using the evidence base of the revised *Health for All Children* report (Hall & Elliman, 2006). The specialist skills and knowledge which health visitors have working with families and communities has been recognised with the new service vision of health visiting being involved in:

- improving public health;
- developing community resources;
- maximising family resources (supporting families);
- bridging family services and primary healthcare services;
- accessing specialist services (DH, 2010b).

There will be an emphasis on health visitors, providing family health services, with more contacts and additional tailored packages of care and support where required.

Vision for public health

It is of interest that for England public health leadership will be returned once again to local authority, placing public health specialists alongside environmental health and housing. Directors of Public Health (DPH) will provide the strategic leadership for tackling health inequalities. There will be an established professional public health service 'Public Health England' which will be part of the Department of Health. The purpose of this service is to strengthen the response to health protection and national emergencies, for example a flu pandemic. By 2012, Public Health England will have assumed the responsibilities and powers of the Health Protection Agency (HPA) and National Treatment Agency for Substance Misuse (NTA) (DH, 2010c). Whether health visitors in some parts of the UK will also return to employment under the local authorities, where historically they were established, is not yet clear.

The envisaged public health role of the health visitor has never reached its full potential and there are probably several reasons for this. The declining number of full-time equivalent (FTE) health visitors, is one possible reason. Since 2005 health visitors have declined by nearly 2000 (DH, 2011). Even if we look at data over a 12-month period from October 2009 to October 2010, the number of FTE health visitors dropped from 8262 to 8098 (NHS Information Centre, 2011). In addition the increased health visitor's role in child protection and safeguarding children involving multi-agency working is time consuming and leaves little time for other work.

Health visitors are one of the few health professionals who receive training in public health. Because of the planned increase in numbers of health visitors and with public health high on the government's priorities there will be a renewed attempt to get health visitors involved in the public health agenda. Health visitors have played a key role in health needs assessment (HNAs) and community profiling. The reaffirmation of the public health role of the health visitor in recent policy (DH, 2010c, 2011) places them in a key position to improve health outcomes. Health visitors have a role in helping communities to improve their health and well-being for example, in increasing immunisation uptake, reducing obesity and tackling health inequalities.

The number of public health priorities which need to be tackled (DH, 2010c) are growing and lifestyle consequences such as obesity and substance misuse are highly prevalent. The Public Health White Paper (DH, 2010c) takes into account the Marmot Report, *Fair Society, Healthy Lives* (Marmot et al., 2010) for setting out its framework for tackling the wider social determinants of health. Marmot et al. (2010) state that health inequalities will require action on:

- giving every child the best start in life;
- enabling all children young people and adults to maximise their capabilities and have control over their lives;
- creating fair employment and good work for all;
- ensuring healthy standard of living for all;
- creating and developing healthy and sustainable places and communities;
- strengthening the role and impact of ill health prevention.

There is recognition that determinants of health often do not fall within the remit of the NHS and therefore partnership and local area agreements for tackling some issues: for example, teenage pregnancies and smoking are a necessity. The established Association of Public Health Observatories (APHO) has provided some of the infrastructure needed in public health. The APHO represents a network of 12 public health observatories (PHOs), working across the UK and the Republic of Ireland. The PHOs are key to providing information and data about people's health and health care.

Health visitors have always been in a position to work with families early on in the ante-natal and postnatal period assisting parents with providing children with the best start in life. The preventative health care aspect of the health visitors' role needs to be recognised as important if work is to extend beyond crisis visiting. Health promotion and assessing the health needs of the community, including understanding and interpreting health data are necessary skills even in undergraduate nurse education, which is now the norm, given by 2012, nursing will be a graduate entry profession.

Working with communities

The focus on communities is very much a part of the government's agenda, with the 'Big Society' and one of the key priorities is to empower communities, with plans for groups or volunteer associations to run organisations such as children's centres, libraries etc. In the *Health Visitor Implementation Plan 2011-2015*, we see that health visitors will have a role in building community capacity so that families and communities help develop new ways of providing services as part of the Big Society (DH, 2011). It is important that health visitors with their knowledge of the community undertake such things as HNAs and contribute to joint strategic needs assessment (JSNA) (DH, 2007), which help plan services more efficiency and effectively for the health and wellbeing of the local community.

New edition

The First and Second Editions of this book were well received and were reprinted several times and became the leading text for health visitor courses. Twenty years has passed since the Second Edition and it has to be said that the promise of moving towards community health nursing has not yet been realised. This new edition is called *Health Visiting: A Rediscovery*, and the health visitor is being placed once again at the forefront of supporting and working with children and families, ensuring the child has the best possible start in life. Public health now has a more distinctive place in the NHS agenda since it is one route into mediating inequalities that adversely affect the health and wellbeing of the population. It is therefore our expectation that health visitors will be able to realise and enhance their public health function.

This is an ideal time to launch this Third Edition. The structure of the book is similar to the other editions, however the content has changed considerably from the last edition. This change has been necessary to keep pace with the developments in health policy, public health priorities and health visiting practice. The chapter on information technology and role of the health visitor has been replaced with a chapter on safeguarding children. This is because

'NHS Connecting for Health', which maintains and develops the information technology infrastructure is continually evolving with new developments, such as the electronic health record and writings in this area would become quickly out of date. With the central role that health visitors have with child protection, a chapter on safeguarding children is an important addition to this Third Edition. There are some new authors for this edition, some who are teaching public health and health visiting and others who are practising as public health specialists, ensuring that this Third Edition is relevant to meet the needs of those training to become health visitors and those who are practitioners working with and in the community.

Chapter 1, 'Managing Knowledge in Health Visiting', previously examined the nature of knowledge and practice of working in the community and in some senses the material included was futuristic and has not been superseded. However, with the emphasis and importance of evidence-based practice, this chapter explores the concept of managing knowledge in health visiting. The concept of evidence-based practice is debated with reference to case studies. The demands on the health visitor to understand the different forms and sources of knowledge in order to ensure the delivery of evidence-based practice is discussed. The issues surrounding use of guidelines and protocols in practice are highlighted. The concept of communities of practice (CoP) is debated as to how they can assist practitioners in working to improve their own practice. In addition generating and managing knowledge in practice using reflective practice is discussed before moving on to the perspective of the clients in terms of what they know and how they know it, drawing attention to the use of social networking sites.

Chapter 2, 'Health Visiting: Context and Public Health Practice', which previously focused on health visiting and the community (some of which is now covered in Chapter 3) explores the specialist and public health role of the health visitor in working with families. It examines the tensions between the demands of the health visiting role with children and families and the public health role. The public health role of the health visitor needs to become more clearly defined with a focus on reducing health inequalities and giving every child in the community the best start in life (Marmot *et al.*, 2010) and this is explored in the section specifically about 'Health inequalities'. This chapter also examines the evidence for health inequities and the contribution health visitors can bring in addressing the wider determinants of health. However, it highlights the importance of good leadership in public health and challenges for health visitors in engaging with a public health role.

Chapter 3, 'The Community Dimension', discusses the concept of 'community' (some of which was covered in the previous edition in Chapter 2) but also explores the current role that health visitors have in identifying and assessing the health needs of the community using health needs assessment rather than the Second Edition's focus on community health profiling, which is no longer routinely used. It focuses on understanding the social determinants of health and explores the theory supporting community working and the skills required for community level work, including how to measure community participation within a locality. With the renewed focus on working with communities, this chapter will provide health visitors with the knowledge and understanding to participate in building community capacity.

Chapter 4, 'Approaches to Supporting Families', previously looked at assessing individual and family health needs, with a discussion of models of interventions in family life which were topical in the 1980-'90s. This new chapter explores the approaches to supporting families and evaluates several child health programmes which are currently in existence. The evidence for successful health visiting interventions to support families, such as the family nurse partnership (FNP), is discussed. The FNP is advocated by the government and provides intensive support and structured visiting. The government has recognised the need for more Family Partnership Nurses delivering this programme to vulnerable first-time young parents from early pregnancy till the child is two years of age and this is being promoted currently. The competing challenges faced by health visitors such as the public health agenda, the level of evidence, and adequate resources in trying to work with these families are debated.

Chapter 5, 'Safeguarding Children: Debates and Dilemmas for Health Visitors', is a welcome addition to this book and replaces the previous chapter on information technology. This new chapter focuses on safeguarding and the enhanced child protection role of the health visitor. The key concepts such as child abuse and significant harm are defined, including highlighting the incidence and prevalence of child abuse. The assessment of vulnerable children using the common assessment framework (CAF) and the graded care profile (GCP) for neglect are discussed. There is a debate on the issues and dilemmas around safeguarding children faced by health visitors and which students may encounter through their practice. Child abuse is a public health issue and the value of the health visitor in safeguarding children is clearly recognised.

Chapter 6, 'Evaluating Practice', was always ahead of its time in previous editions, in so far as everyday health visitors seldom formally evaluate the impact of their work. This chapter has been updated and explores the importance of evaluation in health visiting practice which is a necessity in today's economy, to ensure what health visitors are doing is effective and of value. The tools and sources of information which are now more readily available and will assist health visitors in their clinical practice are described. It is important to ensure that health visitors and other practitioners have the skills and knowledge to identify and critique the available evidence and information in their role in supporting families and communities. Health visitors need knowledge about where to get the best information and the skills to be able to access up-to-date resources, for the delivery of evidence-based practice and this chapter goes some way towards providing this.

New for this Third Edition, for each of the chapters are learning activities referred to throughout and details are found in the Appendices at the end of each chapter. It is anticipated that these activities will help students, health visitors and others to reflect and develop their practice further.

There are many challenges that health visitors will face over the coming years but the vision for high-quality care and improving service provision for individuals and their families makes it an exciting time in health visiting. We hope that this new edition will assist with the 'rediscovery' of health visiting and the contribution health visitors can make to the health and wellbeing of children, families and communities which will ultimately have an impact on achieving better outcomes for health.

References

Department of Health (2007) *Guidance on Joint Strategic Needs Assessment*. Department of Health, London.

Department of Health (2009) *Healthy Child Programme: Pregnancy and the First Five Years of Life*. Department of Health, London.

Department of Health (2010a) *Equity and Excellence: Liberating the NHS*. Department of Health, London.

Department of Health (2010b) *Service Vision for Health Visiting in England*. CPHVA conference, 20–22 October 2010. DH, London.

Department of Health (2010c) *White Paper – Health Lives, Healthy People: Our Strategy for Public Health in England*. Department of Health, London.

Department of Health (2011) *Health Visitor Implementation Plan 2011-15: A Call to Action February 2011*. Department of Health, London.

Hall, D.M.B. & Elliman, D. (2006) *Health for All Children*, 4th edition, revised. Oxford University Press, Oxford.

Marmot, M., Atkinson, T., Bell, J., *et al.* (2010) *Fair Society, Healthy Lives. The Marmot Review*, Marmot Review Team, University College London.

NHS The Information Centre Workforce and Facilities Team (2011) *NHS Hospital and Community Health Services Workforce Statistics in England*. The Health and Social Care Information Centre, London.

Nursing & Midwifery Council (2004) *Standards of Proficiency for Specialist Community Public Health Nurses*. NMC, London.

Unite/CPHVA (2010) *Professional Briefing: Public Safety and Statutory Regulation of Health Visiting*. Unite/CPHVA, London.

1

Managing Knowledge in Health Visiting

Kate Robinson
University of Bedfordshire, Luton, UK

Introduction

The mantra of evidence-based practice is now heard everywhere in health-care. This chapter will explore what it might mean, both theoretically and in the context of everyday health visiting practice. Is it a way of enhancing the effectiveness of practice or yet another part of the new managerialism of guidelines, targets, and effectiveness? Why might evidence-based practice be an important ideal? Arguably, when a practitioner intervenes in a client's life the outcome should be that the client is significantly advantaged. In health visiting that advantage could take many forms – the client could have more and better knowledge, they might feel more capable of managing their affairs, they might better understand and cope with difficult thoughts, feelings and actions – the list is extensive and later chapters will detail the ways in which health visiting can lead to better outcomes for clients and communities. However, the proposition that there should be an advantage derived from the practitioner's intervention is particularly important in the context of a state financed – i.e. taxpayer funded – healthcare system. If an individual wishes to spend their money on treatments or therapies of dubious or unexplored value offered by unregulated practitioners, then that is entirely a matter for them, provided that they have not been mislead or missold! However, when the state decides to invest its resources in the development of a particular service and associated interventions then arguably there has to be some level of evidence or collective informed agreement which gives confidence that the choice is justified. In addition, of course, all health visitors must be able to account for what she/he does and doesn't do to the Nursing and Midwifery Council (NMC), if required.

Health Visiting: A Rediscovery, Third Edition. Edited by Karen A. Luker, Jean Orr and Gretl A. McHugh.
© 2012 Blackwell Publishing Ltd. Published 2012 by Blackwell Publishing Ltd.

Chapter 6 explores how health visiting might be assessed, measured and evaluated. Here the emphasis is on how we choose, individually or collectively, to develop particular services and perform particular actions which we know with some degree of certainty should lead to better outcomes for the client. But how do we know things with any certainty? How can we define the knowledge we need to make good choices? Although there are very many different ways of categorising or describing forms of knowledge, for our purpose here it will be sufficient to make some simple distinctions. First, knowledge can be categorised by type. For example, Carper's (1978) categorisation of knowledge as empirical (largely derived from science), aesthetic (or artistic), ethical and personal, is well known and used in nursing. Or we might categorise it by source and ask where it comes from - books, journals, other people, personal experience, etc.? Or we might use the simple but important distinction between knowing *that* and knowing *how* (McKenna *et al.*, 1999). For example, I can know that swimming pools are places people go to and engage in swimming and other water sports, although I need not have experienced it; I can only say I know how to swim if I can do it. In the case of the former I can probably explain how I came by that knowledge but in the case of the latter, I may not be able to explain how I know how to swim or what I am doing when swimming, but the knowledge statement *I know how to swim* is dispositional: its truth is determined by my ability to swim. Such 'knowing how' knowledge is sometimes called tacit knowledge, in contrast to explicit knowledge or knowing that. Our concern here is less about how theoretically you might define knowledge - that's really a question for philosophers - but about the question of what sort of knowledge *should* health visitors be using - and who says so - and what sort of knowledge *are* they using. You will not be surprised to know that there is substantial controversy as various factions argue that *their* type or source of knowledge is the most important. And the outcome of what might be argued to be a fight to define the 'proper' knowledge basis for practice is important as it has the potential to impinge directly on the health and safety of the client as well as the degree to which health visiting can be said to 'add value' to clients.

In later sections of this chapter we will look more closely at evidence-based practice, which is currently the dominant knowledge protocol in the NHS, and try to establish what forms of knowledge it valorises and why. The chapter will also look at reflective practice, an alternative protocol for generating and managing knowledge about practice which is supported by many institutions and individuals within nursing, and also the idea of knowledge being generated and managed within communities of practice, an idea which is currently more popular in education and some other public sector service organisations. Each of these can be viewed as a social movement with enthusiastic supporters trying to 'capture' the support of key health organisations and institutions, as well as the hearts and minds of individual practitioners. And we will also look at what is known about the types and sources of knowledge which healthcare practitioners actually use in practice - which proves to be somewhat different from any of the 'ideals' promoted by these social movements.

But before examining any of these 'ideal' types of knowledge management it will be useful to remind ourselves about the practice of health visiting. For evidence-based health visiting or reflective health visiting or any other imported concept to be a reality it must be integrated into the taken-for-granted, existing ways in which health visitors go about their business.

Defining health visiting practice

The review of health visiting, *Facing the Future* (Department of Health (DH), 2007), aims to highlight key areas of health visiting practice and skills. It is interesting to note that this is not a research-based document – and makes no claims to be, although there are some references to research. Rather, 'this review is informed by evidence, government policy and the views of many stakeholders' (DH, 2007: section 1). The decisions about what health visiting should be about are therefore largely presented as decisions for the community of stakeholders in the context of stated government priorities. Key elements of the decision-making process can be seen as pragmatic and commonsensical – in the best sense. For example, the review argues that the health visiting service should be one which someone will commission, i.e. pay for; it needs to be a supported by families and communities, i.e. is acceptable to the users of the service; and it needs to be attractive enough to secure a succession of new entrants, i.e. there will be a workforce of sufficient size and ability.

In terms of the future skills of health visitors, the review is clear that they will be expected to be able to translate evidence into practice – although it is less specific about what sort of evidence will count and how the process will be managed. However, at the national level it recommended that the relevant research findings to support a twenty-first-century child and family health service must be assembled. There is also some indication that future practice will be guided by clear protocols, 'Inconsistent service provision with individual interpretation' will be replaced by 'Planned, systematic and/or licensed programmes' (DH 2007: recommendation 8). As we shall see, the reduction in variations in practice is one of the key aims of the evidence-based practice movement. In terms of evidence underpinning practice, the document also draws specific attention to the expanding knowledge base in mental health promotion, the neurological development of young children, the effectiveness of early intervention and parenting programmes and health visiting. Clearly this is a very broad base of evidence derived from a range of academic and practice disciplines.

So, while the review (DH, 2007) is not about the evidence or knowledge base of health visiting and how it might be used, many of the relevant themes in debates about evidence-based practice begin to emerge, for example:

- What is the role of the practitioner in assembling and assessing evidence?
- How can evidence be translated into practice?
- What counts as evidence?
- How can other bodies support the practitioner by generating and assembling evidence?

- How can any practitioner be conversant with developing knowledge bases in a wide variety of other disciplines?
- What will be the role of protocols, guidelines and 'recipes' for practice?

A previous document on health visiting, the *Health Visiting Practice Development Resource Pack* (DH, 2001) raised similar issues, but perhaps gave more emphasise to the importance of evidence-based practice. It drew attention to national statements of 'good' practice such as the National Service Frameworks and suggested that health visitors should 'read widely, keep up to date and engage in debates about what does and doesn't work' (DH, 2001: 34). However, it is relatively silent on the debates and controversies surrounding evidence-based practice, which impinge directly on the possibility and effectiveness of individual practitioners relying on reading to keep up to date in the midst of an exploding healthcare literature.

What do health visitors do – and where do they do it?

However, before we examine how evidence can and should be used in health visiting practice it is important to consider the actual practice of health visiting; that is, what health visitors do on a day to day basis. Unfortunately, relatively little is known – other than by those who do it – about the realities of everyday health visiting practice. That such practice is rarely seen as a valid subject either for scientific research or practice narratives, is well expressed in a very exciting article about social work (Ferguson, 2010). He argues that current research is focused on systems and interprofessional communication, which: 'leaves largely unaddressed practitioners' experiences of the work they have to do that goes on beyond the office, on the street and in doing the home visit,' (Ferguson, 2010: 1100).

In his work he is trying to refocus on actual practice and further argues:

> Reclaiming this lost experience of movement, adventure, atmosphere and emotion is an important step in developing better understandings of what social workers can do, the risks and limits to their achievements, and provides for deeper learning about the skilled performances and successes that routinely go on.
>
> (Ferguson, 2010: 1102)

Of course, this is just as true for health visiting where a significant part of the practice is leaving the office, driving to the client, thinking about how the visit will work, knocking on the door, and so on. Ferguson's account of the excitement and fear of walking through disadvantaged neighbourhoods and of managing to negotiate home visits with disobliging clients is focused on social workers working in child protection, but it must resonate with all practising health visitors.

So how would the ever-useful sociological Martians describe health visiting practice? They would be bound to notice that health visiting practice is largely about doing things with words. Note the emphasis on *doing*; talk isn't just something which surrounds the doing, it *is* the doing – praising, blaming, asking, advising, persuading – every utterance is an action produced for a purpose, although the speaker is rarely consciously aware of this at the granular level. The skills involved in talking are so deep that, just like walking, they are not normally subject to constant on-going analysis. Most of us do not consciously think about how to walk – we just do it. But talk is the health visitors' key performative skill, and because doing things with talk is a primary skill, health visitors need a more profound understanding of how it works – just as a ballet dancer would need a more profound understanding of how her body works than the person taking the dog for a walk. Of course, as well as talking, health visitors also make notes and write reports but text is still doing things with language in order to interact with others, just like talk.

In the 1980s there was considerable interest within sociology in researching how interactions, largely based on talk, could constitute various forms of institutional practice. This idea was rather neatly defined in an edited volume of studies called 'Talk at Work'. The editors argue:

> that talk-in-interaction is the principal means through which lay persons pursue various practical goals and the central medium through which the daily working activities of many professionals and organisational representatives are conducted.
>
> (Drew & Heritage, 1992: 3)

Health visiting is one such profession and organisation. Within health visiting, the collection of audiotaped practice has allowed analysis of actual rather than reported practice. Both Robinson (1986) and Heritage and Sefi (1992) recorded the ostensibly 'private' world of health visiting in client homes (at the time it was considered that video recording home visits would be too intrusive, but subsequent work by Lomax and Robinson (1998) within midwifery showed that it was acceptable to practitioners and clients). Their analyses variously looked at entry and exit, topic initiation and story telling (Robinson, 1986) and the giving and receiving of advice (Heritage & Sefi, 1992) but the point to be made here is that the recordings showed that the visits are recognisable as relatively lengthy conversations with both the health visitor and client contributing. The key feature of any conversation is that each party 'takes a turn' and allows the others to do so. It is interesting to note that turn-taking is such a fundamental human skill that it is exhibited by very young babies and is one of the last skills to be lost by people with dementia – the ability to turn take is far deeper than the knowledge of the meaning of words. While the observation that health visitors and clients hold a conversation may seem obvious, contrast this with the rather more regulated style of client–GP interactions in the GP surgery (Heath, 1986) or the way in which classroom teachers may take extended turns and control how and whether pupils can speak (Delamont, 1976). Elements of the conversation could be typical of a non-professional conversation:

Mother (M):	My two little cousins there they were dying to see her weren't they and they were sort of hold[ing her [disturbing her
HV:	Mmm
Father (F):	[Five minutes each
M:	[Yeah
HV:	Oh you've got it down. Yes well done. Yes
M:	And um then it was a bit embarrassing that has to be said as dad says dad said it isn't sort of worse um going out of the room to do it
HV:	Um …

(Robinson, 1986: 107)

However, analysis of the relative distribution of the talk, and in particular the right to initiate and close down talk, showed how the health visitors use the framework of the conversation to achieve certain goals, thus turning it into a professional conversation. For example, extracts from Robinson's data showed how a different style could be introduced by the health visitor.

HV:	How are you feeding her
M:	Breast
HV:	And everything's all right. You're comfortable
M:	Yes
HV:	Lovely. Aren't you going to be a lovely mum
HV:	Yes. You're not on the phone here in the cottage are you
M:	(unclear response)
HV:	It's all right the first visit that I um just to go through the routine (…) things which I know mainly from what you've told me anyway which is um just to see what the labour's like um just to fill in these little bits …

(Robinson, 1986: 99)

Here the health visitor imposes an interrogatory form on the interaction but, interestingly, feels that it requires an explanation 'It's all right …' because it breaches the conversational norm. However, other extracts show how the client need not follow the lead of the health visitor. The health visitors used the devices of making polite but inconsequential remarks about the baby (or occasionally the family pet) and not taking their turn to speak (the figures in brackets are seconds of silence and in conversational talk prolonged silence is unusual and noticeable) to try to encourage the mother to initiate talk about topics of importance to her, but it rarely worked and the health visitors had to fall back on their list of potential problems:

Example 1

HV:	… except it won't be Christmas day. (2.5) She's blowing raspberries (laughs)
F:	She's found herself already.
HV:	Has she (1.5) She's very alert isn't she. She's following round. (5.0) Lovely any rashes or anything anywhere

Example 2

> HV: Yes hello. You are having a good look round. (3.0) Yes. Did you get sore
> having to feed her nonstop (0.5) yesterday morning.

Example 3

> HV: … One day you'll look for it and find it's not there. Yes. Anyway you're beautiful
> aren't you. (3.5) Is she good for you at night.
>
> (Robinson, 1986: 88, 91)

Note: in all cases the transcription has been simplified from the original. Each example refers to individual clients. It is useful for health visitors to consider their own interactions with clients and this is further explored in Activity 1.1 (see Appendix 1 at the end of the chapter).

The argument here is not that any of the talk is 'good' or 'bad'. The important point is that it shows how complex it is to use talk as a primary practice vehicle. Health visitors' common-sense knowledge of talk is fundamental to their practice but it is rarely fully acknowledged as a knowledge requirement for practice. Moreover, it could be argued that the relatively recent enthusiasm in many healthcare curricula for teaching 'communication skills' often fails to deal with the richness and complexity of institutional language use, especially in venues outside the formal control of the health system.

The above examples are samples of actual health visiting practice and provide evidence of the realities of practice within private homes in the context of mothers with new babies. They are evidence *about* health visiting. The fact that health visitors practise within people's homes is a significant defining characteristic of their work. While the issue of locality underpins all healthcare encounters, the home visit brings to the fore questions of the status of the home and the control of that space. Robinson (1986) showed how, in her sample, health visitors (rather than clients) managed both entry to and exit from the clients' homes. However, Luker and Chalmers (1990), using accounts of practice by health visitors, showed how the practitioners saw negotiating entry as problematic and occasionally difficult as can be seen in these extracts from respondents:

> The first time I went the older child was about four and I didn't actually get into the house because she met me coming up the garden path … she said 'we'd had no problems at all and I don't think I need a health visitor' …
>
> I knocked on the door on the 11th day and said 'hello, I'm the health visitor' and she sort of left me on the door step …
>
> (Luker & Chalmers, 1990: 76)

Health visitors also work in clinics, general practitioner (GP) surgeries, children's centres, church halls, social services departments, etc. So a further defining characteristic of health visiting is that it does not have a fixed locality or place of work. There is an interesting literature on the issue of place in healthcare (see, for example, Angus *et al.*, 2005; Poland *et al.*, 2005) and of course it relates to the issue of mobility which is central to Ferguson's (2010) work cited above. Poland *et al.* (2005) argue that, while practitioners are sensitive to issues of place, this has largely been ignored in debates about best practice and evidence-based practice. He argues that:

> Interventions wither or thrive based on complex interactions between key personalities, circumstances and coincidences … A detailed analysis of the setting … can help practitioners skilfully anticipate and navigate potentially murky waters filled with hidden obstacles.
>
> (Poland *et al.*, 2005: 171)

By 'place' Poland *et al.* (2005) mean a great deal more than mere geography. The concept includes a range of issues, notably the way power relationships are constructed and the way in which technologies operate in and on various places. Alaszewski (2006) draws our attention to the risk involved in practising outside 'the institution'. While there are ways in which physical institutions mitigate the risks from their clientele, it is different outside the institution:

> The institutional structure of classification, surveillance and control is significantly changed in the community. Much of the activity takes place within spaces that are not designed or controlled by professionals, for example the service user's own home.
>
> (Alaszewski, 2006: 4)

The accounts above show that everyday health visiting practice is not a simple enterprise. It is not always conducted in premises controlled by the state nor can health visitors wholly control the responses of clients. Indeed, the fact that health visitors themselves need to locate their clients sets the occupation apart from much of adult and children's nursing and places it alongside occupations such as social work and mental health nursing. So how can the concepts of knowledge management such as that of evidence-based practice fit into the everyday realities of health visiting practice – if at all? Or are there better ways for health visitors to manage their knowledge? First, what is evidence-based practice?

Evidence-based medicine

What has come to be known as evidence-based practice had its foundations in the evidence-based medicine (EBM) movement which started in the United Kingdom (UK) in the early 1990s. There was increasing dissatisfaction among some key individuals in the medical profession, notably (Dr (now Sir) Muir Gray, who was an NHS Regional Director of Research and Development) that, within medicine, treatments which had been proven to be effective were not being used. Similarly, treatments which had been shown to have no or little beneficial effect continued to be used despite considerable efforts to change practice. For example, the GRIPP project (Getting Research into Practice and Purchasing), which was developed in the Oxford NHS Region, looked at four treatments:

- the use of corticosteroids in preterm delivery;
- the management of services for stroke patients;
- the use of dilation and curettage (D&C) for dysfunctional uterine bleeding;
- insertion of grommets for children with glue ear.

Activity 1.2 (see Appendix 1 at the end of the chapter) enables further exploration of the evidence around interventions which health visitors deliver.

Good research evidence was available to underpin decisions in all these areas of practice and health authorities within the Oxford Region sought to ensure that practice adhered to the research-based recommendations. However, variations in practice proved difficult to eradicate and it was felt that more needed to be done. Did the practitioners not understand the research? Did they need motivating to change from their traditional ways of practice? Perhaps a more widespread and coordinated effort to base practice on research needed to be developed.

The fundamental proposition of the subsequent EBM movement was that practice should take account of the latest and best research generated evidence to underpin both individual clinical decision-making and collective policy-making. At its heart is the idea that EBM provides a vehicle by which the practitioner can continually examine and improve their individual practice by testing it against scientifically validated external evidence and importing proven treatments. Sackett *et al.* (1997) define EBM as consisting of five sequential steps:

- identifying the need for information and formulating a question;
- tracking down the best possible source of evidence to answer that question;
- evaluating it for validity and clinical applicability;
- applying it in practice;
- evaluating the outcomes.

So, for example, a doctor, faced with a patient with a severe infection, might ask 'which antibiotic will best cure this infection?' and look to the literature on drug trials to provide an answer. Thereafter they would evaluate the validity of the trial and its relevance to their patient, administer the drug (or not) and see what happened. Or, to use one of the examples from the GRIPP project, the doctor treating a child with 'glue ear' might ask 'will surgery to insert grommets make a difference in the long term compared with conservative treatment?' A search of the literature would indicate that surgery to insert grommets is not necessarily cost-effective in the long run in terms of outcome. But this example illustrates the complexity that the rational model of EBM does not necessarily deal with. At the point that the doctor opts for conservative treatment, what message is conveyed to the parent with a child who has suddenly gone deaf and who is losing speech (and friends at playgroup)? The research evidence on cost-effectiveness may not fully acknowledge the social issues surrounding the clinical problem. Evidence-based medicine is essentially a linear model for change which assumes that clinicians should make rational choices based on the scientific evidence available to them. It does not necessarily take into account the choices which clients make which might be equally rational for them. Activity 1.3 (see Appendix 1) will be helpful in gaining some experience in the practice of EBM.

Evidence-based medicine defines the best source of evidence as the randomised control trial (RCT), or better still a group of RCTs, which can then be systematically reviewed and analysed. Early on in EBM the idea was that clinicians would get involved in all the stages of this process, including the search for and evaluation of the evidence, and there were – and are – various manuals and training programmes to help them do that. In practice, a cadre of specialist and largely university based 'experts' has grown up to manage the searching for and evaluation of the scientific evidence and produce specifications for practice which are then disseminated through various fora. These specifications for practice are known by a number of names, including clinical guidelines, care pathways, etc. and their use will be explored later in the chapter. The degree to which any specification will constitute a suggestion or an instruction to practitioners may largely depend on the importance of the topic and the costs of that area of practice.

As we shall see below, the EBM movement has been, and continues to be, subject to considerable debate and criticism. However, there is a danger that it is criticised for ideas which it does not wholly espouse. First, the enthusiasts did not suppose that the use of research evidence would entirely override clinical judgement but rather that it would work in conjunction with it:

> External clinical evidence can inform, but can never replace, individual clinical expertise and it is this expertise that decides whether the external evidence applies to the individual patient at all and, if so, how it should be integrated into a clinical decision.
>
> (Sackett *et al.*, 1997: 4)

Second, while it is true that a hierarchy of evidence was proposed, which placed that derived from RCTs at the top as the 'gold standard', it did not assert that other forms of evidence were not of some value and neither did it entirely ignore evidence derived from qualitative research (Glaszious *et al.*, 2004). However, while this might express the views of the founders, some followers may be more zealous in promoting the 'gold standard' of the RCT.

Early evidence-based medicine was an enthusiasts' movement. Subsequently a whole industry has grown up around these early beginnings and it is now central to government health policy and is spreading into other occupations. So who is supporting the development of EBM and its promotion in new disciplines such as nursing, social work and education – and why? First, there is a lobby from researchers. After all, if no-one uses their work then why should government continue to fund it? Healthcare research is now a substantial industry forming a significant part of many university budgets. New journals have sprung up to explore the issues and, of course, publication is the lifeblood of academics. Gerrish (2003), citing Estabrooks (1998), argues that EBM has generated a shift in power and prestige in healthcare from experienced expert clinicians to researchers.

Second, there is the government which is increasingly committed to the development of evidence-based policy-making in many spheres but certainly in health. It has established a range of organisations to support evidence-based medicine and funds research which is designed to feed directly into practice. The organisations include the Cochrane Collaboration which exists to produce systematic reviews, within England, the National Institute for Health and Clinical Excellence (NICE) and in Scotland the Scottish Intercollegiate Guidelines Network (SIGN), as well as a number of university based units dedicated to supporting EBM. And within its research programme there has been an increased emphasis on 'impact' as well as validity, reliability, etc. The Research for Patient Benefit (RfPB) programme was explicitly established within the National Institute for Health Research (NIHR) programme to sponsor 'near practice' research, that is research that can be easily applied to practice. There was some initial concern that the projects would be focused on hospital care but the results of the first three funding rounds showed that this was not the case and studies in public health were well represented. Another important characteristic of these projects is that user and practitioner involvement was built in from the start – this programme is clearly trying to get out of the 'ivory tower' and engage in real-life problems. Nevertheless, despite the intentions, it is too soon to know whether such projects make implementation in practice any easier. Activity 1.4 (see Appendix 1) will help you to explore elements of effective health visiting practice.

Third, although there was and is some concern within medicine that EBM would erode the importance of clinical judgement, in professions such as nursing the idea of developing a strong formal and recognised evidence base was seductive. Some decades ago the theory that a profession needed to have certain characteristics became popular in occupations such as nursing, social work and teaching. And while the theory itself was deeply flawed as it largely ignored issues of power and prestige based on class and gender, it did inspire a section of nursing to fight for an independent regulatory body – now the Nursing and Midwifery Council (NMC) – and for graduate entry to the occupation which has now been realised with the 2010 change in NMC regulations. This professionalising agenda has extended to a belief that a 'proper' profession would have – and use – an extensive evidence base from research, that is, it should aspire to be an 'evidence-based' profession. Consequently, some nursing constituencies have vigorously championed the development of nursing research and nursing's inclusion in multidisciplinary research – and indeed there has been a very rapid expansion of nursing research, although much of it remains small scale and relatively little of it uses RCTs.

Fourth, there is the consumer who increasingly wants the 'best' treatment available and is intolerant of variations in practice – or 'postcode lotteries'. This may in part be fuelled by media reports of research 'breakthroughs'. However, the consumers' attitudes are at best ambivalent – the extensive and growing use of 'alternative' therapies, many of which have a research evidence base which is slight at best, shows that the consumer also wants to decide for themselves what works. Activity 1.5 (see Appendix 1) enables this to be explored further.

So we can conclude that powerful forces have fuelled the development of the EBM movement and have vested interests in its success. More fundamentally, like any social movement, it had to be in the right place at the right time. A number of factors seem to have been crucial. Importantly, the oil crisis of the mid 1970s forced Western industrial societies into financial crisis. Muir Gray acknowledges the importance of this economic crisis in the development of EBM (cited in Traynor, 2002). Never again would the price of something not matter and state-funded healthcare represents a massive part of government expenditure. If doctors were undertaking operations for glue ear with no proven benefit then that was no longer just their decision. And partly as a result of the economic crisis, society was also changing. Traynor (2002) defines key products of this new emphasis on fiscal control as the rise of managerialism, the increased use of audit and an increased emphasis on R&D. In addition, society was increasingly conscious of risk but wary of the power and authority of both science and professions to provide solutions. How did EBM fit into this landscape? In theory, having sufficient research evidence to specify 'best practice' allowed managers greater control over individual practitioners, and audit systems ensured that this control was maintained. Although EBM is based on a science embedded in experimental work, it was not a scientific 'grand narrative', rather it provided 'recipes' for best practice which would, in theory, reduce variations in practice and control risk. A further key element in the success of EBM – and the fact that it is a worldwide phenomenon – is the exponential growth in information technology. Without the ability to search electronic databases worldwide EBM would be a much reduced enterprise.

The concepts behind EBM have spread to other healthcare occupations, and subsequently beyond healthcare into management, education and social work and it is commonplace now to describe the movement as evidence-based practice (EBP). In 2008 NICE was given a remit for work in public health, including disease prevention and health promotion. In so doing, changes have had to made to the way in which EBM operates even within the heartland of EBM. Kelly *et al.* (2010) offer an 'insider's' perspective of some of these challenges as they work within NICE on the public health agenda – which of course goes beyond healthcare into education, social welfare, etc. and depends on disciplines such as sociology, anthropology, etc. In moving into new areas, institutions such as NICE have had to move beyond biomedicine with its relatively simple causal models and engage with very different academic and practice disciplines which have their own distinct ways of generating and validating knowledge. A fundamental problem is that the EBM methodology for generating evidence, which gives superiority to RCTs, is not going to work. First, there are few such trials conducted outside of biomedicine, and second, much of the knowledge in social science disciplines is generated by the use of theories and models, which are not amenable to the sort of meta-analysis to which trials can be subject:

> Theories and models require a different way of encapsulating their form and content, their provenance, their ideological dispositions and so on. They are not facts in the sense that someone's occupation or systolic blood pressure are

facts. Theories are ways of organising ideas, usually designed to make observable facts clearer or more coherent, or to offer some kind of explanation for
the particular way the facts are, or appear to be.

(Kelly *et al.*, 2010: 1059)

If these differences in the way in which knowledge is generated and validated
could not be acknowledged then much of the knowledge of these disciplines
would be disregarded as of lower status or including bias. A further problem is
that in many public health issues there is a long causal pathway between an
intervention and the change it is designed to create, and this creates conceptual
complexity not encountered when testing drug A against drug B. Kelly *et al.*
(2010) outline some of the ways in which they are engaging with these issues,
which include both creating new methodologies, such as developing logic
models to manage methodological pluralism, and also trying to use experts in
the field to generate consensus. This is very far from where EBM began.

So despite its success in embedding itself into national structures, and in
spreading into new fields, EBP remains a highly contested concept and an evolving practice. Even within EBM there were many concerns which were articulated
early on in a useful summary document called *Acting on the Evidence* (Appleby
et al., 1995) produced by York University. This summarised the EBM movement
as: 'the movement away from basing healthcare on opinion or past practice and
towards grounding healthcare in science and evidence' (Appleby *et al.*, 1995: 4).
This document raises a number of issues. First, it argues that insufficient
account is taken by EBM of the uncertainty of clinical practice. Second, it argues
that it is impossible to generate information for everything – a key issue for
health visiting which exists in a highly complex epistemological and social context. Third, it notes that information about clinical effectiveness generated by
RCTs is about populations, whereas clinicians deal with individuals:

How rigid do we expect the doctor to be in reconciling the scientifically
derived probabilities of clinical effectiveness with the situation of the individual patient?

(Appleby *et al.*, 1995: 30)

While the debates about EBP generate great heat on all sides, it could be
argued that we still await a proper analysis of it as a social movement.
Mykhalovskiy and Weir (2004) argue that social science's response to EBM,
and by implication EBP, remains immature. They define EBM as: 'the project of
reshaping biomedical practice by creating an organising presence for clinical
research within medical decision making' (Mykhalovskiy & Weir, 2004: 1059).
They define two critical approaches to EBM, one coming from social scientists
focusing on the political economy, where EBM might, for example, be seen as
part of a movement to restrict the autonomy of clinicians. Alternatively, they
identify the critique from social scientists using a medical humanism perspective which suggests that 'In this reading, EBM strips patients of their stories
and the meaning of their experience, reducing them to passive recipients of
doctor-centered communications' (Mykhalovskiy & Weir, 2004: 1062). They

argue that social science's response to EBM remains at the macro level and more studies are needed about how it operates in practice.

The current landscape of evidence-based practice

As we look across the new occupations engaging in EBP we can see three interesting responses to the original concept, each of which will be explored more fully in the following sections. First, there are theoretical objections to EBM and particularly to its export into other areas, which are probably best exemplified in a published 'dialogue' between Iain Chalmers, a key figure in the EBM movement, and Martyn Hammersley, a leading figure in the sociology of education and research methods, which is described below. Second, there are those who are quite enthusiastic about EBP but dismayed that it just doesn't seem to change practice. This has produced what might be called the 'barriers' literature, which attempts to identify and eradicate the reasons why it doesn't work. Third, nursing in particular has responded to these issues in a very interesting way. It has criticised the technological model of knowledge used in EBM, and has acknowledged that the linear model of research evidence utilisation may not be wholly appropriate to nursing practice, but in order to stay within the 'evidence-based' fold – and thereby retain status and government approval – it has built on the existing critique of EBM as having a very narrow view of evidence and has redefined the notion of acceptable evidence more broadly.

Refuting evidence-based practice

From within the discipline of education, Martyn Hammersley has produced one of the most accessible critiques, engaging directly with the arguments of major supporters of EBP, notably Iain Chalmers who wrote an article in support of EBM entitled: 'Trying to do more good than harm in policy and practice: the role of rigorous, transparent up-to date evaluations' (Chalmers, 2003). Hammersley's response is direct: 'Is the evidence-based practice movement doing more good than harm? Reflections on Iain Chalmers' case for research-based policy making and practice' (Hammersley, 2005). Hammersley seeks first to establish common ground. He suggests that there should be broad agreement about the following propositions:

- Practitioners occasionally do harm in their professional work.
- Research can help provide practitioners and policy-makers with useful information.
- Not everything presented as research is either reliable or indeed research.

Further, Hammersley agrees that research needs to be mediated before it can be used by individual practitioners:

> the results of research should be presented to lay audiences through reviews of the available literature, rather than the findings of individual studies being offered as reliable information

(Hammersley, 2005: 87)

However, Hammersley goes on to argue, first, that the methodologies favoured in evidence-based practice – the randomised control trial and the systematic review – are themselves subject to methodological critique and should not be assumed to produce bias free evidence: 'research findings must always be interpreted and are never free from potential error' (Hammersley, 2005: 88). This is not an argument about quantitative and qualitative methods, but rather that *all* forms of research are socially constructed and all research is generated and read within a particular context of experience and judgement.

Second, he argues that Chalmers, and by extension other evidence-based practice proponents, believe that research can *arbitrate* in areas where there are debates about what counts as good practice. By implication he suggests that Chalmers has gone beyond the originally proposed 'partnership' between external research evidence and clinical judgement to valorise the external evidence. He refutes the idea that RCTs should have a privileged status above other kinds of knowledge and be used to resolve disputes.

Third, he argues that judgement is fundamental to good practice because, 'practice is necessarily a matter of judgement, in which information from various sources (not just research) must be combined' (Hammersley, 2005: 88).

He asserts that that the role of professional judgement may differ between different forms and arenas of practice. He argues that downplaying the importance of professional judgement in favour of research evidence could, in some contexts, reduce the quality of practice rather than enhance it.

The dialogue continued with Chalmers's (2005) response: 'If evidence-informed policy works in practice, does it matter if it doesn't work in theory?' which claims that Hammersley misrepresents his views. Interestingly, Chalmers cites a specific example, familiar to health visitors, of research findings changing the previous 'commonsense' recommendations about the way a baby should sleep – on its front or back – as one of the key pieces of evidence supporting the importance and impact of EBM:

> These and countless other examples should leave little doubt that it is irresponsible to interfere in the lives of other people on the basis of theories unsupported by reliable empirical evidence.
>
> (Chalmers, 2005: 229)

Hammersley is, of course, not the only critical commenter of the evidence-based medicine movement. For example, Kerridge *et al.* (1998), writing from a basis in health ethics, argue that EBM has serious ethical flaws. First, they argue that, while EBM is concerned with outcomes, there are many aspects of outcomes which cannot be properly measured. They cite as examples, pain, justice and quality of life.

Second, they argue that in EBM it is difficult to decide between the competing claims of different stakeholders. While it potentially downgrades the power and authority of individual doctors, who should be replacing them in that position? Is it managers; is it patients? And if the latter, how can that be managed? Third, they argue that EBM interventions may transgress common morality because it is concerned only with evidence of efficacy. They raise issues about the ethical status of trials - on the one hand there are now strict criteria which might be seen as 'good' but these criteria shift over time. Kerridge et al. also argue that RCTs in themselves are subject to ethical questions about 'the selection of subjects, consent, randomisation, the manner in which trials are stopped, and the continuing care of subjects once the trials are complete' (Kerridge et al., 1998: 1152).

The literature on evidence-based medicine and practice is full of such claims and counter claims. But while such debates may be exciting and energising for those involved in them, they may be somewhat bewildering or even daunting to lay (i.e. nonresearch) practitioners. But they are important in terms of practice. Kerridge et al. (1998) also cite the Australian health minister as saying that '[we will] pay only for those operations, drugs and treatments that according to available evidence are proved to work' (Kerridge et al., 1998: 1153) and in the UK we are familiar with battles between patient groups and the government (via NICE) about the withdrawal of funding from treatments which the recipients believe work.

So does it work – and if not, why not?

From a purely practical point of view, what is the evidence that research findings, even when expertly mediated through the Cochrane Collaboration, NICE or other guideline systems, are, or indeed can be, directly applied to practice in the linear model implied by the evidence-based practitioners? There is considerable evidence that it is not being applied directly as anticipated, which suggests that we need to think of the relationship between research and practice in more complex terms. In order to examine and explain the problems, a literature developed exploring what were known as the 'barriers' to utilising research. If we could just identify and remove those barriers, the argument went, all would be well. Grimshaw and Thomson (1998) argued that, 'Despite the considerable resources devoted to biomedical science, a consistent finding from the literature is that the transfer of research findings into practice is a slow and haphazard process' (Grimshaw & Thomson, 1998: 20). Grol and Wensing found the same thing:

> One of the most consistent findings in health services research is the gap between best practice (as determined by scientific evidence), on the one hand, and actual clinical care, on the other.
>
> (Grol & Wensing, 2004: S.57).

They studied barriers to change and proposed that they occur at six different levels - for example, the nature of the innovation itself (which is sometimes neglected in the barriers debate), the individual, the social context, the patient, the wider context - really just about anything. These debates are international; there is a very interesting and accessible workshop report from Australia where the National Institute of Clinical Studies (NICS) - their equivalent of NICE - brought together a range of participants to explore how research can be brought into practice (Sweet, 2004). One of the most interesting proposals was the creation of an evidence SWAT (special weapons and tactics) team which would work, not just with practitioners, but with the media and the public to raise awareness of good evidence.

In the UK, Gerrish (2003) explored some of the barriers to introducing research into nursing based on a study within a large acute hospital. She groups them into factors relating to the organisation, the way research is communicated, the quality of the research, and the nurse. Again it seems difficult to identify anything which might not constitute a barrier. Clearly some of these may include barriers to introducing any kind of change; healthcare organisations are very large and complex and the healthcare sector is highly regulated and risk averse. Others are specific to research based knowledge and Gerrish argues that the way in which the research is conducted and the type of knowledge generated may be important. The traditional model of evidence-based practice, as we have seen, assumes the superiority of a-contextual technological knowledge and a linear model of utilisation. She argues that other research models such as the enlightenment model or action research might have substantial value. Activity 1.6 (see Appendix 1) explores further, barriers to implementing research evidence in health visiting.

Redefining evidence-based practice

There is a substantial constituency in nursing which has embraced the concept of evidence-based practice, and a supportive power base of journals, professional bodies and university units has been established. This might seem surprising in an occupation which has fought to defend the importance of qualitative research and does not have a substantial tradition of conducting RCTs or systematic reviews (an important exception in the context of health visiting is the work of Elkan *et al.* (2000) in systematically reviewing the evidence on the effectiveness of domiciliary health visiting). Parker (2002), former director of the Victoria Centre for Evidence Based Nursing in Melbourne, provides an interesting perspective on why nursing should embrace EBP in an editorial in *Nursing Inquiry* in which she feels she has to defend her personal support for EBP, not least because she has a reputation for engaging in research in a different epistemological tradition which focuses on experience and narrative. She argues first, that its time has come because of a range of economic, political and market imperatives. She draws attention to the way in which it helps society manage risk, reduce costs and provide accountability. In addition she argues that:

> It provides investigative and justificatory tools to manoeuvre the morass of uncertainty in situations where decisions must be made without knowing the consequences and where many of the comforting routines of the past have fallen away.
>
> (Parker, 2002: 140)

But other researchers have taken a somewhat different path in reconciling engagement with EBP with their value base. Rycroft-Malone *et al.* (2004), in an interesting study called 'What counts as evidence in evidence-based practice?', suggest that nurses can reconceptualise evidence-based practice by greatly broadening the kinds of evidence which are embraced by the movement in order to make it both more acceptable and more useful. They explore the potential for using four types of evidence: that derived from research; clinical experience; the knowledge of patients, clients and carers; and the local context and environment. The last is somewhat of a 'catch-all' term and includes information from audit and performance, as well as patient narratives, organisational knowledge, local policies, etc. They pose two challenges. First, whatever the source, for knowledge to count as evidence it needs to be examined and tested in some way. So, for example, 'in order for an individual practitioner's experience and knowledge to be considered credible as a source of evidence, it needs to be explicated, analysed and critiqued' (Rycroft-Malone *et al.*, 2004: 84). Second, they argue that we need to develop our collective understanding of how these various evidences are integrated to generate effective practice. It is important to note that this reconceptualising of acceptable evidence goes far beyond the work to expand the evidence-based outlined by Kelly *et al.* (2010). While they are looking to see how other 'sciences' can be incorporated, Rycroft-Malone *et al.* (2004) are developing the concept of useful evidence as coming from outside traditional science.

In the next section, these themes are further explored through case studies of practice showing real instances of how knowledge is generated and used by practitioners at all level. However, before we move on to them it may be helpful to note an important study which defined the sources of knowledge which nurses currently use and which illustrates some of the themes in the last two sections. Estabrooks *et al.* (2005) explored the sources of knowledge which nurses used through two major ethnographic studies in hospitals in Canada. They found that nurses categorised their sources of knowledge into four broad grouping: social interactions, experiential knowledge, documentary sources, and *a priori* knowledge. Importantly, they note that the category of social interactions dominated their findings. They report that when nurses have immediate and practical concerns they will turn first to their peers who can give both information and reassurance, as illustrated by one of their respondents: 'If one of my colleagues says you know what, D, I have seen that happen time and time again...don't worry about it, I will be reassured by that' (Estabrooks *et al.*, 2005: 464). The nurses had a hierarchy of knowledge but it was not consistent with EBP:

> The high regard for experience also caused nurses occasionally to reject advice from clinical nurse specialists, educators, and physicians when they believed that the advice was inconsistent with their own experiential knowledge. Also nurses sometimes rejected evidence-based patient care protocols in favour of those practices they consider effective based on experience.
>
> (Estabrooks *et al.*, 2005: 468)

Hopefully, this sets the scene for a discussion of how knowledge is managed in particular instances.

Managing knowledge and evidence in practice

Much of the debate in both EBM and EBP utilises an 'ideal' model of the linear movement of research findings into practice. But how is knowledge actually managed in practice? In this section, five 'case studies' (not all of them are defined as such by the authors), will be examined, which are derived from primary research, which look at how evidence is used for decision-making in practical situations. The first two are at the national policy level, the third describes the development of local guidelines by GPs, the next looks at the use of protocols by nurses in a diabetic clinic and a cardiac medical unit, and the last looks at the practice level within primary care, mainly focusing on GPs and practice nurses.

> ### Case study 1.1: National policy-making in relation to inequalities in health
>
> In 1997 the government commissioned a review of information on inequalities in health which was asked to make recommendations for policy development. Seventeen topics were identified and experts were asked to provide papers to the scientific advisory group in order to demonstrate the relevant knowledge in the area. In addition, a group of very skilled and influential figures in evidence-based practice was asked to form an evaluation group to look at the quality and adequacy of the evidence presented. This comprised Sally Macintyre, Director of the Social and Public Health Sciences Unit; Iain Chalmers, Director of the UK Cochrane Centre; Richard Horton, Editor of *The Lancet*; and Richard Smith, Editor of the *British Medical Journal* (*BMJ*). They represented a formidable group of supporters of evidence-based practice and its extension into public health.
>
> They developed a methodology for evaluating the policy recommendations which is included here because it presents quite a challenge to those who see supporters of evidence-based policy-making as being concerned *only* with the research evidence to the exclusion of other important issues. Their criteria investigated the following issues:
>
> - 'Supported by systematic, empirical evidence;
> - Supported by cogent argument;
> - Scale of likely health benefit;
> - Likelihood that the policy would bring benefits other than health benefits;
> - Fit with existing or proposed government policy;
> - Possibility that the policy might do harm;
> - Ease of implementation;
> - Cost of implementation.'(Macintyre *et al.*, 2001: 223)
>
> *(Continued)*

Case study 1.1:   (Continued)

It is obvious that they consider that research is one, but only one, of the things which should be considered when making health policy. They argue that: 'Research on the effectiveness of policies will never be more than one of the factors that must be considered by policy makers.' (Macintyre et al., 2001: 223) What was published later in the BMJ is not their report to the enquiry but a subsequent commentary on the issues raised, first, they found that there was little empirical evidence about the effectiveness of the strategies proposed:

> Many of the submissions to the enquiry...consisted of wish lists of potentially useful interventions without evidence of their effectiveness in practice.
>
> (Macintyre et al., 2001: 223)

Second, they found that none of the input papers had a methods section explaining the inclusion/exclusion criteria. In other words, it was impossible to know why some studies had been included and others not and they noted some instances of partial or selective use of evidence. Third, there was little reference to the potential harm the proposed policy might cause, or to costs and opportunity costs. Fourth, there was better evidence for studies related to interventions at the level of the patient or client then there were about policies relating to interventions in communities. Fifth, there was very little reference to policy implementation being monitored. Macintyre and her colleagues concluded that much more needs to be done to create a systematic knowledge base for public health and to keep it up to date. They noted that there were three relevant reviews produced in 1995 but inevitably they were of limited use by 1998. Importantly, one of the key characteristics of the Cochrane Collaboration is that it is committed to keeping all systematic reviews updated.

Case study 1.2:   Introducing new technology

This case study (May, 2006) relates to the potential introduction of telehealthcare systems and explores how policy-makers and researchers engaged with each other over a practical issue. The data in May's case study is derived from a series of public and private meetings held between 1998 and 2004 and two sessions of the UK House of Commons Health Committee in 2001 and 2005. The meetings involved a very wide range of participants – senior health service managers from every NHS level, social care managers from the public and voluntary sectors, policy-makers from a number of UK government departments and from the Welsh Assembly and the Scottish Office, university researchers, and representatives of service providers and manufacturers. May was involved in the meetings as a participant – as an expert advisor from a sociological perspective.

At the beginning of the process the proponents of telehealthcare, the NHS managers and the policy-makers were all agreed that they need the robust evidence RCTs and systematic reviews could provide. However, as time went on there was increasing dissatisfaction with using trials. A senior clinician said:

> Trials are vital, they give us the evidence, but the evidence is always arguable and it doesn't influence policy makers as much as we would like. *They suffer from evidence fatigue* ...
>
> (May, 2006: 519; original emphasis)

Trials began to be disparaged for one of their defining characteristics; they are a-contextual in order that they are generalisable, so by definition cannot provide evidence about the practicalities of innovation in a specific service context. As respondents noted, trials may advantage researchers but they do not reflect what happens in 'normal' practice.

So, while researchers wanted to do clinical trials – they got funding to do them and published their results which could lead to increased funding for their university – managers who actually wanted to get on and solve their problems were disenchanted. Clinical trials did not provide the 'workability' evidence that they needed. By the meeting in 2004 clinical trials had ceased to be of interest and managers and policy-makers were looking to working with service providers to set up local demonstration projects. Interestingly, the providers themselves had moved away from providing telehealthcare, which involved clinical practice at a distance, to telecare, which involved safety systems to support people in their own homes, with a commensurate reduction in the need for research evidence of clinical safety and levels of risk.

May (2006) identifies a number of issues in the organisation and reception of knowledge produced within a Health Technology Assessment model of formal quantitative knowledge generation. He argues that:

> In practical terms the division between research elites and local managers is expressed by the latter seeking more flexible modes of knowledge production ... In the world of service provision, such highly medicalised models of research practice have been by-passed or displaced by different kinds of institutional actors as they seek to rapidly implement new models of service provision.
>
> (May, 2006: 528–529)

He also argues that formal research methods provide a 'flavour' of science to support decisions which are essentially political. In terms of the science, he concludes that evidence is always socially constructed within specific contexts.

Case study 1.3: Creating guidelines in primary care

This study by McDonald and Harrison (2004) looked at the process of developing local clinical guidelines on the treatment of patients with actual or potential heart disease by GPs. At the time of the study, the GPs were linked into a Primary Care Group (PCG) (which were replaced by Primary Care Trusts, which again have been replaced by commissioning groups of GP practices). It was a participant observation study as one of the authors was an expert adviser to the group in the field of economics and finance. The study is largely based on field notes made at a series of meetings between 1997 and 1999.

The impetus for the development of the local guidelines was in part the imminent publication of the National Service Framework on Coronary Heart Disease and in part concern about the costs of existing practice. Statins, a drug for treating or preventing heart disease, are relatively cheap drugs, but the number of potential recipients is large so the overall cost could be significant. The PCG had an existing cardiac focus group which included the Health Authority's Pharmaceutical Advisor, the local consultant cardiologist and a number of GPs. This group was charged with making recommendations to all the GPs about managing patients with cardiovascular disease.

The first part of their work focused on developing a statin prescribing guideline. The group used a number of sources of evidence, including the results from a number of significant RCTs, which clearly showed statins could be effective in reducing mortality, an article from the *BMJ* which discussed the cost-effectiveness of prescribing strategies in relation to statins, guidelines published by the Standing Medical Advisory Committee (SMAC), and information from pharmaceutical companies.

What issues concerned the group? First, the GPs complained that they didn't understand the SMAC guidelines or the RCT results: 'There was general agreement on the difficulties of making informed choices, particularly when faced with "evidence" from pharmaceutical company representatives' (McDonald & Harrison, 2004: 228). They were confused by the risk tables attached to the SMAC guidelines and felt there were key issues missing, such as family history. The Pharmaceutical Advisor – who was presumably keen to limit prescribing – suggested that it might be best to concentrate on patients with coronary heart disease because they were high risk. The group then debated what constituted high risk, with a number of GPs giving examples from their patient population. Importantly: 'The discussions of risk perception revealed that GPs each had their own ideas about what constituted risk' (McDonald & Harrison, 2004: 228), which largely centred around their views on the importance of lifestyle and smoking. A major discussion focused on the age cut-off for prescribing statins. While the Pharmaceutical Advisor urged a focus on younger patients, a number of the GPs cited particular cases of elderly patients who they believed 'deserved' statin therapy and the advice was not taken. There were further debates about, for example, which test should be used to establish cholesterol levels. At one point the economic advisor produced a substantial paper modelling the costs and benefits of options for change, but she was politely told that the GPs were 'simple souls' who couldn't understand it. However, the group did eventually agree a guideline, but it was clear that it was guidance rather than prescription. The result of all the work is interesting: before the guideline was produced there was huge variation in prescribing; afterwards there was huge variation in prescribing!

McDonald and Harrison (2004) were interested at the start of the study about whether guidelines were the tools of management or of a professional elite. Their conclusion is that it is really more complicated than that – localities, people and histories all play a part. The GPs relied on reference to individual cases: 'I had a patient in the other day' (McDonald & Harrison, 2004: 228); managers who were concerned about the outcomes of the project tended to move on to other jobs before the work was complete; and while the GPs agreed with the consultant when he was there they ignored his views after he had left the meeting. However, McDonald and Harrison (2004) argue that while the guidelines here did not seem to alter practice, an increased government focus on guidelines subsequent to this study may have made adherence to guidelines more likely. But in terms of the way in which local guidelines might be developed, a conclusion from this study must be that the introduction of technical research solutions into practice is not a simple linear process and practitioners rely heavily on their own knowledge and experience.

Case study 1.4: Protocol-based decision-making in nursing

This case study (Rycroft-Malone *et al.*, 2009) looked at nurses' decision-making in two contexts – a diabetic and endocrine unit and a cardiac medical unit. Using a variety of data collection methods, including participant and nonparticipant observation, interviews, field notes, and existing documentation, they sought to determine how nurses reached decisions, and in particular whether and how they used protocols. As they note, standardised care approaches can have a variety of names, including protocol, care bundles, care pathways, and clinical guidelines. However they all have a similar aim of standardising practice through the provision of a 'best care' recipe. This is intended to ensure that 'best

(Continued)

Case study 1.4: *(Continued)*

care' is given but also to simplify decision-making for practitioners. In each of the research sites a number of protocols were available, although interestingly, a number of them were put away in the office.

They found that there were four major sources of information used in decision-making: interaction with colleagues, standardised care approaches, instinct, and patients. They found that: 'Decision making was a social activity, especially during a shift with nurses of mixed experience and knowledge' (Rycroft-Malone *et al.*, 2009: 1494) and nurses would often look to more senior or experienced nurses for advice. While protocols were used, this was not in an obvious and systematic way. The nurses in the cardiac medical unit thought they were too busy to refer to protocols and, in any case, they believed that they were impersonal and did not necessarily define best practice. In the diabetic clinic the nurses were aware that the patients had a lot of knowledge about their own condition and any protocol would have to be 'flexed' to accommodate this. In general, the knowledge derived from the protocol became 'intertwined with experience' and indistinguishable in everyday decision-making. Where protocols were thought to be useful was in teaching, in 'new' situations, and in order to support the nurses' decision-making post-hoc, should there be a query.

Importantly, the study noted that nurses make a lot of decisions, from medication and treatment to time management, and that protocols could not possibly be available for every decision. They report that:

> Some nurses described the mental processes during decision-making as following steps or a mental flowchart or checklist, not necessarily linked to a particular guideline or protocol.
>
> (Rycroft-Malone *et al.*, 2009: 1494)

As we shall see, this concept, as well as the notion of authority figures, resonates with some of the conclusions of the final case study.

Case study 1.5: Knowledge management in primary care

Gabbay and le May (2004) conducted a substantial ethnographic study looking at knowledge management in primary care based in two practices. They were interested in how research evidence might pass into practice, and particularly at how – and if – this was managed at the level of the individual practitioner and/or the level of the collective, and how the two were connected. They did not find evidence to suggest that research findings were feeding directly into decision-making:

> We found that the individual practitioners did not go through the steps that are traditionally associated with the linear-rational model of evidence based health care - not once in the whole time we were observing them. Neither while we observed them did they read the many clinical guidelines available to them ...
>
> (Gabbay & le May, 2004: 3)

In contrast, they found a more complex picture of practitioners using a variety of sources of information, notably professional journals (not research journals) and networks of other practitioners, to build up their knowledge. Within their professional networks some people were thought of as 'authorities' who could be relied on to give reliable advice. For example, in this case the local Primary Care Trust (PCT) pharmaceutical advisor was considered to be such a reliable source. They present an example of how in one practice a local protocol for heart failure was generated. The doctor who was asked to develop the protocol used the local hospital guidelines (where the cardiologist was another respected 'authority'), and integrated this with two other published guidelines and with her own experience. The result was presented to the practice team which largely left the scientific basis unquestioned - after all, it was based on trusted sources. Their concerns were much more about whether the protocol was workable and would advantage the practice both in terms of financial and quality measures.

Gabbay and le May (2004) coin the term 'mindlines', in contrast to 'guidelines', to convey the way in which practitioners use such sources, as well as their training and their experience, to generate personal internalised tacit knowledge to guide their practice. These 'mindlines' are not static but will be progressively negotiated and changed through various interactions - for example practice meetings, discussions with colleagues and interactions with patients. They argue that, if research is to affect practice, it will be via these processes and not through an idealised model of rational adoption. Further, they draw attention to the importance of locality - clinicians practice in a particular context of colleagues, managers and histories. Consequently they propose that

> the real skill of the practitioner might be expected to be that of learning reliably from the knowledge of trusted sources either individually or through working in a community of practice.
>
> (Gabbay & le May, 2004: 6)

Lessons from the case studies

The brief summaries above cannot do justice to the richness of data and analysis contained in each case study and they would reward further reading. They paint a rich picture of how things get done - in effect, telling 'stories' about how the participants make sense of their world. The studies all relate to key issues of importance to health visiting – how is national and local policy determined, how are guidelines constructed and used, and how does a group of people on the 'front line' manage its knowledge base? This literature does not support the ideas of a linear model of research being unproblematically imported into practice. Neither does it support the concept of 'barriers' to research utilisation, a concept which of course still depends on a rational linear model of research integration into practice. While a debate raged about the theoretical, political and practical aspects of EBP, the actors involved in these case studies did not seem to engage with that but just went about their business in ways which seemed sensible to them and which would achieve the outcomes they wanted. That is not to say that they did not understand that knowledge is both contested and situated. Key messages from the case studies include the notion that research is never value free; that its relevance and applicability are as important as issues of research design, and that in practice, both managers and practitioners have to decide what to do in conditions of uncertainty and in the context of patient expectations. Because knowledge is contested so must be one of its important manifestations in healthcare – the protocol or guideline. Hutchinson and Shakespeare (2010) argue that

> Wherever a protocol is generated – and it may be at the highest governmental level of standard setting and regulation – it is operationalised by individuals working in contexts that shape their own practice and identity. Therefore, while protocols may appear to be straightforward unambiguous statements of practice matters, there is an infinite range of possible application.
>
> (Hutchinson & Shakespeare, 2010: 75)

The nurse respondents in Traynor *et al.*'s (2010) study also referred to protocols when describing the nurses' decision-making. The study, which is based on nurses' accounts of their practice, describes a dichotomy between technical knowledge and indeterminate knowledge. Clearly the former relates to formal sources of knowledge, including protocols, whereas the latter was related to terms such as instinct and intuition. Their descriptions of technical knowledge – guidelines, manuals, protocols and evidence – acknowledged them as valid but of little use in practice. Traynor *et al.* suggest that

> participants constructed a balanced, but professionally defendable position. On one hand, they acknowledged and appreciated formalised instruments for being helpful and in some cases necessary in clinical decision-making … On the other hand, the instruments were also something obviously (in practical and ethical terms) impossible to adhere to fully in practice, and therefore they need constant modification according to the clinical situation.
>
> (Traynor *et al.*, 2010: 1589)

Activity 1.7 (see Appendix 1) enables you to explore the use of guidelines in practice. Whether protocols, guidelines, care pathways, etc. are locally or nationally constructed they will be mediated in practice by the practitioner and, Hutchinson and Shakespeare (2010) argue, by the context in which the practitioner is operating. They look particularly at how this works in a community of practice, a concept which was contained in the last case study which suggested that they are fundamental to the way in which practice – and knowledge management – gets done. So what are communities of practice?

Communities of practice

The current interest in the concept of communities of practice (CoP) has largely come from the work of Lave and Wenger (2001). Wenger (2006) proposes that 'Communities of practice are groups of people who share a concern or a passion for something they do and learn how to do it better as they interact regularly' (p. 1). The primary focus, and why it is of interest and potential use in healthcare, is in how we learn and how learning takes place in ways that are not dependent on 'teaching'. They therefore have the potential to create a mechanism through which practitioners can work to improve their own practice. A community of practice can occur in any sphere of social activity but it will have the following attributes:

- a shared domain of knowledge;
- a group willing to share ideas and to interact;
- a shared practice.

So a classroom could be a CoP, as could the staff working in a GP practice, as could a group of health visitors and nurses working around a clinic. Such communities do not need to correspond to institutional boundaries – for example, although all the health visitors in a particular district or city might be brought together in a meeting organised by management, this would not automatically constitute a community of practice, although it might be managed so that it does. Key to a community of practice is the mutual engagement of the participants and their willingness to work together in developing their practice through a variety of activities including (Wenger, 2006):

- collaborative problem-solving;
- asking others about their experiences and seeking information from them;
- reusing the knowledge assets of the group;
- coordination and synergy;
- discussing developments and innovations;
- documenting projects;
- mapping knowledge and identifying gaps.

The end result of these activities will be 'a shared repertoire of ideas, commitments and memories' (Smith, 2003, 2009).

While it is obvious that such communities are arenas of shared learning and development, it should not be assumed that they will have the same interests and goals as either other communities or their employers. For example, Wenger (1998) refers to schools in which communities of practice organise their knowledge in opposition to that proposed by institutional curricula. Each community will have its own ideas about what constitutes knowledge and competence. Neither should it be assumed that all the participants think and act the same, rather they are engaged in a shared enterprise. Each participant might have a very different view of what constitutes valid knowledge, but they are prepared to discuss and negotiate until they achieve workable solutions. Communities are also not just about managing knowledge, they are vehicles for social engagement, making work meaningful and developing identity. The resources which a community will use are not all, or even largely, locally generated. Language is the most obvious example of a resource which is imported from outside, although communities may nuance language to reflect their particular history and circumstances. Research knowledge and national and local protocols for practice will also be imported, but because a community is a negotiated enterprise their meaning and use will differ between communities.

There are many communities of practice which together will generate a *landscape* of practice. The communities will intersect and interact in various ways. Wenger (1998) argues that the participant at the periphery of a community can sometimes bring new ideas into the group because they are still able to see beyond the taken for granted knowledge of the group. Newly qualified practitioners could take this role – bringing resources from the 'old' community of practice – the classroom or placement – into their 'new' community of work, which of course may or may not welcome them!

Hutchinson and Shakespeare (2010) draw our attention to Wenger's ideas about the ways in which sources of professional knowledge and expertise have been associated with particular institutions:

- universities are connected with theory and research;
- workplaces are connected with experience and local practice;
- regulatory agencies produce prescriptions of best practice;
- professional bodies are concerned with local management and professional identity.

Each of these institutions will have many communities of practice. Researchers in universities, for example, largely enjoy similar contractual obligations and rights related to their employment, but they are likely to belong to different communities of practice related to their research interests and methodological affiliations. This produces a 'landscape' of practice in which different communities of practice overlap and interact and communities of practice could cross these institutional boundaries. Academics interested in reflective practice, for example, may be more likely to be in a community of practice with practitioners using reflective practice than with fellow academics who embrace RCTs. Negotiation takes place within communities about what sort of knowledge is to be valorised. Practitioners may despise 'university' knowledge as irrelevant to practice; university practitioners may see health service practice as largely a source for recruitment for research. However, Andrew *et al.* (2008) offer a very practical example of a working CoP in nursing which crosses these institutional boundaries. They describe how a group of 30 practising nurses and university academics throughout Scotland operated as a CoP within the framework of the Gerontological Nursing Demonstration Project. They interacted regularly, both on-line and in real time, and explored their practice in an environment of mutual respect and support. A number of best practice statements were produced which have subsequently been disseminated more widely. They argue that

> In nursing, CoPs have the potential to allow practitioners and academics to collaborate to challenge and change practice ... this way of working has the potential (to) create a vibrant work and learning environment. The fluidity of the framework encourages practitioners and academics, to integrate incrementally, the dimensions of research, education, clinical practice and user experience to respond to the increasing demand for wider institutional and professional awareness.
>
> (Andrew *et al.*, 2008: 251)

An example of a community of practice within social work is a project called *Making Research Count*. This brings together on a regular basis academics from ten different universities and associated groups of social work practitioners and managers working in approximately 60 agencies. While much of the focus is on getting research into practice, the fact that the agencies, which provide funding for the programme, can define their needs and set the agenda, and that the research is discussed in the context of actual practice needs, seems to take this beyond some of the constraints of EBP. In addition, practitioners are encouraged to generate evidence from their own practice and are taught how to use appropriate tools. It could be argued that this is an effective 'evidence focused' community of practice.

Reflective practice

Another way of both generating and managing knowledge in practice is through what is known as reflective practice. Just like evidence-based practice this started as an enthusiasts' movement but has now become institutional-ised within nursing - and is used within other occupations, particularly within healthcare. The basic concept is relatively simple:

> Reflection is more than just thinking, it is an intentional practice based learning activity that focuses on improving future actions in clinical practice by looking back at what has already happened or is happening.
>
> (Driscoll & Teh, 2001: 102)

It is intended to help the practitioner unearth and explore her knowledge about her practice, with a view to moving beyond routinised actions into new ways of thinking and doing. Because it is not easy to 'just reflect' on your practice, various methodologies have been produced to assist the practitioner.

These essentially offer a series of 'prompts' or questions to help the practitioner structure her thinking. In addition, practitioners are encouraged to keep a reflective diary or journal in which they describe and explore their practice. Reflective practice has been adopted by institutions within nursing as a way of ensuring and evidencing that practitioners continue learning and are therefore eligible for re-registration, and it is being taken up within medicine and other healthcare occupations for the same reason. It has also been adopted by many universities and associated regulatory agencies and built into many education curricula at both pre and post registration levels.

However, while its proponents and supporters remain enthusiastic about the power of reflective practice, it has not been without its critics. Jennifer Greenwood (1998), from the University of Western Sydney, entitled an editorial, 'On nursing's "reflective madness"'. She argues that reflection requires adequate time and proper training and that, in the absence of these, it will result in poor learning. More profoundly, she argues that, although the theories supporting reflection were intended as an antidote to the valorisation of technical rationality, they themselves support the idea that 'intelligent action requires conscious thought' and fail to understand that much of the tacit knowledge the practitioner uses to deal with complex practice is inherently unavailable to them. Mackintosh (1998) argues that the theoretical basis of reflective practice remains unclear despite acknowledged links to educational theorists, particularly Schön (1983). A further issue is that reflection has come to focus on the individual practitioner's thoughts, values and beliefs. So, for example, Somerville and Keeling (2004) say that:

> Reflection is the examination of personal thoughts and actions. For practitioners this means focusing on how they interact with their colleagues and with the environment to obtain a clearer picture of their own behaviour. It is therefore a process by which practitioners can better understand themselves in order to be able to build on existing strengths and take appropriate future action. (p. 42)

Consequently, it tends to downplay a number of important aspects of practice. First, by focusing on the non-technical-rational aspects of knowledge such as the personal and ethical aspects, it may not help practitioners understand how they might integrate technical-rational knowledge. Second, the patients and clients may in these accounts become passive recipients of practice rather than active participants in a joint enterprise. Third, by focusing on the personal it may ignore the social aspects of knowledge management. And perhaps the most important issue is that it does not focus on the outcomes for the patient or client.

Looking back at Case study 1.5 and on the discussion on communities of practice, it could be argued that we need to focus more on how groups and communities manage knowledge, and even within individual reflection we could ask the practitioner to reflect explicitly on her community of practice and her place within it. Is it a community which encourages managed innovation? Is it a community which values knowledge coming from external sources – and, if so, which ones? Is it a community which values the knowledge base of the client and looks at their individual circumstances? How are protocols discussed and integrated into practice by the community? In each of these – and many other examples – the practitioner can explore her relationship with the group, deciding whether she is satisfied that it is a community of practice which supports her learning and what she might do to improve her practice. Poland *et al.* (2005), in their discussion of place, suggest that reflection could usefully see practice through the 'lens' of place which again would offer a fuller understanding of the social environment of practice.

A further important criticism of reflective practice is that the resources available to the individual practitioner through recollection cannot reflect the reality of practice. Recall is rarely accurate – as anyone engaged in the judicial system will affirm. Here we need to return to the comments at the beginning of the chapter about the complexity of health visiting practice and the focus on the central importance of language. Taylor and White (2000), writing about social work and community nursing practice, agree with reflective practice in so far as it provides a potential response to the technical-rational approach embedded in EBP which they agree cannot deal with the complexities and ambiguities of practice. However, they propose that engaging in *reflexive* practice offers a remedy to the problems of memory and recall. They argue that:

> We are not interested simply in what we have done and how we have gone about things when we reflect on our practice, we must also concern ourselves with the (tacit) assumptions we are making about people, their problems and their needs when we apply knowledge about child development, mental health, learning disability and so forth.
>
> (Taylor & White, 2000: 35)

By this they mean that practitioners must produce hard evidence (they propose audiotape recordings) about their practice in order to analyse it rigorously. This will allow them to determine what they actually did rather than what they can recall. Their 'tacit' knowledge may not be available for recall but it will appear and will be available for analysis in the record of what they actually said. They are proposing that practitioners can themselves undertake the kind of analytic work about institutional practices which can be seen in Drew and Heritage (1992) and in the discourse analysis of health visiting which was described above:

> by analysing transcripts of their own talk as part of a regular self-audit, professionals can be made more aware of the embedded alternative readings, so that they may judge for themselves whether those readings are or were worth pursuing.
>
> (Taylor & White, 2000: 135)

Taylor and White (2000) provide useful ideas about how this transcript analysis can be done; for example, they suggest a number of analytic questions including how authority is conveyed, how control is managed, how facts are defined and by whom, etc. And while clients may be relatively absent in reflective practice, within reflexive practice they become both visible and expert practitioners in their own right:

> Patients are not docile and passive recipients of advice and treatment. They use the resources at their disposal to show their moral adequacy, to resist being undermined, to attempt to define 'the facts' and to make themselves worthy of sympathy.
>
> (Taylor & White, 2000: 115)

Clients: what do they know and how do they know it?

So far, the focus has largely been on how the practitioner accesses and assembles knowledge and what might be useful sources of valid and reliable evidence for them. In the past, access to such knowledge would have been largely limited to practitioners and this created an important differential between practitioner and client and arguably was part of the power base of the practitioner who was seen as the 'expert'. However, this differential in the ability to access knowledge has largely been eroded by the explosion of electronic media. In terms of text based knowledge, clients have *access* to the same sources of knowledge as most practitioners. Whatever is on the web is available to everyone. Wilson (2002) tells us that: 'A poll in August 2001 concluded that almost 100 million Americans regularly go on line for information about health care' (p. 598.) And she also tells us that over 100 000 sites offer health advice – and this was in 2002; it is unlikely that this number has diminished subsequently. Health visitors can see this as a threat or a challenge – but either way they cannot ignore it.

The general public can now access a range of formal sources of knowledge: the Cochrane Library, NICE guidelines, other guidelines, original research reports and all the media responses to them. Many research and professional journals are also now available free electronically. Government websites provide national and local data on public health statistics (discussed further in Chapter 6). There is absolutely no possibility that access to these data sources can be controlled. Access is also free to a number of less formal sources of knowledge such as wikis. Any search engine, such as Google, will access lists of knowledge sources. Some of these sources will be formal – such as journals – but they will also include media reports, advertising sites, etc. Wikipedia is one of the best known knowledge access sites – what is perhaps less well understood is that the knowledge posted on Wikipedia is not subject to the same process of expert contribution, rigorous review and guarantee as that in a conventional encyclopaedia.

There is, as you might predict, a lively debate about the quality of the advice on these sites and whether they should be quality controlled in some way.

A study of health information in relation to managing fever in children at home (Impicciatore *et al.*, 1997) found 41 relevant web pages (there may well be more today) but only four which adhered closely to published guidelines for the home management of childhood fever. Wilson (2002) suggests that there are a number of possible mechanisms for 'controlling' information:

- a self-applied code of conduct or quality label;
- user guidance systems;
- filtering tools which accept or reject sites;
- quality and accreditation labels applied by third parties.

Codes of conduct do exist but, of course, it is easy to write a code but much harder to enforce it and third party accreditation systems are extremely expensive. An alternative approach is to say that the general public copes with books and will learn to cope with the internet. So one argument is that:

> The greatest challenge is not to develop yet more rating tools, but to encourage consumers to seek out information critically, and to encourage them to see time invested in critical searching as beneficial.
>
> (Wilson, 2002: 600)

What is the role of the health visitor in this debate? What advice should she give clients about the information on the web? How might she explain the relative validity of various websites?

Social networking sites

Social networking sites now represent a major source of information for a number of client groups, but especially mothers. These new forms of electronic communication have allowed us to move away from the role of passive recipient of information and into a role as an active participant in a dialogue. There are vast numbers of social networking sites which may be used synchronously or asynchronously. An internet forum, message board, Usenet group, etc. is essentially asynchronous. It is not a live conversation. Two of the most obvious examples are *Mumsnet* and *Netmums*. Whereas once the new mother might depend on the local mother and toddler group – and may well still – today she also has access through websites such as *Mumsnet* and *Netmums* to a vast community of people experiencing the same rites of passage and tackling the same problems as herself. Not only can she access that knowledge, she can specifically seek answers to her questions – and is very likely to get responses – and can contribute her own experiences. It can be argued that these sites are essentially large communities of practice – they are clearly focused on the practice of motherhood, and many participants are keen to engage and contribute, although many others may be content to watch from the periphery. Certainly both of these sites provide enormous resources of advice and experience, which may not be verified in any formal fashion but are undoubtedly very influential. Again, it is worth asking what the relationship of individual health visitors and of the occupation should be to these sites. Could health visitors join with clients to create a CoP transcending professional boundaries?

If access to electronic sources of knowledge is a major part of how knowledge is transmitted and acquired in the early twenty-first century, it might be argued that the role of the health visitor is twofold. First, to ensure that all her clients have access to these sources; and second to help each client understand their use and validity. With regard to the first, the government has made it clear that access to digital information is a right of every citizen. With regard to the second, the practitioner needs a sophisticated understanding of how all kinds of evidence are promoted and disseminated electronically.

The internet has been called 'A Postmodern Pandora's Box' (Kata, 2010). Kata looked in particular at internet sites in the USA and Canada which were opposed to vaccination. She found that these sites offered only one version of 'truth' – that vaccination was unsafe, ineffective, unnatural (compared with alternative medicines) and a threat to civil liberties (in some parts of North America vaccination is required before entry to the public school system). Furthermore, some sites asserted that the diseases which vaccination was designed to prevent were either not serious – an example was smallpox – or caused by other agents – polio, for example, was thought to be caused by eating too much sugary food, notably ice-cream, hence it was prevalent in the summer. In terms of the style of the websites, personal testimonies, mostly narratives from parents who felt their children had been damaged by vaccines, were the most common means of generating a response.

Given that such sites will continue to proliferate in a democratic society increasingly dependent on electronic communications, an obvious response might be to offer a strong refutation based on the scientific evidence and to increase the focus on educating parents. Kata (2010) argues strongly that this cannot be an effective response:

> The post-modern perspective questions the legitimacy of science and authority. Traditional controversy dynamics, with 'audiences' needing to be 'educated' by 'experts' no longer apply. Confidence in the power of expertise has sharply declined; appeals to experts are often considered manipulative.
>
> (Kata, 2010: 1715)

She argues that we need to understand the discourses and ideologies which underpin people's beliefs in order to enter into a meaningful dialogue with them.

The controversy over the measles, mumps and rubella (MMR) vaccine offers a useful example of how some of these issues are managed by parents in a real situation. In the late 1990s a research paper was published which suggested a link between the MMR vaccine and the development of autism and inflammatory bowel disease (Wakefield *et al.*, 1998). While not many parents read *The Lancet*, the media picked up on the potential importance of the issue and it became headline news. The take-up of the combined vaccine fell from over 90% to a low of 58% in some parts of the country and there were outbreaks of measles and mumps (Hilton et al., 2007). Evidence from a study of parental views using focus groups (Hilton et al., 2007) demonstrates that parents have serious concerns about who to trust in such situations. Five main sources of information were cited by parents but their credibility varied. The government had little credibility, possibly because of its position on previous public health scares including the Bovine Spongiform Encephalopathy (BSE) outbreak. The degree to which the media was trusted varied widely but the amount of media coverage and the fact that the media tried to show both sides of the story, and thereby raised the profile of the work of Wakefield et al. (1998) fuelled concerns about the vaccine's safety. Views about the trustworthiness of health-care professionals were again mixed but doubts were raised as they were perceived to be part of 'the system' and therefore bound to support the government 'line'- and possibly also securing a financial advantage by meeting targets. A common theme in the parents' responses is that they:

> did not know to what extent their own GP or health visitor was acting in their child's best interest, as opposed to acting in their role as an advocate of public heath policy.
>
> (Hilton et al., 2007: 8).

While the health professionals were often seen as having entrenched positions, Wakefield himself was admired by some as having dared to bring the issue out into the open. He was seen as a principled 'whistleblower'. Interestingly, the most trustworthy source was defined as other parents who were perceived as just telling it like it is. Even within the media coverage:

> Parents spoke of feeling particularly drawn to anecdotal stories involving real people, and spoke about finding other parents' stories more convincing than statistics and reassurances from scientists and politicians …
>
> (Hilton et al., 2007: 9)

As we have seen, by using the website parents can access for themselves a rich source of other parents' stories and concerns.

Hilton et al. (2007) also raise the issue of the expectations parents may have of health services which may be different from the role the health visitors feel they can perform. The BBC News health website (BBC, 2008) quotes a mother as saying she wants a guarantee that there is no danger, specifically she is reported as wanting: 'Some documentation, or reliable medical information from GP surgeries or the government to prove that there is no link whatsoever.' While clients may want certainty, very little research can provide it, certainly not at the level of the individual. This issue has been well explored by the proponents of EBM, see, for example, Gray (1997) who acknowledges that RCTs can only ever deal in generalities over a given population. And the fact that in a study population of, say, 2000 there was one case of negative effects, cannot be extrapolated to define the risk to any single individual as one in 2000. The specific risk to the individual is largely unknowable so in all one-to-one discussions with the client the practitioner must rely on her own experience and skills as well as evidence 'imported' from outside and she should also rely on the experience, beliefs and skills of her client.

The debate

At various points in this chapter we have looked at how we can obtain and use evidence *for* practice, evidence *about* practice, evidence about *your* practice and the *client*'s evidence base. Two of these have received much more attention than the others because they are supported by substantial groups of enthusiastic followers and, more importantly, have become embedded in institutions and policies at every level. Evidence-based practice focuses on evidence *for* practice and despite serious critiques from both those willing it to succeed and those opposed to it in principle and practice, it is fully embedded into the NHS quality assurance systems at all levels, despite the fact that it absorbs considerable resources. While, in general, the emphasis is now on the prescription of protocols for practice – the use of which may determine the funding formula of providers – some nurses are still enjoying the spirit of the early days of EBP when individual practitioners were exhorted to find and evaluate the evidence and change their practice. An anecdotal review of curricula for health visiting suggests that despite the critiques – and the lack of actual success in changing practice – the focus remains on evidence *for* practice, and the idea that individual practitioners can and should review and evaluate the importance of research studies and decide to change their practice on the basis of them remains a prevalent model. Hopefully, it is clear from the argument above that, for a number of reasons, this is not a sustainable or indeed a safe model for practice. First, it is impossible for any practitioner, or even group of practitioners, to keep up with the range and volume of relevant research. Second, evaluating research is a very skilled and specialised practice and the methodological variety of relevant studies makes evaluation of the full range impossible. Third, very many of the studies in nursing and health visiting are conducted on a small scale and, while these are often stimulating and interesting, they cannot provide the necessary evidence needed to underpin practice change. Lastly, and rather importantly, there is a growing body of evidence on the 'barriers' to using research which shows that it just doesn't work!

However, practitioners are the focus of a massive array of protocols. Many of them, such as those produced by regulatory bodies, seek to define the identity of the practitioners either directly or through specifications for education. Protocols are a way of communicating between all the different layers of practice, management and regulation (Hutchinson & Shakespeare, 2010). The protocols which come, or purport to come, from rigorous scientific research assert that they have a particular scientific warrant which gives them a privileged status. But in practice, as has been shown, they may be of dubious scientific provenance and embedded in particular political or managerial positions. Practitioners should always explore, and if necessary challenge, these prescriptions for practice.

The other focus, certainly within nursing but increasingly in other groups, has been on generating evidence of *your* practice through reflective practice. As with EBP, a whole industry of journals, books and 'experts' has flourished and the movement – evangelical again – has become embedded in curricula and re-accreditation processes. Mackintosh, writing in 1998, asserted then that reflection was a passing fad and would be gone in ten years – how wrong she was! Interestingly, there is far less debate and fewer critiques of reflective practice than of EBP – perhaps because its power base is in nursing rather than medicine, rendering it less interesting to external academics and commentators. But this may well also be due to the lack of any clear formulation of what reflective practice really is. This has rather left a vacuum where supporters and practitioners of reflective practice can assert that it improves practice without any serious evidence, other than their own anecdotes. Much of the writing about reflective practice focuses on it as a methodology rather than on its outcomes.

Within nursing curricula these two great knowledge ideologies tend to be separated – perhaps because those who support the one rarely support, and probably would find it difficult to teach, the other. This is unfortunate because we should be bringing them together as different facets of evidence in practice and generating a dialogue between them. But the two most neglected aspects of evidence in practice are evidence *about* practice, and the *client*'s evidence base. With regard to the latter there is a very substantial body of work in sociology about how prospective or actual patients and clients think about health, illness and care (see, for example, Radley & Billig, 1996). Some reference is made to it and there is some interest from researchers – for example, Rycroft-Malone *et al.* (2004) argue that knowledge from patients, clients and carers is one of the four important sources of evidence for practice. However, within much of current practice it has lost the conceptual depth and clarity of the sociological literature and has been conceptualised as 'the patient experience', which is largely captured through routinised satisfaction surveys and reviews of complaints, and used by managers as evidence of good practice (or not).

With regard to evidence *about* practice, at the very beginning of this chapter it was argued that we have very little primary evidence about practice – about what it looks like; where and how we might have expected this body of evidence to grow and it has not. Indeed, simulated environments have been developed to serve as adequate proxies. There may be a number of reasons for this. It is often difficult to get ethical permission to record – using audio or video – actual practice. While this is understandable, it is interesting in a country where CCTV cameras follow your every move! The rich data which recording produces sets a real challenge to researchers both in the time it takes to analyse and in publishing accounts which contain enough of the primary data. But the vision of Taylor and White (2000) of a workforce continually recording and analysing their practice is a compelling one. Traynor *et al.* (2010) infer that a parallel strategy may be useful – that of asking practitioners to produce narratives about their practice and then subjecting these to the sort of rigorous discourse analysis which Taylor and White use for primary data. Certainly the health visiting knowledge base lacks a database of rigorous narratives about practice which are available for analysis and debate.

A central theme of this chapter has been that all knowledge is contestable. While the example of the anti-vaccination websites might constitute an extreme example of the rejection of scientific evidence, it is clear from the case studies that in everyday practice all kinds of experience and knowledge are brought forward alongside science as justification for practice. As May (2006) notes:

> Struggles about the facts - what they are, who they are made and recognised by, and how they are played out in different kinds of political arena - are ubiquitous in the conditions of late modernity. (p. 513)

Summary

Practising in a post-modern world, therefore, demands of the practitioner a sceptical and sophisticated understanding of the different forms and sources of knowledge generation from the national to the local level. However, a further key theme of the chapter is that the practitioner need not, and indeed should not, grapple with these issues alone. Practice takes place in a complex social environment of networks, 'authorities', experienced practitioners, clients' experience, etc., all of which can be effectively utilised as rich sources of knowledge. The effective practitioner, it can be argued, is not one who adheres to simple models for practice derived from any source, but rather is one who works with colleagues in examining, contesting, negotiating and exploiting all the knowledge sources available to her - and contributes generously to the knowledge needs of others.

References

Alaszewski, A. (2006) Managing risk in community practice: nursing, risk and decision-making. In: *Risk and Nursing Practice* (ed. P. Godin), pp. 24–41. Palgrave, London.

Andrew, N., Tolson, D. & Ferguson D. (2008) Building on Wenger: communities of practice in nursing. *Nurse Education Today*. **28**, 246-252.

Angus, J., Kontos, P., Dyck, I., McKeever, P. & Poland B. (2005) The personal significance of home: habitus and the experience of receiving long-term home care. *Sociology of Health and Illness*, **27**(5), 161-187.

Appleby, J., Walshe, K. & Ham C. (1995) *Acting on the Evidence*. National Association of Health Authorities & Trusts, Birmingham.

BBC News (2008) 'MMR: Mothers divided'. Available from: http://news.bbc.co.uk/1/hi/health/1804665.stm (accessed 3 March, 2011).

Carper, B.A. (1978) Fundamental patterns of knowing in nursing. *Advances in Nursing Science*, **1**(1), 13-23.

Chalmers, I. (2003) Trying to do more good than harm in policy and practice: the role of rigorous, transparent, up-to-date evaluations. *Annals of the American Academy of Political and Social Science*, **589**, 22-40.

Chalmers, I. (2005) If evidence-informed policy works in practice, does it matter if it doesn't work in theory? *Evidence and Policy*, **1**(2), 227-242.

Delamont, S. (1976) *Interaction in the Classroom*. Methuen, London.

Department of Health (2001) *Health Visitor Practice Development Resource Pack*. Department of Health, London.

Department of Health (2007) *Facing the Future. A Review of the Role of Health Visitors*. Department of Health, London.

Drew, P. & Heritage, J. (eds) (1992) *Talk at Work*. Cambridge University Press, Cambridge.

Driscoll, J. & Teh, B. (2001) The potential of reflective practice to develop individual orthopaedic nurse practitioners and their practice. *Journal of Orthopaedic Nursing*, **5**, 95-103.

Elkan, R., Kendrick, D., Hewitt, M. *et al.* (2000) The effectiveness of domiciliary health visiting: a systematic review of international studies and a selective review of the British literature. *Health Technology Assessment*, **4**(13), i-v, 1-339.

Estabrooks, C. (1998) Will evidence based nursing practice make practice perfect? *Canadian Journal of Nursing Research*, **30**, 15-36.

Estabrooks, C., Rutakumwa, W., O'Leary, K. *et al.* (2005) Sources of practice knowledge among nurses. *Qualitative Health Research*, **15**(4), 460-476.

Ferguson, H. (2010) Walks, home visits and atmospheres: risk and the everyday practices and mobilities of social work and child protection. *British Journal of Social Work*, **40**, 1100-1117.

Gabbay, J. & le May, A. (2004) Evidence-based guidelines or collectively constructed 'mindlines?' Ethnographic study of knowledge management in primary care. *British Medical Journal*, **329**, 1013 (30 October).

Gerrish, K. (2003) Evidence-based practice: unravelling the rhetoric and making it real. *Practice Development in Health Care*, **2**(2), 99-113.

Glaszious, P., Vandenbroucke, J. & Chalmers, I. (2004) Assessing the quality of research. *British Medical Journal*, **328** (3 January), 39-41.

Gray, J.A.M. (1997) *Evidence-based Healthcare*. Churchill Livingstone, Edinburgh.

Greenwood, J. (1998) On nursing's 'reflective madness'. *Contemporary Nurse*, **7**(1), 3-4.

Grimshaw, J.M. & Thomson, M.A. (1998) What have new efforts to change professional practice achieved? *Journal of the Royal Society of Medicine*, **S35**(91), 20-25.

Grol, R. & Wensing, M. (2004) What drives change? Barriers to and incentives for achieving evidence-based practice. *The Medical Journal of Australia*. **180**, 15 March, S57-S60.

Hammersley, M. (2005) Is the evidence-based practice movement doing more good than harm? Reflections on Iain Chalmers' case for research-based policy making and practice. *Evidence and Policy*, **1**(1), 85-100.

Heath, C. (1986) *Body Movement and Speech in Medical Interaction*. Cambridge University Press, Cambridge.

Heritage, J. & Sefi, S. (1992) Dilemmas of advice: aspects of the delivery and reception of advice in interactions between health visitors and first-time mothers. In: *Talk at Work* (eds P. Drew & J. Heritage), pp. 359-417. Cambridge University Press, Cambridge.

Hilton, S., Petticrew, M. & Hunt, K. (2007) Parents' champions vs. vested interests: who do parents believe about MMR? A Qualitative Study. *BMC Public Health*, 7, 42, published online 28 March, doi 10.1186/1471-2458-7-42.

Hutchinson, S. & Shakespeare, P. (2010) Standard setting, external regulation and professional autonomy: exploring the implications for university education. In: *Education for Future Practice* (eds J. Higgs, D. Fish, I. Goulter, S. Loftus, J. Reid & F. Trede), pp.75-84. Sense, Amsterdam.

Impicciatore, P., Pandolfini, C., Casella, N. & Bonati, M. (1997) Reliability of health information for the public on the world wide web: systematic survey of advice on managing fever in children at home. *British Medical Journal*, **314**, 1875 (28 June).

Kata, A. (2010) A postmodern Pandora's box: anti-vaccination misinformation on the internet. *Vaccine*, **28**, 1709-1716.

Kelly, M., Morgan, A., Ellis, S., Younger, T., Huntley, J. & Swann, C. (2010) Evidence based public health: a review of the experience of the National Institute of Health and Clinical Excellence (NICE) of developing public health guidance in England. *Social Science & Medicine*, **71**, 1056–1062.

Kerridge, I., Lowe, M. & Henry, D. (1998) Ethics and evidence based medicine. *British Medical Journal*, **316**, 11 April, 1151–1153.

Lave, J. & Wenger, E. (2001) *Situated Learning, Legitimate Peripheral Participation*. Cambridge University Press, Cambridge.

Lomax, H. & Robinson, K.S.M. (1998) Evidence base practice: a dilemma for health visiting? In: *The Sociology of the Caring Professions* (eds. P. Abbott & L. Meerabeau), 2nd edn. Routledge, London.

Luker, K.A. & Chalmers, K.I. (1990) Gaining access to clients: the case of health visiting. *Journal of Advanced Nursing*, **15**, 74–82.

McDonald, R. & Harrison S. (2004) The micropolitics of clinical guidelines: an empirical study. *Policy and Politics*, **32**(2), 223–239.

MacIntyre, S., Chalmers, I., Horton, R. & Smith, R. (2001) Using evidence to inform health policy: a case study. *British Medical Journal*, **322**, January 27, 7280.

McKenna, H., Cutliffe, J. & McKenna, P. (1999) Evidence-based practice: demolishing some myths. *Nursing Standard*, **14**(16), 39–42.

Mackinlosh, C. (1998) Reflection: a flawed strategy for the nursing profession. *Nurse Education Today*, **18**(7), 553–557.

May, C. (2006) Mobilising modern facts: health technology assessment and the politics of evidence. *Sociology of Health and Illness*, **28**(5), 513–532.

Mykhalovskiy, E. & Weir, L. (2004) The problem of evidence-based medicine: directions for social science. *Social Science and Medicine*, **59**, 1059–1069.

Parker, J.M. (2002) Evidence-based nursing: a defence. *Nursing Inquiry*, **9**(3), 139–140.

Poland, B., Lehoux, P., Holmes, D. & Andrews, G. (2005) How place matters: unpacking technology and power in health and social care. *Health and Social Care in the Community*, **13**(2), 170–180.

Radley, A. & Billig, M. (1996) Accounts of health and illness: dilemmas and representations. *Sociology and Health and Illness*, **18**(2), 220–240.

Robinson, K.S.M. (1986) *The social construction of health visiting*. PhD thesis, CNAA, Polytechnic of the South Bank.

Rycroft-Malone, J., Seers, K., Titchen, A., Harvey, G., Kitson, A. & McCormack, B. (2004) What counts as evidence in evidence-based practice? *Journal of Advanced Nursing*, **47**(1), 81–90.

Rycroft-Malone, J., Fontenla, M., Seers, K. & Bick, D. (2009) Protocol-based care: the standardisation of decision -making? *Journal of Clinical Nursing*, **18**, 1490–1500.

Sackett, D.L., Richardson, W.S., Rosenberg, W. & Haynes, R.B. (1997) *Evidence Based Medicine. How to Practice and Teach EBM*. Churchill Livingstone, Edinburgh.

Schön, D. (1983) *The Reflective Practitioner: How Professionals Think in Action*. Temple Smith, London.

Smith, M.K. (2003, 2009) Communities of practice, *the encyclopaedia of informal education*. Available from: www.infed.org/biblio/communities_of_practice.htm (accessed 19 November, 2010).

Somerville, D. & Keeling, J. (2004) A practical approach to promote reflective practice within nursing. Available from: www.nursingtimes.net/204502.article (accessed 3 March, 2011).

Sweet, M. (2004) Development of strategies to encourage adoption of best evidence into practice in Australia: workshop overview. *Medical Journal of Australia*, **180**(6) Supplement, S45–S47.

Taylor, C. & White, S. (2000) *Practising Reflexivity in Health and Welfare*. Open University Press, Buckingham.

Traynor, M. (2002) The oil crisis, risk and evidence-based practice. *Nursing Inquiry*, **9**(3), 162–169.

Traynor M., Boland, M. & Buus, N. (2010) Autonomy, evidence and intuition: nurses and decision-making. *Journal of Advanced Nursing*, **66**(7), 1584–1591.

Wakefield, A.J., Murch, S.H., Anthony, A. *et al.* (1998) Ileal-lymhoid-nodular hyerplasia, non-specific colitis, and pervasive developmental disorder in children. *Lancet*, **351**, 737–641.

Wenger, E. (1998) *Communities of Practice, Learning, Meaning and Identity*. Cambridge University Press, Cambridge.

Wenger E. (2006) *Communities of Practice*. Available from: http://www.ewenger.com/theory/index.htm (pp. 1–5; accessed 4 August, 2010).

Wilson, P. (2002) How to find the good and avoid the bad or ugly: a short guide to tools for rating quality of health information on the internet. *British Medical Journal*, **324**, 9 March, 598–602.

Appendix 1 Activities for Chapter 1

Activity 1.1

Analysing health visitor – client interactions

With a colleague, role-play an interaction with a health visitor and client. Tape record this and listen and analyse the conversation. Focus on the detail of the words and silences and what they are achieving. What can you learn from this? There is some excellent guidance in Taylor and White (2000).

Activity 1.2

Finding the supportive evidence

Identify two common health visitor interventions and provide the evidence which a commissioner would use in deciding whether to pay for them. Do you find the evidence convincing? If the commissioner had to choose between them, which one should take priority?

Activity 1.3

Practising evidence-based medicine (EBM)

Identify what is the best treatment for sore nipples by completing the table below using the steps of EBM.

Steps to EMB	Example
Identify the need for information and formulate question	What is the best treatment for sore nipples?
Track down best possible source of evidence to answer question	
Evaluate it for validity and clinical applicability	
Compare the evidence you have with the practice you have seen. Does It support it? If not, how would you argue for a change in practice?	
How would you evaluate the outcome?	

Activity 1.4

Assessing the effectiveness of your practice

Identify a question about the effectiveness of health visiting practice. Search the organisational websites such as NICE (http://www.nice.org.uk/); SIGN (http://www.sign.ac.uk/) or Cochrane Collaboration (http://www.cochrane.org/) to collect your evidence. How easy are they to use to find the evidence? Did they help you answer your question?

Activity 1.5

Identify and evaluate the evidence base

Think of an alternative therapy for example, reflexology and explore the evidence base and if a client asked about the effectiveness of this treatment what would you tell them?

Activity 1.6

Implementing research evidence

Using the categorisation of barriers as suggested by Gerrish (2003) (i.e. factors relating to the organisation, the way research is communicated; the quality of research, and the practitioner) explore the barriers in your own practice context.

Activity 1.7

Use of guidelines

Identify in your practice a guideline currently in use. Discuss the sources of evidence that underpin it. You might like to use the 'The AGREE Collaboration. Appraisal of Guidelines for Research & Evaluation (AGREE) Instrument' (available from: www.agreecollaboration.org) for appraising the quality of the guideline, asking such questions as: has the overall objective of the guideline been described?; have the clients' views and preferences been taken into account?; has the criteria for selecting the evidence been clearly described?

2
Health Visiting: Context and Public Health Practice

Martin Smith
Mersey Deanery School of Public Health, Liverpool, UK

Maria Horne
The University of Manchester, Manchester, UK

Introduction

Health visiting has long been recognised as providing the model for public health nursing in the UK. However, for a number of decades it has found itself having to respond to a fast-moving world of policy change and contrasting political views of public health. The result of which has left the profession constantly having to adapt to the prevailing political ideology in order to ensure its survival. To its credit – if not relief – the profession has responded well to these challenges. Indeed, since the late 1990s there has been an implicit assumption in UK policy that health visitors have a key public health role to play in the support of children and families (Home Office, 1998; DH, 1999, 2010a; HM Government, 2006). It could be argued that such policies arose less in the interests of health visiting and more as a means to securing the economic potential of the future adult population, as Glass (1999) suggested was the case with Sure Start. Nevertheless, these and a plethora of other policies at both global and national level have resulted in health visiting becoming increasingly associated with an early years' intervention model for practice and framed within a public health context through working with individuals, families and communities (DH, 1999, 2003, 2011).

What is less clear is exactly what the public health context means for health visiting. The origins of health visiting are said to be firmly rooted in a public health approach (Frost & Horner, 2009) and indeed, its beginnings as an occupation are said to have aligned closely with the public health movement (Cowley & Frost, 2006). However, public health itself is recognised as a contested concept (Verweij & Dawson, 2009) with different and often

Health Visiting: A Rediscovery, Third Edition. Edited by Karen A. Luker, Jean Orr and Gretl A. McHugh.
© 2012 Blackwell Publishing Ltd. Published 2012 by Blackwell Publishing Ltd.

conflicting interpretations of its meaning. This chapter aims to articulate the concept of public health for the practice of health visiting. To do so will expose public health as a social construct with a range of perspectives on what it means and some of the consequent tensions and ambiguities that exist between policy and practice. It is therefore an analytical text rather than a description of 'how to do' public health nursing. This is important for two reasons. Firstly, as Craig (2000) highlights, the range of perspectives on what public health nursing is, does have a direct impact on how that role is practised. Secondly, it is important for practitioners to consider these tensions because their own understanding of public health, and their role as specialist community public health nurses (SCPHNs) will frame the decisions they make concerning their own health, the approach they take to the interpretation of policy, and the promotion of health with others.

This exploration of the connection between health visiting and public health is particularly relevant for contemporary practice and a policy context which focuses the role on families and young children. This analysis will therefore take account of a broad child health policy framework that covers both international and national policy and legislation. Globally, UNICEF has reported continuing concerns over the plight of children subjected to the forces of poverty and inequities in health (UNICEF, 2009). This UNICEF Report was published twenty years after the United Nations Convention on the Rights of the Child (UNCRC) (UNICEF, 1989). The UNCRC highlights the rights of children to life and health, and yet globally one billion children are still deprived of food or shelter, clean water or healthcare, with thousands of children under the age of five dying every day from preventable causes (UNICEF, 2009). The UNCRC is the world's most ratified convention of which the UK government is a signatory. Furthermore, the UK government was a signatory along with other UN member states to the Millennium Declaration in 2000 (UN, 2000). This Declaration set out eight goals to be achieved by 2015, two of which were concerned with reducing child mortality (reduce by two-thirds, between 1990 and 2015) and improving maternal health (reduce maternal mortality by three-quarters, between 1990 and 2015). Again, despite the aspirations of governments to these goals and perhaps as a consequence of the limited power and authority of the United Nations, the evidence to date suggests much work is still to be done (UNICEF, 2010).

A concern for the health and wellbeing of children is also particularly important nationally at a time when the UK government grapples with the outcomes of a global recession and a political strategy to stimulate economic growth through a reduction in public services. Indeed, recession or not, the constant pressure for cost efficiency within health and social care services means that the ongoing political rhetoric for reducing child poverty and improving the health and life chances for children presents significant challenges on the one hand but opportunities for health visiting on the other. This was clearly evident in the Marmot Review of health inequalities which set out the disproportionate impact of poverty on the lives of children and called for a policy objective of 'Giving every child the best start in life' as their highest priority with health visitors having a key role (Marmot *et al.*, 2010: 15). From a policy perspective, health visitors are clearly at the forefront of supporting these goals through leading the Healthy Child Programme (DH, 2009) and also through strong links to Sure Start Children Centres (Lansley, 2010). Additionally, the recent *Health Visitor Implementation Plan* is clearly focused on a role designed to give children and their families a healthy start (DH, 2011).

This chapter, therefore, will offer an analysis of the health visiting role with children and families and will consider how this sits with a public health approach to practice. This is important as it has been argued that a focus on children rather than addressing health needs across the whole population does not fit a public health approach (Symonds, 1991). However, children are a distinct population within the population and as will be demonstrated from a lifecourse perspective poor social circumstances in early life can have lasting influences (Davey Smith *et al.*, 1997). Lifecourse theory therefore suggests that children are exposed to health and environmental factors that subsequently are connected to the development of disorders, disability, and death in adulthood. Consequently health visitors are in a prominent position to maximise the health and wellbeing of children who will subsequently become the adult population with children of their own.

The Marmot Review (Marmot *et al.*, 2010) recognised this and saw health visitors as critical to the success of any programme that aimed to improve the life chances of children and highlighted concerns at the falling numbers of health visitors. The Review was not a lone voice in highlighting the depleting health visitor workforce and its capacity to respond to the needs of children and families with calls for significant investment (HSC, 2009; UKPHA, 2009; UNITE, 2009). However, despite these calls and an expedient political rhetoric on the importance of health visiting (DH, 2007, 2009; DH/DCSF, 2009) it appeared that future prospects were bleak.

The advent of a new UK coalition government in 2010 brought significant changes for health visiting. So ironically, at a time of economic and social austerity the profession finds itself at the dawning of a new era with significant investment on the horizon that will result in a 50% increase in the workforce by 2015 (DH, 2010b). This investment will come at a price with health visitors facing challenges in enacting government policy that, it will be argued, diverge from the four principles that underpin health visiting (CETHV, 1977) and which are explored in detail in this chapter. Consequently, meeting these challenges will mean that health visitors have to make full use of each of the four principles in order to optimise any possibility of success.

Throughout the discussion, the terms 'health visiting' and 'public health nursing' will be used interchangeably. This is not to assume that the terms mean exactly the same thing. Indeed, Craig (2000) has already given an enlightening deconstruction of the concept of 'public health nursing' and what this means for UK health visiting. However, for the purposes of this chapter the analysis will remain focused on the context of health visiting for a public health role and not on the relationship between health visiting and nursing per se.

Public health

Before examining the relationship between health visitors and the public health function, it is important to consider and understand what is meant by 'public health' and the language and frameworks commonly used. The term 'public health' is widely recognised as a contested concept (Baggott, 2000; Orme *et al.*, 2007; Verweij & Dawson, 2009). As a result, several terms are used which describe or help to explain the need for public health and public health initiatives. In the first instance, and to support the analysis, it may be useful to consider the two underlying terms related to public health separately; that of 'public' and 'health'.

Defining public

Verweij and Dawson (2009) suggest the term 'public' may be interpreted in two ways. Firstly, as an aggregate (sum) of the health experiences of individuals that make up a population to determine the public's 'health'. Examples of populations in this context can be seen in Box 2.1. You may also find Activity 2.1 useful (see Appendix 2 at the end of the chapter).

Box 2.1   Examples of defined populations for health visitors

- Geographically determined, e.g. GP registered practice list; geographical area
- Settings, e.g. workplaces, schools, prisons, nurseries
- Characteristics, e.g. homeless, travelling families, asylum seekers

---

And secondly, how 'public' reflects collective and organised action either by the state or groups of people. Therefore, 'both the interventions and objectives of public health are "public" and go beyond the level of individuals' (Verweij & Dawson, 2009: 21). The concept of 'public' is important for health visitors as much of their work is with individual people. However, an understanding of the health of those individuals can be aggregated to a population level to support a broader understanding of health need and the social context within which clients live their lives. Furthermore, the notion of collective or organised action can mean two things for health visitors:

- The *organisation* of a response for care based on the health visitor understanding the aggregate need within the 'population' of clients. For example, the development of a postnatal support group in response to an increasing demand for postnatal mental health support.
- Facilitating and supporting *collective* action either with or on behalf of groups or communities to tackle local issues that affect health. For example, supporting a resident's association in articulating the health impact of poor housing in a community or seeking political support to prevent the closure of a nursery.

Understanding the concept of 'public' through work that is substantially with individuals does present challenges for health visitors. The process of contact and care with one individual or family, followed by another, fragments the perception of population in day-to-day practice. SmithBattle *et al.* (2004) were aware of this difficulty that inexperienced Public Health Nurses (PHNs)[1] in Canada were finding as they came to terms with the transition from nursing to public health nursing. This finding arose from a qualitative study that was designed to consider knowledge and skill acquisition of PHNs through their experience. The study demonstrated how through experiential learning, the PHNs developed a perceptual grasp of the 'bigger picture' through experience. There was a shift by the PHNs from a reliance on a nurse focused agenda with predetermined frameworks and protocols to follow, to a 'situated understanding of practice' (SmithBattle *et al.*, 2004: 96). In other words, through their experiences with individuals and families they were increasingly able to recognise the larger patterns and subtle cues that were embedded within the social context of clients' lives. The PHNs demonstrated a shift from viewing client contact as a narrow, clinical situation to one in which the PHNs instinctively began to see patterns that required a community response. As one of the PHNs stated: 'Individuals in a community are as healthy as their community is, and vice versa …You can't address one without addressing the other' (SmithBattle *et al.*, 2004: 99). The study was therefore clear in its view that 'individual and family level experience was a crucial foundation for aggregate-level practice' (SmithBattle *et al.*, 2004: 99).

So for health visitors, the concept of 'public' as something that reflects collective and organised action (Verweij & Dawson, 2009) may be likely to develop with experience, as health visitors gain a perceptual understanding and readiness to respond to the broader issues surrounding complex situations in families.

Defining health

Defining 'health' is equally complex. How it is defined is determined by the underlying perspectives and values of those that seek to explain what health is. Earle (2007) highlights how health can therefore be categorised into three broad areas:

- Health as the absence of disease. This reflects a negative (i.e. absence of disease) narrow biomedical interpretation of health.
- Broader interpretations of health concerned with health as wellbeing in its widest, positive sense. For example, the frequently cited World Health Organisation (WHO) defined health as a 'state of complete physical, social

[1] Public health nurses in Canada have a similar role to health visitors in the UK.

and mental wellbeing, and not merely the absence of disease and infirmity' (WHO, 1946).

- Health as a resource suggesting that health is embedded in the processes and actions of everyday life. For example, WHO (1986) define health as: 'a resource for everyday life, not the object of living. It is a positive concept emphasising social and personal resources as well as physical capabilities'.

Cowley and Frost (2006) refer to the challenges of attempting to define the value of health and refer to work done by health visitors in 1992 that considered the value of health and its practicability through health promotion from a health visiting perspective. This working group identified seven underpinning beliefs to inform health visiting practice:

1. *Rights and responsibilities*: Through a fundamental right of all to an optimum state of health, health visitors take on a responsibility to address health inequality and inequity.
2. *Health in context*: Health cannot be separated from the socioeconomic and cultural context from which it is experienced. It is the health visitor's understanding of the individuals, their families and their communities that takes account of the wider influences on health.
3. *Choice and blame*: Health must be regarded in broad holistic terms, encompassing individuals and families within their personal situation. Health visitors need to utilise their skills to promote an environment in which individuals, families and communities are able to make healthy choices. To do so, health visitors will also need to consider who in society has responsibility for health beyond the individual, to minimise the risk of 'blaming the victim' (Ryan, 1976).
4. *Positive health*: Health promotion involves finding ways to create resources for health. This requires health visitors to think innovatively with families and communities about how to maximise their social and personal resources to effect health improvement.
5. *Health improvement*: Health visitors work to enable people to make full use of their physical, emotional and social capacities to improve health. The focus is on working with the active participation of clients to address those factors that influence their health in the broader context.
6. *Empowerment*: Enabling people to recognise that through active participation, they have the power to achieve health for themselves and to shape their own lives and those of their families. Health visitors therefore need to recognise the importance of facilitating people to engage in decision-making about their health. In particular, those groups in the population, e.g. those on low incomes, from ethnic minority groups or with mental health problems who are frequently marginalised and excluded and known to make less use of services.

7. *Community partnership and participation*: Healthcare services should be readily acceptable and accessible, and involve full community participation. This requires health visitors to work together with individuals, families and communities and alongside other professionals in order to maximise the opportunities and capabilities for improving health.

(adapted from Cowley & Frost, 2006: 13-14)

From the analysis undertaken by the working group that Cowley and Frost refer to, it is evident that the concept of health requires health visitors to be adaptable and responsive to the needs of the most disadvantaged and socially excluded in society. The health visitor role becomes one that seeks out ways to promote health that takes account of the environment in which people live in, alongside enabling people to actively participate and shape their own lives. Activity 2.2 (see Appendix 2) may be useful in helping you to explore your own underpinning values for health promotion.

Defining public health

By recognising the diverse nature of 'public' and 'health' and the competing perspectives that can occur in those explanations, it is not surprising then, that to interpret 'public health' presents significant challenges. Verweij and Dawson (2009) highlight how interpretations of public health fall into two main categories: narrow and broad, much as the above definitions of health do. The narrow perspective sees public health in terms of how long people can remain free from disease. In contrast, the broad perspective sees public health in terms of not only protecting the health of the population but also in a broader role of health promotion and disease prevention (Verweij & Dawson, 2009). This broader view of public health is said to be 'anticipatory, geared to the prevention of illness rather than simply the provision of care and treatment services' (Baggott, 2000: 1). However, taking a broad approach presents a key difficulty for the concept of public health. Perspectives that are packaged to be so inclusive and capture the broad issues across society result in a concept that is so ambiguous they risk collapsing into a confusing set of ideas that are devoid of any useful purpose. The temptation to define public health in narrow terms is strong, to address a specific problem or disease but then risks focusing on treatment and provision of care without taking account of the broad range of factors that can influence health. You may wish to undertake Activity 2.3 (see Appendix 2) at this point.

Different perspectives on public health will reflect what society sees as the priorities for improving the health of the public (Baggott, 2000). Baggott highlights that 'Different interests favour their own particular interpretations of public health and their interplay establishes its meaning … it is essentially a political process' (Baggott, 2000: 2). As highlighted in the introduction, the political process of public health has clearly had an impact on health visitors and their health promoting work with children and families in recent decades. Baggott goes on to suggest three broad ideological perspectives on public health that reflect the key ideological debates surrounding freedom and responsibility between the individual and the state. Table 2.1 summarises Baggott's interpretation of these ideologies and also includes an application of these ideologies and the implications for children and families.

It is clear from the table that the prevailing political environment has an impact upon how services for families with children are delivered. Indeed, current UK policies are designed to recover savings as a result of a recession through a reduction in public sector spending. This will have an impact on children and families, with cutbacks in services and benefits. Health visitors will therefore increasingly face the outcomes from these cutbacks and be working with families with reduced or limited incomes where services may no longer be available for family support. It is therefore important at this point to consider public health more specifically in relation to health visiting.

A frequently cited definition of public health is that of the UK Commission for Inquiry into the Public Health Function undertaken in the late 1980s: 'The science and art of preventing disease, prolonging life and promoting health through the organised efforts of society' (DH, 1988). It is often referred to as the 'Acheson definition' as Sir Donald Acheson, the Chief Medical Officer at the time, chaired the committee. This definition clearly presents a broad interpretation of public health and encompasses some of the difficulties in interpretation highlighted above. It also reflects much of the collectivist ideology in Table 2.1. Beaglehole and Bonita (1997) have also suggested that the definition emphasises the main components of public health:

- population perspective;
- collective responsibility for health and prevention;
- role of the state linked to a concern for underlying socioeconomic determinants of health as well as disease;
- multidisciplinary basis which incorporates quantitative and qualitative approaches;
- emphasis on partnerships with populations served.

These components see health improvement through action with populations that take account of the wider social determinants of health, much as Cowley and Frost's (2006) seven underpinning beliefs for health promotion in health visiting mentioned earlier seek to demonstrate. One of the key phrases within the Acheson definition is the 'science and art of preventing disease'. This phrasing reflects not only a scientific perspective that uses epidemiological evidence and research to determine the causes of ill health, but also suggests public health is concerned with innovation and action through public health delivery. For health visitors, this is a key aspect of practice in not only being able to understand the needs of the population through the process of health needs assessment (discussed more in Chapter 3), but also how to 'create' a response to those needs in practice at a local level. For example, following cuts within the welfare system, working jointly with local welfare rights agencies to make welfare rights and benefits information accessible in a local clinic.

Table 2.1 Ideological perspectives on public health.

Collectivist/socialist perspectives	Liberal individualist perspectives	Environmental and green perspectives
• Emphasise the role of the state and other collective arrangements	• Individuals free to pursue activities without interference from the state providing no harm to others	• Oppose the destructiveness of industrial society
• Mutual approaches and co-operatives – organising people together	• Suggest that the socialist perspective coerces and disempowers citizens.	• Place an emphasis on the role of individuals and small, local groups in promoting the local environment
• Questions the ability of individuals to produce their own solutions to complex social problems	• Individual freedom should not be sacrificed for an elusive common good	• An ecological model of health – environmental influences
• Equity in health is a key element of social justice	• Emphasises individual responsibility for health; individuals should make informed choices rather than be told what to do by the 'nanny state'	• Many health problems linked to pollution – viewed as the product of human exploitation of the environment.
• individuals have little incentive to contribute to population health improvement – the prevention paradox	• Negative liberty – the freedom to pursue activities without interference from the state	• Structure of industrial society is damaging in view of its tendency to create unhealthy lifestyles and working patterns, as well as to produce socioeconomic inequalities that undermine health.
• Positive liberty: extent to which individuals are in control of their own fate & free from circumstances that limit opportunities		• Holistic solution required – sustainable development, balancing economic, social and environmental considerations.

| **Implications for children and families** | • Development of national policy programmes, e.g. Healthy Child Programme; immunisations; Sure Start; Family Nurse Partnerships
• Legislation to minimise the impact of advertising, e.g. tobacco, fast food, alcohol
• National policy to support healthy lifestyles; Child health Strategy; Healthy Start; National healthy School Standard
• State legislation to protect children from abuse
• Policy to constrain the disciplining of children
• Provision of parenting programmes
• Tackling poverty through state provided benefits for families with children
• Making services accessible in response to the disproportionate impact of health inequalities on children
• Family and child friendly working practices in the workplace | • Reduction of state involvement in all but essential health protection initiatives, e.g. immunisation and screening
• Freedom from state involvement in how parents utilise their resources and capacity to parent their children
• Freedom from interference by the state in the family – limiting the involvement of public services
• Freedom to choose how and when to access services
• Access to income through personal venture to gain employment to support the family
• Reduction in state benefits leading to reduced taxation and greater levels of income for meeting children's needs
• Freedom to discipline children in a way parents feel appropriate | • State policy programmes for supporting children and families, but considering the health impact of policies e.g. energy; transport; business and commerce
• Emphasis on reducing health impact in the environment on children, e.g. air quality; industrial and domestic waste; energy usage
• Legislation to minimise the influence of industry that seeks profit through unhealthy lifestyles, e.g. tobacco, fast food, alcohol
• State legislation to protect children from abuse
• Making services accessible in response to the disproportionate impact of health inequalities on children
• Family and child friendly working practices in the workplace
• Local, community based campaigns for health improvement, e.g. road safety for children; healthy eating initiatives; safer play areas |

Source: Aapted from Baggott (2001) and applied to children and families.

Human rights and public health

Beaglehole and Bonita's (1997) analysis of the Acheson definition highlights collective responsibility, concern for socioeconomic determinants of health and the importance of partnerships for public health. These also suggest an underlying significance of human rights for health. Sirkin *et al.* (2005: 538) are very clear that healthcare professionals 'have a responsibility to protect and promote human rights'. The reasons for this are twofold. Firstly, those human rights that are violated (e.g. being subjected to torture or deprived of an education) can have health consequences. And secondly, that the process of promoting and protecting human rights can be the most effective means to securing health (Sirkin *et al.*, 2005). Health visitors therefore have a responsibility to protect and promote human rights as a means to optimising the health of communities and to reducing the impact of health inequalities. Indeed, as employees of a public service, health visitors are required to comply with the UK Human Rights Act 1998 and to international legislation that the UK government has ratified. This includes:

- the Universal Declaration of Human Rights (UDHR) (UN, 1948);
- the International Covenant on Economic, Social and Cultural Rights (ICESCR) (UN, 1966);
- the European Convention on Human Rights (ECHR) (Council of Europe, 1950);
- the United Nations Convention on the Rights of the Child (UNCRC) (UNICEF, 1989).

These declarations of human rights contain series of 'articles' that reflect rights of freedom and rights of protection; what Fromer (1981) refers to as option rights and welfare rights respectively. As Sirkin *et al.* (2005) allude to above, if the ideal health outcomes in the WHO definition of health are to be acknowledged, then health will underpin all human rights. Conversely, this could be on occasion when in the interests of public health, other human rights may be restricted. For example, in circumstances when someone is detained against their will for a highly infectious disease or risk of harm to the self or others.

Despite the UK Government having ratified these conventions, in relation to human rights there is only the Human Rights Act 1998 that is enshrined in UK Law and is therefore the framework that makes the UK Government directly accountable for human rights. However, international covenants of human rights are referred to in legal processes and are accepted as part of legal argument to determine case law. Interestingly, the UK Human Rights Act and its parent human rights framework, the ECHR do not contain a specific article on the right to health, thereby removing any explicit accountability for that right from national legislation. If health visitors therefore wish to use the UK Human Rights Act to argue the right to health, they need to articulate that right through deprivation of rights under the available articles within the Act, much as Sirkin *et al.* (2005) highlight above in the process of promoting and protecting human rights.

Box 2.2   Article 24 of the United Nations Convention on the Rights of the Child (UNICEF, 1989)

1. States Parties recognise the right of the child to the enjoyment of the highest attainable standard of health and to facilities for the treatment of illness and rehabilitation of health. States Parties shall strive to ensure that no child is deprived of his or her right of access to such health care services.

2. States Parties shall pursue full implementation of this right and, in particular, shall take appropriate measures:
   (a) To diminish infant and child mortality;
   (b) To ensure the provision of necessary medical assistance and health care to all children with emphasis on the development of primary health care;
   (c) To combat disease and malnutrition, including within the framework of primary health care, through, inter alia, the application of readily available technology and through the provision of adequate nutritious foods and clean drinking-water, taking into consideration the dangers and risks of environmental pollution;
   (d) To ensure appropriate pre-natal and post-natal health care for mothers;
   (e) To ensure that all segments of society, in particular parents and children, are informed, have access to education and are supported in the use of basic knowledge of child health and nutrition, the advantages of breastfeeding, hygiene and environmental sanitation and the prevention of accidents;
   (f) To develop preventive health care, guidance for parents and family planning education and services.

3. States Parties shall take all effective and appropriate measures with a view to abolishing traditional practices prejudicial to the health of children.

4. States Parties undertake to promote and encourage international cooperation with a view to achieving progressively the full realisation of the right recognised in the present article. In this regard, particular account shall be taken of the needs of developing countries.

In the case of the UN Declarations, member states are required to submit reports to the UN of their performance against the articles in the declarations, but again, without explicit national legislation accountability is limited. There is further discussion on human rights legislation and its impacts for health visiting in Chapter 5, particularly in relation to the United Nations Convention on the Rights of the Child. However, it is suffice to say at this point that the UNCRC does contain a specific article on the right to health for children that has relevance to health visiting and a public health role (see Box 2.2).

Article 24 of the UNCRC in Box 2.2 sets out a comprehensive statement about the rights of the child to health that takes account of the wider determinants and in particular the right of access to healthcare. The article also makes reference to the concept of 'progressive realisation'. This is an acknowledgement of the governmental obligations to the UNCRC, and that the rights may be difficult to achieve in a short timescale. However, this does mean that governments are required to demonstrate through their reporting to the UN, that they are taking steps towards 'realisation' of the right to health (Gruskin & Tarantola, 2004). It is also clear that achievement or otherwise of the remaining articles of the UNCRC will each have a profound impact on securing the health of children. You may wish to explore this further in Activity 2.4 (see Appendix 2).

The UNCRC also needs to be viewed within the context of the WHO definition of health, the Universal Declaration of Human Rights (UDHR) (UN, 1948) and the International Covenant on Economic and Cultural Rights (ICESCR) (UN, 1966) which also contain rights to health. The UDHR was noteworthy as the first articulation of the right to health. However, the ICESCR holds particular significance for public health and health visiting. The Covenant under Article 12 'recognises the right of everyone to the enjoyment of the highest attainable standard of physical and mental health' (UN, 1966) and also makes specific reference to a reduction in child mortality and the healthy development of children under this Article. The Covenant also places a particular emphasis on the social and economic context to people's lives and reflects how in the absence of rights of freedom and protection the infrastructure for health is lost. The United Nations have affirmed this with the statement that under Article 12 of the ICESCR:

> States must protect this right [the right to health] by ensuring that everyone within their jurisdiction has access to the underlying determinants of health, such as clean water, sanitation, food, nutrition and housing, and through a comprehensive system of healthcare, which is available to everyone without discrimination, and economically accessible to all.
>
> (CESCR, 2000)

The United Nations is very clear therefore, through the ICESCR and the UNCRC, that not only do the underlying social and economic determinants of health need to be addressed in order to realise an attainment of health but also that member states need to recognise the unfair distribution of those determinants and that they should take steps to reduce the impact of health inequalities. Health visitors therefore need to recognise how this international framework of legislation can be used to support their role as an advocate for local children, families and communities.

Not only is there a legislative requirement for health visitors to uphold human rights, but also it could be argued from an ethical standpoint that health visitors have a moral duty to promote and protect human rights as a means to securing health. Indeed, the Code of Conduct (NMC, 2008) requires nurses, midwives and health visitors to 'work with others to protect and promote the health and wellbeing of those in your care, their families and carers, and the wider community' (NMC, 2008: 2). This statement clearly resonates with the role of health visitors. Furthermore from an ethical standpoint, health visitors need to have an understanding of how ethical health visiting practice links to a public health approach. Beauchamp and Childress (2001) identified four principles for ethical practice: autonomy, beneficence, nonmaleficence and justice. Table 2.2 highlights the implications of these ethical principles for health visitors in their role of protecting and promoting health:

In summary at this point, the process of defining the underlying concepts associated with public health have demonstrated clear associations with health visiting and their role in promoting health and reducing health inequities. Furthermore, this is supported by an ethical and moral justification for promoting the health of children and their families through consideration of the broad social determinants of health. It is useful therefore, with reference to the above discussion, to progress further to a consideration of the underpinning principles of health visiting that enables an articulation of the public health role for health visiting.

Table 2.2 Principles for ethical health visiting practice.

Principles	Implications for health visiting practice
Autonomy	Supporting freedom to self-determination by building self-esteem of clients and encouraging active participation in how to shape their lives for improving health.
Beneficence	Supporting health improvement with individuals, families and communities through the identification of health needs that takes account of the broader social determinants of health.
Nonmaleficence	Ensuring that health visiting practice uses evidence-based approaches and is undertaken cost effectively for disadvantaged populations. This is important for two reasons: • practice that is delivered inappropriately through outdated methods or without an evidence base could potentially be harmful to clients; • delivering care to populations with fewer needs means a cost to the time and opportunity for addressing the health needs of those who need it most.
Justice	Ensuring that health visiting practice is delivered equitably across the population and is focused on addressing the needs of vulnerable groups in the population and seeking to reduce the impact of health inequalities.

The principles of health visiting

The Acheson definition also views public health in terms of disease prevention and health promotion. There are thus clear and direct parallels here with the role of health visiting defined as 'The promotion of health and the prevention of ill health' (CETHV, 1977). Such an approach clearly draws health visiting into the anticipatory and preventive nature of public health by seeking to prevent illness and improve the health and quality of life for whole populations of people that they work with. Health visitors undertake this work by focusing at various times on individuals, families, groups or communities.

Health visiting itself is underpinned by four principles (CETHV, 1977). These principles were first articulated over three decades ago by the Council for the Education and Training of Health Visitors, the Regulatory Body for Health Visiting at that time. However, they have been reaffirmed more recently by Cowley and Frost (2006) and are said to reflect the knowledge base and process of health visiting (UKPHA, 2009):

- the search for health needs;
- the stimulation of an awareness of health needs;
- the influence on policies affecting health and;
- the facilitation of health-enhancing activities.

Each of the principles are interconnected with each other and form the basis for health improvement with individuals, families and communities. They reflect a philosophy of health visiting (rather than specific activities per se) that focuses intervention with those people identified as in greatest need and therefore aim to reduce health inequalities. The UKHPA (2009) highlight the importance of these principles for children and families; particularly the most disadvantaged who become socially excluded and who suffer comparatively poorer levels of health. The principles of health visiting are also clearly action focused which again reflects the art of preventing disease, prolonging life and promoting health aspect of public health. A consideration of each of the principles demonstrates they have distinct features that are embedded within a public health approach.

The search for health needs

The search for health needs is viewed as an essential starting point for health improvement (Cowley & Frost, 2006). Whilst it forms the basis of an assessment process with populations in order to develop a plan to improve health, often in the form of a health needs assessment, it also frames the search for health need within a positive interpretation of health. Health needs assessment will be considered in more detail in Chapter 3 but suffice to say at this point that searching for health needs broadens the horizon within which the health visitor views the people they work with and the factors to take into account when making an assessment. The emphasis is on what needs can be fulfilled to maximise health rather than what the health problem(s) is/are. Searching out need therefore goes beyond the individual client to the context within which they live their lives, e.g. their access to material resources and services, income and employment.[2] Searching for health needs therefore aligns with a public health approach as a preventive process that takes account of the wider determinants of health.

However, it has to be acknowledged that meeting health needs will be a challenging area of health visiting practice, given the increasing pressures and likely cuts in public and voluntary sector services (BBC News, 2011). There is a risk of minimising those health needs that the health visitor perceives may require additional assistance or referral and prioritising a focus on the client changing their individual behaviours. Given the account above on the client's rights to health and the duty of the health visitor to respond to those rights, health visitors need to think creatively about how they respond to unmet health needs. For example, utilising an asset based community development approach (Kretzmann & McKnight, 1993) with peer- or group-based approaches can be an empowering process for clients to finding solutions to needs through a collective approach. Searching out health needs is therefore a challenging but important process for opening up the social determinants of health in client's lives. This is in contrast, as Cowley and Frost (2006) point out, to other primary healthcare professionals who will be framed by the presence of illness or disease and will be constrained by a focus on the health problem to be treated or rectified.

The stimulation of an awareness of health needs

The knowledge and understanding that health visitor's gain from searching for health needs is a rich resource for raising awareness to determine an appropriate public health response. For example the health visitor's awareness of the extent of domestic abuse occurring in the community, and the associated impacts on families and the community as a whole, are important pieces of information that warrant some form of action. What is less clear is whose awareness is to be stimulated. Cowley and Frost (2006) suggest three different levels to engage awareness raising in order for an issue to be recognised as a priority. These have been applied to the issue of domestic abuse below:

- *With individuals and communities*, e.g. building trusting relationships and focusing on attributes and capability to promote self-esteem in people suffering from domestic abuse and to be able to explore with them the unseen impact of domestic abuse on their health and the health of children. Such an approach can stimulate awareness of health as a positive resource.
- *With commissioners and providers of services*, e.g. to raise their awareness of the extent of domestic abuse as an often hidden and unmet need. The purpose is to give a richer understanding about the barriers and challenges that exist for health service managers when attempting to meet key health improvement targets in local areas. For example women experiencing domestic abuse are more likely to smoke, have an alcohol dependency or suffer from depression. In this situation, the approach to improving health targets means also investing resources in to tackling domestic abuse.

[2] Material resources in this context refer to those living materials that are considered essential, e.g. adequate shelter, heating, washing and cooking facilities, healthy food or safe toys and play facilities.

- *With politicians and policy-makers*, e.g. raising awareness of politicians about proposed cuts in services for people experiencing domestic abuse and the subsequent impacts for individuals, society and the economy.

Health visitors should therefore be prepared to employ all of these levels in order to maximise the opportunities for improving the health of individuals, their families and communities. To do so will require the health visitor to think critically as to whom the most appropriate audience to engage with is and raise full awareness of health need.

The influence on policies affecting health

Influencing policy development has been perceived as the most challenging of the principles for most health visitors (Cowley & Frost, 2006). The political nature of public health suggests that perspectives on public health and healthcare policy should be challenged to recognise the needs of the most vulnerable in society. In effect, the practitioner becomes an advocate for those with health needs to challenge and support policy-making in ensuring that policies have a positive health impact. Cowley and Frost (2006) suggest that this principle has three underpinning mechanisms for health visiting:

- *Health intelligence:* a recognition of timely local population evidence, often ahead of official statistics can be useful in determining a local policy response or service development. For example, health visitors are able to use their up-to-date knowledge of the community through the process of health needs assessment (HNA) and other ways (explored in Chapter 3), to gather qualitative information to highlight health needs.
- *Innovation and change:* being an active participant in change; challenging current practice and becoming involved in new approaches. An example of this could be as a member of a project steering group to develop a breastfeeding policy in a Local Authority Children's Centre.
- *Acting as a resource:* either:
  - directly
    - undertaking and disseminating robust research to support policy-makers in identifying best practice to underpin new policies;
    - getting involved in policy development which may include redesigning local service delivery;
    - informing or responding to policy proposals;
  - indirectly
    - enabling community groups or pressure groups to access and interpret information on health and health services;
    - enabling colleagues and other services to interpret the health impact of policies to ensure their actions are conducive to good health. An example of this could be raising awareness within a school about the unhealthy nature and contradictory messages of having a vending machine containing snack foods and sweets – and to consider alternatives.

The political nature of public health and the extent to which it is dependent upon the values of those that make policy means that this is arguably one of the most important areas of health visiting practice to become involved in. It is the capacity to influence service redesign and policy-making that will determine the extent to which the population will be able to maximise their health potential.

The facilitation of health enhancing activities

Milio (1986) offered the phrase 'making the healthier choice the easier choice'. To do so suggests a focus on addressing the environment within which families and communities live as a means to achieving improvements in their health. Clearly, there are strategies that individuals can be supported in, in changing their health behaviours, but to do so isolates the underlying factors that may be contributing to those behaviours. It is therefore the emphasis on facilitating change in the environment that this principle was originally intended (Cowley & Frost, 2006). Focusing on individual behaviour places clients under substantial pressure to change their lifestyles when they may not have the capacity or resources to do so. Indeed, estimates have suggested that of the gap in health outcomes between the most and least wealthy, only 10–30% may be explained by differences in health-related behaviours (Lantz et al., 1998). This suggests that the remaining 70–90% of the gap is determined by other factors in the individual's social environment. There is therefore a high a risk of failure with the individual behaviour approach that can stifle health-enhancement.

Facilitating health focuses on multidisciplinary approaches to enable people to actively participate and shape their own futures. Giddens (2006: 8) highlights how the 'social contexts of people's lives are not just random assortments of events or actions; they are structured, or patterned in distinct ways'. This social patterning across populations is built on access to income and employment, cultural and community patterns and norms, adequate housing and access to education and healthcare services. Tackling inequalities in health is therefore at the core of facilitating health-enhancing activity. Health inequalities will be discussed further below, but at this point, the key issue is for health visitors not to focus solely on the health behaviours of clients but to see their role within the broader context of social determinants of health. Activity 2.5 (see Appendix 2) may be useful in helping you to explore the principles of health visiting further.

The four principles described above set out the underpinning values and process of health visiting. They resonate with public health principles and form the basis for health visitors to view their practice in a broad context that can promote health-enhancement for the most disadvantaged. The emphasis through the principles is of a population understanding of health and the wider determinants that impact upon people's lives. Success is best placed through a process of enabling people and communities to determine how they can shape their lives to maximise their health experience by prioritising the issues that matter to them. The principles themselves have endured for over thirty years and whatever the political landscape, they have to date, and need in the future, to remain as the bedrock for health visiting practice.

The principles of health visiting are also included in the current Standards of Proficiency for Specialist Community Public Health Nurses produced by the Nursing and Midwifery Council (NMC) (NMC, 2004). As the regulatory body for health visiting, the NMC sets the standards for entry to that part of the NMC register that is concerned with public health nursing and provide the framework which regulates health visitors. Health visitors are not alone on this part of the NMC register which includes school nurses, occupational health nurses, family health nurses in Scotland and nurses practising in a variety of settings including sexual health and health protection. The four principles, (referred to rather ambiguously as 'domains' in the NMC document) are mapped against ten key areas for public health practice (see Box 2.3).

Box 2.3   Ten areas for public health practice (Skills for Health, 2004)

1. Surveillance and assessment of the population's health and wellbeing;
2. Promoting and protecting the population's health and wellbeing;
3. Developing quality and risk management within an evaluative culture;
4. Collaborative working for health and wellbeing;
5. Developing health programmes and services and reducing inequalities;
6. Policy and strategy development and implementation to improve health and wellbeing;
7. Working with and for communities to improve health and wellbeing;
8. Strategic leadership for health and wellbeing;
9. Research and development to improve health and wellbeing;
10. Ethically managing self, people and resources to improve health and wellbeing.

The ten areas for public health practice were developed as national occupational standards for public health practice (Skills for Health, 2004), the purpose of the ten areas being to identify the necessary standards required for the public health workforce to practise within and be measured by.

The Standards of Proficiency were thus developed in 2004, following the creation of the third part to the NMC Register. In a controversial move, health visiting was removed from statute in 2001 at the creation of the NMC in 2002 (UKPHA, 2009). Removal from statute signalled a lack of government support for the profession (Unite/CPHVA, 2009). Previously as a profession in its own right, health visiting had been under the auspices of a regulatory body since 1962. However, since 2004 its status has been that of a post-registration nursing qualification. As discussed above, the preventive nature of public health does not sit easily with a philosophy of healthcare that focuses on managing and caring for individuals with health problems and diseases, as is the case in nursing. The concern was that health visiting risked being increasingly diluted and constrained into a nursing rather than public health model of delivery and regulated within a framework that prevented people from backgrounds other than nursing from being able to join the profession. Indeed, the *Standards of Proficiency for Specialist Community Public Health Nurses* document (NMC, 2004) does not give a context or the origins of the underpinning theoretical framework and its association with public health. There are also gaps particularly around public engagement and the significance of leadership which are both important for effective public health practice.

Current policy suggests a stronger role with children and families by improving and safeguarding health and through leading, managing and delegating programmes of work. Maintaining a public health focus through the regulatory framework will clearly require efforts to preserve an approach that recognises the social determinants of health to reduce health inequalities. Indeed, it is to the issue of health inequalities that the discussion now turns.

Health inequalities

During the nineteenth century public health efforts were concentrated on addressing the appalling living, sanitary and working conditions of the population and the impact of diseases such as cholera, smallpox and tuberculosis (Ashton & Seymour, 1988). Improvements in the environment such as housing, sanitation and water supplies during the late nineteenth century are said to have been the main factors associated with a reduction in deaths from infectious diseases. This became known as the environmental phase of public health (Ashton & Seymour, 1988). The origins of health visiting are said to have lain in this era (Frost & Horner, 2009). However, as Frost and Horner indicate, the greater focus of health visiting was to come at the end of the nineteenth century with the rise of the maternal and infant welfare movement.

Indeed, the early twentieth century saw the influence of public health measures begin to narrow with advances in medicine and scientific knowledge, e.g. the discovery of bacteria and viruses and the development of anaesthesia and antibiotics (Ashton & Seymour, 1988). The result of this was a greater focus on treating the individual and the rise of personal health education. Indeed, as Caraher and McNab (1997) highlight, a focus and concern for health visitors in providing education and teaching to poor families. The increasing emphasis on providing healthcare and clinical interventions, coupled with rapid technological advances in medicine particularly after the Second World War resulted in more attention to treating the unwell rather than addressing the social conditions that prevent illness (Graham, 2007). McKinlay (1975, cited in Graham, 2007: 101) used the metaphors of 'upstream' and 'downstream' to reflect the story told to him by the sociologist Irving Zola, of a doctor jumping in a river to rescue drowning people with no time to look 'upstream' to see why people are falling in the river in the first place. McKinlay suggests that 'downstream', relates to the delivery of medical care whilst 'upstream' thinking challenges us to think of the wider and prevailing set of influencing factors that shape the experience of health.

A series of influential critiques of health policy at the latter end of the twentieth century highlighted the significance of the social determinants of health (Graham, 2007), and as a result the need for a greater emphasis on upstream thinking. Figure 2.1 describes layers of influence that exists within the social structure to form the main determinants of health (Dahlgren & Whitehead, 1991). The most inner layer of the diagram is (arguably) fixed with age, sex and hereditary factors being predetermined. Moving outwards from the inner layer, there is an emphasis on health being partly as a result of individual lifestyle behaviours such as tobacco use, diet and exercise. The diagram then draws attention to the networks and relationships that exist within the family, friends and others in the community that determine cultural norms and beliefs. The following two layers of living and working conditions and the broader socioeconomic, cultural and environmental conditions both relate to the 'upstream' determinants of health. It is here that powerful forces shape health experience. For example, the political landscape and governmental change, industry and business, wealth, access to services, the welfare and taxation system all have an influence on people's lives and the capacity for them to experience good health.

What is less evident from Figure 2.1 is that these layers interact with each other to magnify further poor health experience. For example, unemployment or low pay results in an income that prevents people from sustaining adequate housing arrangements which cause family upheaval and stress. Low income

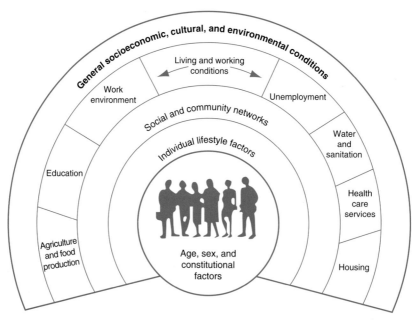

Figure 2.1 The main determinants of health.
Source: Dahlgren & Whitehead (1991), Institute for Futures Studies, Stockholm. (Reproduced by kind permission.)

also impacts on the quality of food consumed and the capacity to engage fully with social and community networks, all of which can compound further levels of stress and anxiety for individuals.

These determinants of health therefore result in variations or inequalities in health experience. However, Whitehead and Dahlgren (2006) contend that these variations are not just unequal. For example, health experiences are different between men and women or across different age groups. They also suggest that some variations are unfair or inequitable. They suggest further that there are three features that underpin health inequities. Firstly that they are systematic; that they do not happen randomly but show a consistent social gradient, i.e. of poor health across societies heavily influenced by socioeconomic status. Essentially, the social gradient refers to the lower an individual's socioeconomic position the worse their health (WHO, 2011). The emphasis is on the word 'gradient' as it is not just the difference between the most and least disadvantaged, but also those in between; that poor health and different levels of income are spread across the population. Hence the steepness of the gradient becomes important too. Secondly, health inequities are socially produced and therefore can be changed e.g. as Whitehead and Dahlgren (2006: 2) highlight, 'No Law of Nature, for instance, decrees that the children of poor families should die at twice the rate as that of children born into rich families.' Thirdly, that health inequity is unfair on the basis of being unjust. For example, all children should have the opportunity to be breastfed, regardless of the socioeconomic status of the parents.

On many levels, tackling health inequities is a fundamental aspect of public health and health visiting practice. From an ethical and human rights perspective and as a duty as a health professional health visitors should undertake their practice with a clear focus of ensuring that whilst ensuring a continuing universal service for all, health visitors focus their work to those most in need. This is what the Marmot Review referred to as 'proportionate universalism' (Marmot *et al.*, 2010: 16). The purpose being to reduce the steepness of the social grading, i.e that tackling health inequities is proportionate to the level of disadvantage.

Recognising that socioeconomic status is a key determinant of health has led some writers to suggest pathways that provide an explanation for health inequalities (Graham, 2007). One such pathway suggests that people's health is influenced over time; through the course of their lives – known as the lifecourse perspective. The lifecourse perspective suggests that disadvantage starts before birth and accumulates throughout life. As the Marmot Review observed:

> From the time of birth, the individual is exposed to a wide range of experiences – social, economic, psychological and environmental … It is the accumulation of these influences, their effects and the interactions that 'cast a long shadow' over subsequent social development, behaviour, health and well-being of the individual.
>
> (Marmot *et al.*, 2010: 40)

In other words, poor health in adulthood may lie in childhood disadvantage. Indeed, there is growing evidence that the circumstances in which children are conceived, born and grow up may reflect later socioeconomic inequalities in the health of adults. Work carried out by Barker (1992) known as the foetal origins hypothesis, suggested that impaired fetal growth during pregnancy (using low birth weight as an indicator) may contribute to disease in adulthood including cardiovascular disease and its precursors such as diabetes, high lipid values and high blood pressure. This indicates that maternal health through pregnancy is a concern; the suggestion being that maternal poverty and disadvantage can affect fetal development (Earle & O'Donnell, 2007). Indeed, disadvantaged mothers are more likely to have babies of low birth weight (Jefferis *et al.*, 2002) and are more likely to be exposed to stress, poor diet, alcohol, tobacco and drug misuse during pregnancy (Marmot *et al.*, 2010). Furthermore, Davey Smith *et al.* (1998) found in their prospective cohort study[3] that poor childhood circumstances increase the risk of death from stroke, heart and respiratory disease in later life. You may find Activity 2.6 (see Appendix 2) useful at this point.

With its emphasis on childhood disadvantage, there are clearly ramifications for the role of health visitors in supporting disadvantaged families with young children. Furthermore, the lifecourse perspective gives a strong indication of the public health interventions that are required with increased attention to the importance of maternal nutrition, breastfeeding and smoking cessation. Consequently, the Marmot Review (Marmot *et al.*, 2010) frames much of its analysis through the lifecourse perspective and not surprisingly identifies health visitors as important to any success in reducing health inequalities to disadvantaged families through their focus on families with infants and young children. The review highlights some key findings through the analysis of material available:

- People living in the poorest areas of England die seven years earlier than those in the most affluent areas.
- The average disability-free life expectancy is 17 years, i.e. people from disadvantaged areas may not only die sooner, but they will also spend more of their later years with a disability than those in affluent areas.
- One in four deaths of infants under the age of one would be avoided if all births had the same level of risk as infants born to those women who are least disadvantaged.
- There are higher rates of smoking and obesity amongst low income groups and higher rates of drug use and alcohol related admissions amongst people living in disadvantaged areas.
- There is a strong social gradient associated with the prevalence of postnatal depression.

---

[3] A prospective study involves taking a cohort of subjects (e.g. a group of people born at the same time) and watching them over a long period to look for outcomes, such as the development of a disease. The intention is to see if this relates to any other factors that are present or not, in those that have the disease or not.

- A child's physical, social, emotional and cognitive development during the early years strongly influences her or his school-readiness and educational attainment:
  - ○ Children with a high cognitive score at 22 months but with parents of low socioeconomic status do less well (in terms of subsequent cognitive development) than children with low initial scores but with parents of high socioeconomic status.
  - ○ Children of educated or wealthy parents can score poorly in early tests but still catch up, whereas children of worse-off parents are extremely unlikely to do so.

The Marmot Review of health inequalities is a report that health visitors will find particularly useful for understanding more about health inequalities and the impact on children, families and communities. It also presents a challenge to health visitors to reflect on and consider appropriate, evidence-based responses to addressing the public health priorities identified in the report. For this reason, you may find it useful to undertake Activity 2.7 (see Appendix 2).

The advent of a new UK coalition Government in 2010 brought about significant policy changes for public health and health visiting (DH, 2010a, 2010b, 2011). The NHS White paper set out arguably the most radical reforms for the NHS in its 60-year history with proposals for structural changes that meant commissioning of services would largely be driven by GPs in primary care. The public health budget was to be ring fenced with a new 'health premium' to promote action in tackling health inequalities' (DH, 2010b: 5). Health visiting will be delivered and funded under the auspices of a new organisation 'Public Health England' with continuing support for the Family Nurse Partnership (FNP) programme. The FNP programme is explored in Chapter 4. Initially, health visiting will be commissioned through a national NHS Commissioning Board although long term, this will be done locally (DH, 2010b). The Public Health White Paper appears to suggest that the commissioning of health visiting services will draw on decision-making at a local level, taking into account the views of the new GP Consortia, Health and Wellbeing Boards in Local Authorities and the local Joint Strategic Needs Assessments.[4] The purpose of this is to foster stronger links between NHS services such as maternity and primary care and local authority early years' services such as children's centres (DH, 2010a: 60). What is not yet clear is who will employ health visitors long term and/or, whether they will return into a local authority setting after nearly forty years or continue to be based within an NHS setting. However, this will be supported by considerable investment in an additional 4200 health visitors by 2015 (DH, 2011).

---

[4] Joint Strategic Needs Assessment is a process that identifies the 'big picture' in terms of the health and wellbeing needs and inequalities of a local population. It is a joint initiative, usually between health and social care services and the local authority and takes a long-term view to informing future service planning and taking into account evidence of effectiveness.

The subsequent action plan to take forward that health visiting investment (DH, 2011) confirms the additional funding for health visitors that will result in a 50% increase in the workforce till 2015. It also sets out a framework for a new health visiting service and these are further explored in Chapter 3 (see Box 3.5).

Existing health visitors will be encouraged to refresh and develop their skills, taking lessons from the early intervention FNP programme and other evidence-based programmes aimed at helping families with complex needs. Interestingly the plan refers to work undertaken by Field (2010) and Allen and Duncan Smith (2010) with the health visitor action plan being a response to the challenges posed in these reports. Both pieces of work clearly focus on early intervention to improve life chances for children; however, there is less focus on socioeconomic factors and social structure and more about what can be done for children and families at an individual level. Indeed Field comments that he has 'come to view poverty as a much more subtle enemy than purely lack of money' (Field, 2010: 12), focusing on the cycle of poverty and disadvantage that occurs across the generations. From this viewpoint, and other early intervention programmes such as the FNP, the behaviour and characteristics of poor parents come to be seen as the problem and as a result the focus for interventions are the changes in individual behaviour. The intention is to break the alleged cycle of deprivation, much as Clarke (2006) suggests in her critique of the Sure Start initiative. However, as discussed above, focusing on individualistic approaches results in a risk that behaviour change may not occur. Additionally, there is the potential psychological harm that can arise with increased levels of stress for individuals' families and groups who feel powerless to respond to messages of behaviour change. The point for health visitors is that whilst the increased investment will be very welcome to the profession, it will come at a cost. Health visitors will have to deliver a government policy that promotes individualised approaches to improving health and minimises the scope for health visitors to address the broader social context.

Focusing on individual behaviour is reflected further in the Public Health White Paper (DH, 2010a) with an emphasis on health improvement and tackling health inequalities through approaches such as 'nudging' people to change health behaviour. Nudging is a phrase coined by Thaler and Sunstein (2008) who suggest that people are more likely to respond to instant reward for benefit now rather than the future. They refer to 'libertarian paternalism' and systems of human thought that lead to instinctive or automatic responses and base the notion of nudging on the premise that it is legitimate to influence behaviour (paternalism) to promote health, but that people should not be compelled to change that behaviour (libertarianism). The cues for people making healthy choices are 'architectured' or designed to occur in subtle ways that nudge them, through their sense of freedom, to make the choices for themselves. These might include placing healthy foods in a prominent position in a cafe or designing a building where it is easier to take the stairs than the escalator. It also includes methods such as providing informed comment to targeted groups to dispel myths on behaviour, known as 'social norm feedback'. For example, that most people do not smoke or drink excessively.

Bonnell *et al.* (2011) argue that nudging already happens through social marketing techniques, peer approaches, motivational interviewing that have a more robust theory and evidence base. Marteau *et al.* (2011) refer to nudging as being 'fuzzy' and raise the potential harms, through the lack of evidence available of its effectiveness, highlighting that there is evidence that it works to promote unhealthy behaviours (e.g. the placing of sweets at the eye level for children at supermarket checkouts) but little evidence that it improves health and no evidence of cost effectiveness compared to other interventions. Marteau *et al.* point to the limited effectiveness of self-regulation by the food and alcohol industry who have as much interest in promoting unhealthy as well as healthy nudges. Health visitors may also find that people from more advantaged areas are more likely to respond to nudges or cues to change health behaviours than those from disadvantaged areas, given the increasing evidence that health inequalities can widen when using an individual-behaviour change approach (Capewell & Graham, 2010).

The concept of libertarian paternalism fits well with a conservative/liberal approach, much as Baggott's (2000) reference earlier in the chapter to liberal ideology does, and which emphasises freedom of the individual to make choices without state interference and minimising legislation and regulation. Bonnell *et al.* (2011) highlight that public health is rarely coercive and does seek to influence those processes that support healthy choices being made by people. Nevertheless, it is evident that the 'nudge' approach does not sit well with the principles of public health that identifies more with collective approaches and a readiness of the state to intervene and legislate for health improvement. From a health visiting perspective, there will be expectations from government that 'nudge' initiatives and early intervention approaches through the Healthy Child Programme will be delivered to success. The difficulty as above is that the philosophy of health visiting through its four principles does not sit easily with the individualised approaches proposed, and that at best, policy may limit or worse, deny the opportunity to address socioeconomic and other factors in the social structure.

Good leadership is a fundamental aspect of public health practice. Indeed, the analysis provided in this chapter highlights the challenges that health visiting faces. There is no doubting the complexity of the contemporary role for health visiting when engaging a public health approach in light of current policy. Herein lies the challenge for health visitors at a dawning of a new era for the profession. Leadership in this context is centred on managing the divergence between a policy agenda that focuses practice on changing health behaviour at the level of individuals (whether carried out at individual, family or community level), and in contrast, seeking to maintain a footing in public health principles that promote a collective approach to addressing the main determinants of health. The key is to maximise to the fullest extent all of the principles of health visiting. This will require strength, clarity of thought and vision, and a recognition of human rights as a basis for advocacy, influence and change – whether at a local or national level.

Plastow (2009) points to the large number of health visitors who are using their leadership skills through delegation and risk assessment to lead teams of practitioners as well as undertake health needs assessments, manage the delivery of parenting programmes and behaviour change approaches. This will all be essential to support policy delivery, e.g. the Healthy Child Programme. However, good leadership also demands a capacity to think innovatively and critically about how to respond to the needs of communities and being ready to advocate for, and influence local agendas. This is particularly important recognising the increasing integration that is likely to occur between local authority early years' services and NHS provision for families with young children. There will be opportunities to influence that process, but also challenges of ambiguity, ignorance and conflict to overcome. Developing strategic and political awareness is therefore important for health visitors. There is also evidence through a diverse array of leading roles both within and without health visiting, of leaders using their health visiting principles to support change, for example, specialists working in infant feeding, weight management, and immunisation programmes and those working at a senior level in organisations who have a health visiting background and continue to utilise their health visiting skills, e.g. in public health, commissioning, procurement and quality management of services.

Summary

This chapter has sought to give an understanding of the public health role for health visiting through an analysis of the context and delivery of contemporary practice. History has shown how the development of health visiting arose at a time when public health concerned itself with broader, social determinants of health. However, its development into the maternal and welfare movement resulted in an approach centred in health education and advice for most of the twentieth century. The development of the principles for health visiting has given the profession a broader appreciation of the contribution that it can make to improving health and reducing health inequalities.

The concepts associated with the term 'public health' have been analysed and discussed and a connection has been made with health visiting and its underlying four principles. An analysis of the human rights agenda and the right to health has demonstrated that solutions to tackling health inequities are interconnected with the main determinants of health and not individual behaviour alone. By recognising the wider determinants of health highlights the importance of good partnership working to enable active participation of individuals, families and communities so that they are in a position to shape their health experiences and outcomes. Thirty-four years after their inception, the four principles of health visiting continue to give a sound philosophical footing to health visiting practice and its contribution to reducing health inequalities.

Despite dwindling numbers in the profession it has a number of influential political allies who recognise the added value of health visitors to supporting children and families. Consequently, at a time of economic and social austerity the profession finds itself at the dawning of a new era with significant investment on the horizon. This investment will, however, come at a price with health visitors facing challenges in enacting government policy that diverges from the principles that underpin health visiting and public health. The challenge in addressing these tensions cannot be underestimated. The way forward therefore lies in health visitors taking a fresh approach and exploiting each of the four principles to the full with strong leadership at all levels within the profession and with the support of its political allies. To do so gives the best opportunity for many years for the profession to be able to contribute towards a more fair society and to demonstrate how it truly is able to maximise its approach to promoting health and preventing ill health.

References

Allen, G. & Duncan Smith, I. (2010) *Early Intervention: Good Parents, Great Kids, Better Citizens*. The Centre for Social Justice and The Smith Institute, London. Available from: http://www.centreforsocialjustice.org.uk/default.asp?pageRef=269 (accessed 8 March, 2011).

Ashton, J. & Seymour, H. (1988) *The New Public Health*. Open University Press, Milton Keynes.

Baggott, R. (2000) *Public Health: Policy & Politics*. Palgrave Macmillan, Basingstoke.

Barker, D.J.P. (ed.) (1992) *Fetal and infant origins of adult disease*. BMJ Publishing, London.

BBC News (2011) Cuts 'destroying big society' concept, says CSV head BBC News, London. Available from: http://www.bbc.co.uk/news/uk-politics-12378974 (accessed 8 March, 2011).

Beaglehole, R. & Bonita, R. (1997) *Public Health at the Crossroads*. Cambridge University Press, Cambridge.

Beauchamp, T. & Childress, J. (2001) *Principles of Biomedical Ethics*, 5th edn. Oxford University Press, Oxford.

Bonnell, C., McKee, M., Fletcher, A., Wilkinson, P. & Haines, A. (2011) One nudge forward, two steps back, *British Medical Journal*, **342**, d401.

Capewell, S. & Graham, H. (2010) Will cardiovascular disease prevention widen health inequalities? *PLoS Medicine*, **7**(8), e1000320. Available from: http://www.plosmedicine.org/article/info%3Adoi%2F10.1371%2Fjournal.pmed.1000320#pmed.1000320-McLaren1 (accessed 11 March, 2011).

Caraher, M. & McNab, M. (1997) Using lessons from health visiting's past to inform the public health role. *Health Visitor*, **70**, 380–384.

CESCR (2000) *Substantive Issues Arising in the Implementation of the International Covenant on Economic, Social & Cultural Rights: General Comment No. 14*. Committee on Economic, Social & Cultural Rights, New York. Available from: http://www.unhchr.ch/tbs/doc.nsf/(Symbol)/40d009901358b0e2c1256915005090be?Opendocument (accessed 7 March, 2011).

CETHV (1977) *An Investigation into the Principles of Health Visiting*. Council for the Education and Training of Health Visitors, London.

Clarke, K. (2006) Childhood, parenting and early intervention: a critical examination of the SureStart national programme, *Critical Social Policy*, **26**(4), 699–721.

Council of Europe (1950) *Convention for the Protection of Human Rights and Fundamental Freedoms (amended, 2010)* Council of Europe, Available from: http://conventions.coe.int/treaty/en/Treaties/Html/005.htm (accessed 6 March, 2011).

Cowley, S. & Frost, M. (2006) *The Principles of Health Visiting: Opening the Door to Public Health Practice in the 21st Century*. Community Practitioners' and Health Visitors' Association, London.

Craig, P.M. (2000) The nursing contribution to public health: In: *Nursing for Public Health. Population-based care* (eds P.M. Craig & Lindsay G.M.). Churchill Livingstone, London.

Dahlgren, G. & Whitehead, M. (1991) *Policies and Strategies to Promote Social Equity in Health*. Institute for Futures Studies, Stockholm.

Davey Smith, G., Hart, C., Blane, D., Gillis, C. & Hawthorne, V. (1997) Lifetime socioeconomic position and mortality: prospective observational study. *British Medical Journal*, **314**, 547.

Davey Smith, G., Hart, C., Blane, D. & Hole, D. (1998) Adverse socioeconomic conditions in childhood and cause specific adult mortality: prospective observational study, *British Medical Journal*, **316**, 1631.

Department of Health (1988) *Public Health in England: the Report of the Committee of Inquiry into the Future Development of the Public Health Function*. Department of Health, London.

Department of Health (1999) *Saving Lives: Our Healthier Nation*. The Stationery Office, London.

Department of Health (2003) *Liberating the Public Health Talents of Community Practitioners and Health Visitors*. Department of Health, London.

Department of Health (2007) *The Government Response to Facing the Future: a Review of the Role of Health Visitors*. Department of Health, London. Available from: http://www.dh.gov.uk/en/Publicationsandstatistics/Publications/PublicationsPolicy AndGuidance/DH_075642 (accessed 26 February, 2011).

Department of Health (2009) *Healthy Child Programme: Pregnancy and the First Five Years of Life*. Department of Health, London. Available from: http://www.dh.gov.uk/en/Publicationsandstatistics/Publications/PublicationsPolicyAnd Guidance/DH_107563 (accessed 23 February, 2011).

Department of Health (2010a) *Healthy Lives, Healthy People: Our Strategy for Public Health in England*. Stationery Office, London Available from: http://www.dh.gov.uk/en/Publicationsandstatistics/Publications/PublicationsPolicyAnd Guidance/DH_121941 (accessed 23 February, 2011).

Department of Health (2010b) *Equity and Excellence: Liberating the NHS*, The Stationery Office, London, Available from: http://www.dh.gov.uk/en/Publications andstatistics/Publications/PublicationsPolicyAndGuidance/DH_117353 (accessed 3 March, 2011).

Department of Health (2011) *Health Visitor Implementation Plan 2011-15: Call to Action*. Department of Health, London. Available from: http://www.dh.gov.uk/en/Publicationsandstatistics/Publications/PublicationsPolicyAndGuidance/DH_124202 (accessed 23 February, 2011).

Department of Health and Department for Children, Schools & Families (2009) *Healthy Lives, Brighter Futures – The Strategy for Children and Young People's Health,* Department of Health and Department for Children, Schools & Families, Stationery Office, London. Available from: http://www.dh.gov.uk/en/Publicationsandstatistics/Publications/PublicationsPolicyAndGuidance/DH_094400 (accessed 28 February, 2011).

Earle, S. (2007) Exploring health. In: *Theory and Research in Promoting Public Health* (eds S. Earle, C.E. Lloyd, M. Sidell & S. Spurr). Sage, London.

Earle, S. & O'Donnell, T. (2007) The factors that influence health. In: *Theory and Research in Promoting Public Health* (eds S. Earle, C.E. Lloyd, M. Sidell & S. Spurr). Sage, London.

Field, F. (2010) *The Foundation Years: Preventing Poor Children from Becoming Poor Adults*. Cabinet Office, London. Available from: http://www.frankfield.co.uk/review-on-poverty-and-life-chances/ (accessed 8 March, 2011).

Fromer, M.J. (1981) *Ethical Issues in Healthcare*. CV Mosby, St Louis.

Frost, M. & Horner, S. (2009) Health visiting. In: *Community Health Care Nursing* (eds D. Sines, M. Saunders & J. Forbes-Burford), 4th edn. Wiley-Blackwell, Chichester.

Giddens, A. (2006) *Sociology*, 5th edn. Polity Press, Cambridge.

Glass, N. (1999) 'Sure Start: The development of an early intervention programme for young children in the United Kingdom', *Children and Society*, **13**, 257-264.

Graham, H. (2007) *Unequal Lives*. Open University Press, Maidenhead.

Gruskin, S. & Tarantola, D. (2004) Health and human rights. In: *Oxford Textbook of Public Health* (eds R. Detels, J. McEwen, R. Beaglehole & H. Tanaka), 4th edn. Oxford University Press, Oxford.

Home Office (1998) *Supporting Families: A Consultation Document*. Stationery Office, London.

HM Government (2006) *Reaching Out: An Action Plan on Social Exclusion*. Cabinet Office, Social Exclusion Task Force, London. Available from: http://webarchive.nationalarchives.gov.uk/20061019062131/http://cabinetoffice.gov.uk/social_exclusion_task_force/publications/reaching_out/reaching_out.asp (accessed 4 March, 2011).

HSC (2009) *Health Inequalities: Third Report of Session 2008-09* Health Select Committee, House of Commons, London. Available from: http://www.publications.parliament.uk/pa/cm200809/cmselect/cmhealth/286/286.pdf (accessed 12 February, 2011).

Jefferis, B.J.M.H., Power, C. & Hertzman, C. (2002) Birth weight, childhood socioeconomic environment, and cognitive development in the 1958 British birth cohort study. *British Medical Journal*, **325**, 305.

Knai, C. (2009) What is public health? In: G. Thornbory (ed.), *Public Health Nursing: A Textbook for Health Visitors, School Nurses and Occupational Health Nurses*. Wiley-Blackwell, Chichester.

Kretzmann, J.P. & McKnight, J.L. (1993) *Building Communities from the Inside Out: A Path towards Finding and Mobilising a Community's Assets*. Acta Publications, Chicago.

Lansley, A. (2010) *Health Committee – Minutes of Evidence Responsibilities of the Secretary of State for Health* Question 38. Available from: http://www.publications.parliament.uk/pa/cm201011/cmselect/cmhealth/380/10072004.htm (accessed 1 March, 2011).

Lantz, P.M., House, J.S., Lepkowski, J.M., Williams, D.R., Mero, R.P. & Chen, J. (1998) Socio-economic factors, health behaviours and mortality *Journal of the American Medical Association*, **279**(21), 1703-1708.

Marmot, M., Atkinson, T., Bell, J., *et al*. (2010) *Fair Society, Healthy Lives. The Marmot Review*. Marmot Review Team, University College London.

Marteau, T.M., Ogilvie, D., Roland, M., Suhrcke, M. & Kelly, M.P. (2011) Judging nudging: can nudging improve population health? *British Medical Journal*, **342**, d228.

Milio, N. (1986) *Promoting Health through Public Policy*. Canadian Public Health Association, Ottawa.

NMC (2004) *Standards of Proficiency for Specialist Community Public Health Nurses.* Nursing and Midwifery Council, London.

NMC (2008) *The Code: Standards of Conduct, Performance and Ethics for Nurses and Midwives.* Nursing and Midwifery Council, London.

Orme, J., Powell, J., Taylor, P. & Grey, M. (2007) Mapping public health. In: *Public Health for the 21st Century: New Perspectives on Policy, Participation and Practice* (eds J. Orme, J. Powell, P. Taylor & M. Grey), 2nd edn. Open University Press, Maidenhead.

Plastow, L. (2009) Strategic directions for public health nursing. In: *Community Health Care Nursing* (eds D. Sines, M. Saunders & J. Forbes-Burford), 4th edn. Wiley-Blackwell, Chichester.

Ryan, W. (1976) *Blaming the Victim.* Vintage, New York.

Sirkin, S., Iacopeno, V., Grodin, M.A. & Danieli, Y. (2005) The role of health professionals in protecting and promoting human rights. In: *Perspectives on Health and Human Rights* (eds S. Gruskin, M.A. Grodin, S.P. Marks & G.J. Annas), Routledge, Abingdon.

Skills for Health (2004) *National Occupational Standards for the Practice of Public Health Guide.* Skills for Health, Bristol.

SmithBattle, L., Diekemper, M. & Leander, S. (2004) Moving upstream: Becoming a public health nurse, Part 2. *Public Health Nursing,* **21**(2), 95–102.

Symonds, A. (1991) Angels and interfering busy bodies: the social construction of two occupations. *Sociology of Health & Illness,* **13**, 249–264.

Thaler, R.H. & Sunstein, C.R. (2008) *Nudge: Improving Decisions about Health, Wealth, and Happiness.* Yale University Press, London.

UKPHA (2009) *Health Visiting Matters: Re-establishing Health Visiting* UKPHA, London. Available from: http://www.ukpha.org.uk/media/14945/health%20visiting%20matters%20final%20report.pdf (accessed 26 February, 2011).

UN (1948) *United Nations Universal Declaration on Human Rights,* United Nations, New York. Available from: http://www.un.org/en/documents/udhr/index.shtml#a25 (accessed 6 March, 2011).

UN (1966) *United Nations International Covenant on Economic, Social and Cultural Rights,* United Nations, New York. Available from: http://www.un-documents.net/icescr.htm (accessed 6 March, 2011).

UN (2000) *United Nations Millennium Declaration* United Nations, New York. Available from: http://www.un.org/millennium/ (accessed 28 February, 2011).

UNICEF (1989) *The United Nations Convention on the Rights of the Child.* United Nations International Children's Emergency Fund. Available from: http://www2.ohchr.org/english/law/crc.htm (accessed: 16 January, 2011).

UNICEF (2009) *The State of the World's Children 2009 Report.* United Nations International Children's Emergency Fund. Available from: http://www.unicef.org/sowc09/ (accessed 2 March, 2011).

UNICEF (2010) *Progress For Children: Achieving the MDGs with Equity,* United Nations International Children's Emergency Fund. Available from: http://www.unicef.org/publications/files/Progress_for_Children-No.9_EN_081710.pdf (accessed 2 March, 2011).

UNITE (2009) *Press Release – Fall in Health Visitor Numbers is 'A National Scandal', Nursing Commission Told.* Available from: http://www.unitetheunion.org/news__events/latest_news/health_visitor_crisis_is_a_na.aspx (accessed 1 March, 2011).

UNITE/CPHVA (2009) *Regulatory Issues and the Future Legal Status of the Health Visitor Title and Profession.* UNITE/Community Practitioners' and Health Visitors' Association, London.

Verweij, M. & Dawson, A. (2009) The meaning of 'public' in 'public health'. In: *Ethics, Prevention, and Public Health* (eds A. Dawson & M. Verweij), Oxford University Press, Oxford.

Whitehead, M. & Dahlgren, G. (2006) *Concepts and Principles for Tackling Social Inequities in Health: Levelling Up Part 1,* World Health Organization, Regional Office, Copenhagen. Available from: http://www.enothe.eu/cop/docs/concepts_and_principles.pdf (accessed 6 March, 2011).

World Health Organization (WHO) (1946) *Constitution of the World Health Organization*, New York, 22 July, 1946, World Health Organization, Geneva.

World Health Organization (1986) *Ottawa Charter for Health Promotion*. World Health Organization, Geneva.

World Health Organization (2011) *Social Determinants of Health: Key Concepts*. Commission on Social Determinants of Health, World Health Organization, Geneva. Available from: http://www.who.int/social_determinants/thecommission/finalreport/key_concepts/en/index.html (accessed 7 March, 2011).

Appendix 2   Activities for Chapter 2

Activity 2.1

Populations

What other distinct populations can you identify that health visitors may work with?

Activity 2.2

Health promotion

What do you consider are your underpinning values for health promotion?

Activity 2.3

Defining 'public health'

- How would you define public health?
- Have a discussion with your colleagues from other professional groups or agencies and ask them too, how they define public health.
- Reflect on the value of this activity. Why might gaining different views be helpful?

Activity 2.4

Relevance of UNCRC to public health

Take the opportunity to access the UNCRC online (http://www2.ohchr. org/english/law/crc.htm). Given that 'promoting and protecting human rights can be the most effective means to securing health', what relevance do each of the articles have for public health?

Activity 2.5

Reflection on the principles of health visiting

- The search for health needs;
- The stimulation of an awareness of health needs;
- The influence on policies affecting health and;
- The facilitation of health-enhancing activities

(CETHV, 1977).

- Think critically about the extent to which the principles of health visiting are embedded in local practice.
- What are the strengths, weaknesses, opportunities, and threats to fulfilling the principles in practice? How can you respond to these?

Activity 2.6

Reflection on experiences in childhood

Take some time to think of your own childhood experiences.

- How have they influenced your opportunities in life so far?
- How have they have impacted upon your health?

Activity 2.7

Tackling health inequalities

- Familiarise yourself with any local strategies that contribute to tackling health inequalities.
- What added value can your public health role offer to these strategies?

3

The Community Dimension

Rosamund Bryar
City University London, London, UK

Jean Orr
Queen's University Belfast, Belfast, UK

Introduction

Health visitors are fundamentally community public health workers – they work in communities, they work with communities and they are part of communities. In 2004 the NMC opened the Specialist Community Public Health Nursing Register emphasising in the title of the register and the qualification both the *community* and *public health* role of the practitioners, including health visitors, on that register. In Chapter 2 the case is made that in undertaking community work health visitors are essentially working with individuals, who are part of a community, to address the health of that community (that community's public health) at the level of individual behaviour change. Draper *et al.* (2010) cite O'Dwyer *et al.*'s (2007) systematic review of area-based interventions and comment that the differentiation between these two approaches to working with communities is not often acknowledged:

> The distinction between community-based interventions (programmes that are based in communities, but focus on achieving change in individuals) and community-level interventions (programmes that seek to achieve change in a whole community via participation and other community wide changes) is also rarely made. (p. 1104)

Health visitors in putting into practice the principles of health visiting (Cowley & Frost, 2006) are seeking through such work to influence community level health, through both community-based and community-level interventions, wider public health policies and the main determinants of health (Dahlgren & Whitehead, 1991).

In working with and in communities, health visitors are responding to the identification within the Declaration of Alma Ata (WHO/UNICEF, 1978), reiterated in *Primary Health Care – Now More Than Ever* (WHO, 2008) of the importance of communities to the health of individuals, populations and countries. The *Health for All Declaration* identifies that communities should be involved in the development, provision and monitoring of health services and healthcare is seen as contributing to overall community development. This focus is reinforced in current primary healthcare reforms proposed by WHO (2008) which seek to move health systems towards health for all through services becoming more people-centred, promoting and protecting the health of the public and improving health equity: 'reforms that secure healthier communities, by integrating public health actions with primary care and by pursuing healthy public policies across sectors' (WHO, 2008: xvi). Health visitors are front line public health workers working with local communities and in a prime position to contribute to these reforms.

Before examining the role of the health visitor in and with communities there is a need to explore the definition and meaning of the term community and to consider why communities are important to health.

Defining community

Much confusion seems to surround the usage of the term. This occurs despite the fact that the notion of community is central to the provision of healthcare and to the description of social life in general. To explore your understanding of community before reading on, go to Activity 3.1 (see Appendix 3 at the end of the chapter).

The various meanings and confusion surrounding the concept community occurs because the word is used both in descriptive and evaluative terms. Just think of the many ways we use the word: we talk of community nursing, community spirit, community policing, the European Community, community education and so on. In addition, when the term community is used it often not only describes a range of features in social life but puts these features in a favourable perspective. It is suggested by Greer and Minar (1969) that community refers to a unit of society and to aspects of that society which we value. Unlike many other terms in relation to social organisation, such as state or society, the term community is seldom used in an unfavourable context.

Benson (1976) reinforces this view when he says the word is often used in a strongly evaluative and emotive way. For example, when we talk of community spirit the implication is that this is somehow a 'good thing'. When we talk like this we are not referring to an objectively definable type of social structure, instead we are referring to a vaguely sensed and worthwhile quality of common life which is felt to be valued and is assumed to depend for its existence on a specific type of social structure, such as a small village. Within the concept of community, however, there are negative connotations. By defining an 'in group' making up a community we are, by implication, identifying an 'out group' of those who do not belong. One has only to think of the experience of migrants or the phenomenon of gangs related to a small geographical area to see the reality of such a phenomenon. Furthermore, the existence of a community can result in the use of informal means of social control being exerted to maintain community norms and values.

Many words have both evaluative and descriptive meaning. A word such as 'beautiful', for example, can be used in both ways. It is necessary therefore to be aware of the confusion which can arise with these two kinds of meanings. We must be clear about which descriptive features of a social group are relevant to the value judgments that are made about it. Some words touch on so many diverse phenomena depending on the context in which they are used (Tucker, 1979). Community is such a word because it is prone to multiple connotations and therefore misunderstandings. The term is frequently used both verbally and in writing with the assumption that there is a shared sense of meaning: 'community care', for example, is talked and written about as if there was total agreement among professionals as to its meaning. Such assumptions lead to confusion and make it necessary to formulate a working definition of this term.

The word community has been in common usage since its Latin origin as *communitas*. There are no less than 100 definitions available for the *communis* from which this word was derived (Weaver, 1977). Hillery (1955, 1982) articulated the problems involved when attempting to define the word. One of the major difficulties is the enormous number of contexts and structures to which the term has been applied. It has been used to describe geographical areas and linked to similar concepts like locality and neighbourhood. Hillery (1955) re-examined 94 definitions and found that the most significant areas of agreement among 20 of the definitions were about the 'possession of common ends, norms and means'. The idea of life in common appeared in nine of the definitions, self-sufficiency in eight and consciousness of some kind in seven. In attempting to analyse the word community further, Tönnies (1887) contrasted the concepts of *Gemeinshaft* and *Gezellschaft*. *Gemeinshaft* is described as the most basic form of human grouping characterised by rich and satisfying relationships. *Gezellschaft* on the other hand describes those relationships which are essentially superficial and impersonal. When interpreting Tonnies' view in the context of twenty-first-century values, MacIver and Page (1962) described community as an area of social living marked by some degree of social coherence. The basis of community therefore may be locality and community sentiment. Midwinter (1973), on the other hand, saw a community as being an abstract entity, yet one to which most people see themselves as belonging. Bell and Newby (1971) considered definitions of community as implying the organisation of people, goods, services and commitments in a specific area with a marked emphasis upon sharing both the common good and the locality. Konig (1968) reinforced this view in claiming that in a strictly sociological sense the phenomenon of spatial proximity of neighbourhood is inseparable from the idea of community. An example of this concept is seen in Weiner (1975) when he studied the fragmentation of a community in the

Shankhill area of Belfast. He described the community as a hierarchical structure, beginning with the extended family, moving through street collectives to the whole entity which he described as the Shankhill community. His concern was with the sets of relationships which existed in the area and to which inhabitants attributed great value. This prescriptive use of the word community implies that certain sets of relationships are valued as worthwhile in that they constitute a community. As McNaught (2009) comments: 'What gives the notion of community its strengths is the self-perception and awareness of its members that they are a "community"' (p. 167).

Communities and theories about communities, however, are not static (Crow, 2002), what applied to the Shankill community in 1975 may or may not apply in 2011. The changes in one community over time are made very clear in comparison of the East End community over a period of 50 years. In 1957 Young and Willmott published a classic study entitled: *Family and Kinship in East London* (Young & Willmott, 1957, 2007) which showed the value of the strong relationships in that community to supporting the resilience of that community. Fifty years on a new study of the area, revealingly entitled: *The New East End: Kinship, Race and Conflict* (Dench et al., 2006) found that the community had changed radically and that tensions between different community groups characterised relationships in the area.

These descriptions of the various types of community indicate that it is a complex concept. This complexity is captured in the Young Foundation (2011) definition:

> Community means different things to different people at different times. It can mean a group of friends or family, a local neighbourhood, a virtual network, a school group, a place of worship, a community association, or a cultural network that is spread across the world.

This inclusive approach is also found in the definition used by NICE (2008):

> A community is defined as a group of people who have common characteristics. Communities can be defined by location, race, ethnicity, age, occupation, a shared interest (such as using the same service) or affinity (such as religion and faith) or other common bonds. A community can also be defined as a group of individuals living within the same geographical location (such as a hostel, a street, a ward, town or region). (p. 38)

Considering these definitions it can be seen that health visitors work with a range of different communities, defined by location (e.g. a neighbourhood); by interest (e.g. new mothers); by ethnicity (e.g. a Turkish women's group); and interface with other communities such as those on the internet (e.g. *Netmums*). From the discussion above it can be seen that communities have a central part to play in people's lives and it is therefore important to ask: what is the impact of these communities on the health of individuals, families and on the communities themselves?

Impact of communities on health

The Young Foundation has produced a range of tools brought together in the Community action toolkit (Young Foundation, 2011) to help in understanding and working with local communities, defined by geography as in neighbourhoods or by common interest or by other features of belonging. If we focus on the neighbourhood, the usual workplace for health visitors, the Young Foundation (2010) suggests:

> Neighbourhoods are ultra-local communities of place. Most people feel they intuitively understand what they mean, in the shape of neighbourly interactions, mutual support, gathering places and a friendly, attractive environment – or a 'bad neighbourhood', danger, anti-social interaction, exclusiveness, isolation and dereliction. (p. 9)

They refer to the rule of thumb of planners of new towns that: '....the overall size of a neighbourhood should be dictated by "the maximum walking distance for a woman with a pram"....' (Young Foundation, 2010: 11). The neighbourhood or a group of neighbourhoods form the usual area of practice of the health visitor and health visiting team although in many rural areas these neighbourhoods may be spread over a large area.

The Young Foundation (2010) suggests that our understanding of neighbourhoods brings together three aspects (see Figure 3.1): the administrative wards or geographic boundaries of an area; our personal identification and mental map of our neighbourhood, and the public realm

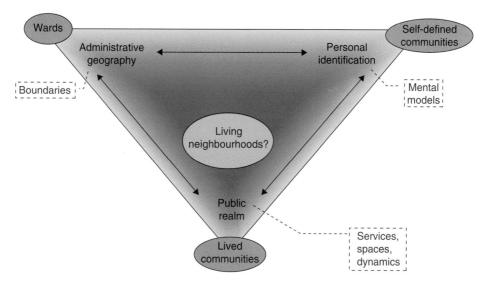

Figure 3.1 Elements of neighbourhoods.
Source: The Young Foundation, 2010: 14. (Reproduced by kind permission.)

including open spaces, services, schools and community centres. The interaction of these three aspects provides a description and understanding of the experience of a neighbourhood. From a health visiting point of view it also indicates the role that local public services, such as health visiting, make to the experience of community and raises questions concerning joint working between different public services to support positive neighbourhood experience.

An individual's experience of their neighbourhood includes feelings of mutual support and relationships within the community, helping their ability to cope with and enhance their health and the health of their families. These subjective elements go to make up what has been called the social climate which affects the quality of life of the individual and community (Moos, 1976). Moos suggests that environments have unique personalities just as people do. Some are supportive, some competitive. This approach, using the environmental-social, rather than the environmental-physical, emphasises impressionistic elements of description (Moos, 2002).

Historically, planners and policy-makers have placed their reliance on objective measures of a community. They have measured such things as housing and unemployment because it is argued that such factors influence people's lives. These types of measures are useful because they enable comparisons to be made between areas and groups and can be a guide to changing socioeconomic conditions. The question, however, remains as to the meaning of these statistics and their relationship to the subjective experience. We can, for example, measure the housing density but what does that tell us about the pleasures or problems of living in a particular estate? According to Campbell *et al.* (1976) the use of social indicators alone is not sufficient and, in order to know the quality of life experiences, one must go directly to the individual for a description of what life is like. Krupat and Guild (1980) examined a number of factors which they suggest could be used to capture the social climate of a city or community. Six meaningful factors emerged by which social climate could be described. These were:

1. *Warmth and closeness*. This first and most important factor contains items reflecting general feelings of security and support which an environment may provide such as: relaxed atmosphere, sense of intimacy, a safe, healthy and peaceful place and friendly people.
2. *Activity and entertainment*. This contains items such as: activity, entertainment, diverse selection, dense population, and an atmosphere of culture. Density is seen as being related to the opportunity for activity and entertainment, and reflects positive aspects of urban life rather than the isolation and anonymity that is often seen to be the case.
3. *Alienation and isolation*. This factor contained items such as: apathy, dirty surroundings, loneliness, distrust, confusion, and violence. This factor predominantly includes items referring to characteristics of people but it also refers to the physical condition of the environment which is seen as something which fosters, or is a result of, a breakdown in interpersonal solidarity.

4. *Good life*. This factor contains items such as: intellectual people, affluent people, liberal people, prestigious place, old ways valued, and people who are interesting because they are not locals. This factor again refers to characteristics of the people but is elitist. Included here is the recognition of spatial mobility and innovation.
5. *Privacy*. This factor includes items such as: gossip, intrusion, ignorance and pettiness. This factor refers to a dimension of life involving privacy and carries a strong negative connotation with the inclusion of items noting pettiness and ignorance on the part of people.
6. *Uncaring*. This factor includes items such as: snobby people, depressing environment, and insensitive people. This factor represents the uncaring aspects of social climate and includes aspects of people's behaviour and feelings about the overall social life.

In their study of self-help in an inner city, Knight and Hayes (1981) found that the social climate placed limits on the likelihood of small groups emerging and operating successfully. They conclude that postwar city planning was geared to solving physical problems rather than interpersonal or communal problems and that the opportunities to involve local people were wasted in part because of the anomie and alienation which exist in inner city areas. In general, the lack of awareness of the concept of social climate meant that little emphasis was given to ameliorating undesirable social conditions because it had not been thought possible to identify these in a measurable way.

The level of support in a neighbourhood indicates the networks and relationships or social capital in that neighbourhood which interact to reinforce a salutogenic approach to health and wellbeing. Such relationships and networks enable people to manage and deal with the challenges in their lives leading to the question, of great relevance to health visitors working with communities, posed by Antonovsky (1996): 'What can be done in this "community" – factory, geographic community, age or ethnic or gender group, chronic or even acute hospital population, those who suffer from a particular disability, etc. – to strengthen the sense of comprehensibility, manageability and meaningfulness of the persons who constitute it?' (p. 16).

Wellbeing extends the idea of social climate (Krupat & Guild, 1980) and has been described by Layard and Dunne (2009) cited by Roberts *et al.* (2009) as resulting from the interaction of seven factors:

- family relationships;
- financial situation;
- work;
- community and friends;
- health;
- personal freedom;
- personal values.

Individual, subjective wellbeing is therefore impacted by the person's health and feelings of being healthy. Mguni and Bacon (2010) define the feeling of wellbeing experienced by an individual as a combination of subjective wellbeing and community wellbeing:

> The focus of our work has been on individual 'subjective wellbeing', how people experience the quality of their lives, alongside community wellbeing – the extent to which local services and infrastructure has the capacity to support or reduce wellbeing. We see this as the most fundamental test of any area: does it provide its citizens with a good life? (p. 11)

These authors illustrate the relationship between community wellbeing and the individual's sense of wellbeing and health in a circular diagram (see Figure 3.2).

When we consider the elements of Figure 3.2 in relation to the discussion of the model of the Main Determinants of Health (Dahlgren & Whitehead, 1991) in Chapter 2 (Figure 2.1, p. 72) we can see how the experience of individuals of, for example, poor access to education and thus job opportunities, interacts to form a community with a reduced sense of

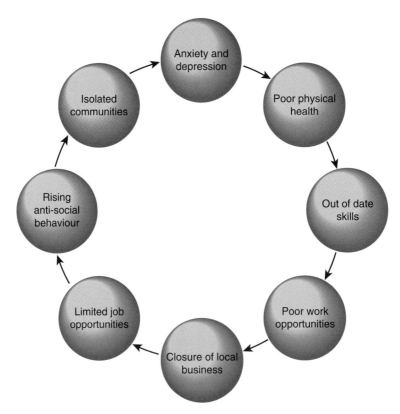

Figure 3.2 How local environments can interact with individual characteristics in harmful ways.
Source: Mguni & Bacon, 2010, Figure 2: How local environments can interact with individual characteristics in harmful ways, p. 12. (Reproduced by kind permission.)

wellness, a poorer sense of social capital (Gilchrist, 2007) and in greater need of inclusion in the Big Society (Mulgan, 2010).

Communities living close together can experience widely different health. The iconic map of the underground system in London provides a graphic representation of the different levels of health of communities within one small geographic area. As shown in Figure 3.3 communities located along the underground system from affluent Westminster in the centre of London to the more deprived Canning Town in the east experience loss of one year in life expectancy for each underground stop further east you move.

Evidence of the impact of the different factors on health and the identification of the needs of a local community enables us to identify where interventions, for example, through children's centres, in supporting parents' sense of wellbeing, social networks and relationships have the potential to change communities, people's experience of their neighbourhood, wellness and health:

> Even when families live in poor housing with inadequate income and experience unemployment and multiple deprivations, finding ways to enhance adult wellbeing can have positive repercussions on the whole family, giving all its members a better chance of constructing a different kind of future.
>
> (Roberts *et al.*, 2009: 13)

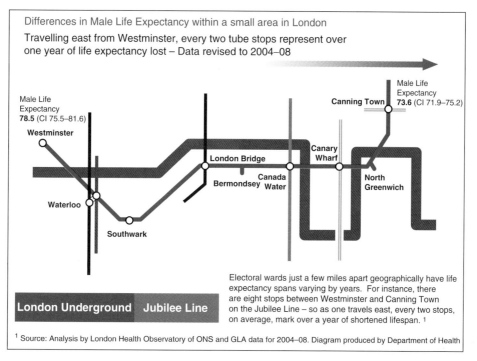

Figure 3.3 Differences in life expectancy: taking the Jubilee Line route to health inequalities.
Source: London Health Observatory. Available online at: www.rho.org.uk/LHO topics/ National Lead Areas/HealthInequalitiesOverview.aspx (accessed 13 May, 2011.)

In 1971 Tudor Hart put forward the concept of the Inverse Care Law that: the availability of good medical (and nursing) care tends to vary inversely with the need for it in the population served (Hart, 1971; Watt, 2002), i.e. people who have greater healthcare needs have less access to good healthcare provision. One way to address this imbalance is through a reorientation of healthcare to an approach which:

- is people-centred;
- includes a focus on health needs and on enduring personal relationships;
- is comprehensive and continuous;
- takes responsibility for the health of the whole community across the lifespan;
- has responsibility for tackling the determinants of ill-health and in which 'People are partners in managing their own health and that of their community' (WHO, 2008: 43);
- integrates public health with primary care provision (Starfield, 1996; WHO, 2008; Bryar et al., 2011).

Public health practitioners, as part of health systems, therefore have a role in enabling the better health of communities and in the following section the role of the health visitor in this regard will be considered.

The role of health visitors with communities

There is a long history of community or public health working in health visiting. Since the establishment of health visiting in 1862 there has been an ongoing tension for health visitors and health visiting services between working at the community or public health level and work with individuals and families on a one-to-one basis. Craig (1995: 5) refers to both the public health role and the role of the health visitor working with individuals in a description of the work of the first health visitor employed in Glasgow in the early twentieth century who worked with the city's first woman doctor: 'to supervise the Milk Depot Scheme and undertake infant consultation sessions'. The tension between a public health/community focus and a focus on individuals is also reflected in public health policy. For example, measures such as the smoking ban in public places (Bauld, 2011) are aimed at changing the exposure of whole populations to tobacco smoke while strategies such as Change4Life are aimed at changing individuals' health behaviours to improve the health of that person and ultimately the health of the whole population.

In relation to the education of health visitors the public health role has long been included in guidance on courses of preparation for student health visitors. One of the functions of the health visitor identified in 1967 was: 'Recognition and identification of need and mobilisation of appropriate resources.' (Council for the Education and Training of Health Visitors, 1967, cited in Robinson & Elkan, 1996: 4). Robinson and Elkan comment that: 'The formalisation of group and population-based health needs assessment by nurses working in community settings can be traced from 1965, when a new syllabus of training for health visitors was introduced (Council for the Education and Training of Health Visitors, 1965' (p. 4). The increasing emphasis on the community role of the health visitor at this time is illustrated in an earlier edition of this book (Luker & Orr, 1992; Orr, 1992) and evident in the Principles of Health Visiting first defined in 1977 (see Chapter 2, p. 66).

In the 1970s-1980s there was a resurgence of interest in the community role of health visitors as Drennan (1988) comments:

> While envisaging a role that responds to present-day society, health visitors have come to look increasingly to group and community work methods of practice, with their emphasis on consumer-expressed definitions of need. Health visitors are not alone in this change of emphasis. Increasingly, the philosophies of the provision of health care are now embracing the notion of partnership between the professional and individual and community at large. More emphasis has been given to client or community perceptions and definitions of need, participation in planning and active involvement in the provision and evaluation of care. (p. 8)

Examples of this type of work are provided by the Stockport Model of Health Visiting (Swann & Brocklehurst, 2004) which emphasised, enabled and required health visitors to engage with the public health elements of the role; the multifaceted public health/community development activities in Glasgow (Craig, 1995; Craig & Lindsay, 2000) and the community development approach used in work in a community health house set up on a council estate in the Welsh Valleys (Bryar & Fisk, 1994).

During the 1990s and into the new century the focus of health visiting work reverted back to a focus on individuals away from work at the community/public health level. This reorientation resulted from a number of changes including the NHS focus on targets, the influence of evidence-based documents which raised questions concerning the efficacy of some of the screening work undertaken by health visitors (Hall & Elliman, 2006) and changes in the regulation of health visitors. The development of Sure Start centres from the late 1990s providing community level activities further reduced the need for health visitors to lead or provide group and community level initiatives. The closure of the health visiting register by the NMC in 2002, which led to a reduction in the numbers of health visitors, further contributed to a reduction in community level work by health visitors. Given these pressures managers of health visiting services required health visitors to prioritise work with individuals at the expense of community focused work. This dichotomy in provision has been perceived as a tension for many health visitors (Craig & Lindsay, 2000). Cameron and Christie (2007) interviewed health visitors in 2003 and one of the respondents, looking back over the previous ten years of her practice (to 1993) in various parts of the UK, illustrates this lack of focus on community/public health work:

> My early experience of health visiting was mainly crisis visiting and coping with a very large 0-5 caseload, with lots of problems and public health was a very small component of the work and only in relation to core under 5 work. I can't remember doing any groups or development work. (p. 84)

At the same time as the retraction in the community role of the health visitor was occurring work on setting competency standards for the wider public health workforce was taking place supported by public health organisations including the Community Practitioners' and Health Visitors' Association. This resulted in the publication of a framework identifying the ten key areas of public health practice, with associated competencies, that could be applied to all public health practitioners. These are found in Chapter 2, Box 2.3, p. 70. You might like to turn to Activity 3.2 (see Appendix 3) to help you explore the use of one of these elements of public health practice to your work with a community.

The application of this framework to the education of specialist community public health nurses including health visitors was then made in the publication by the NMC in 2004 of the 'Standards of proficiency for specialist community public health nurses'. Within this document the standards of proficiency for the ten areas of public health practice are aligned to the four principles of health visiting (termed domains of practice in the document). All the 24 NMC Standards, which guide learning in the university and in practice, can be seen to relate to the development by health visitors of skills in working to promote the health of communities. In Box 3.1 an example is provided of standards in relation to each of the domains of practice (principles of health visiting) with the associated principle (area of public health practice). (As noted in Chapter 2 the use of the terms principle and domains in the NMC document is both ambiguous and confusing.)

Box 3.1 Selected standards of proficiency for health visiting which relate to working with communities

Principle	**Domain:** Search for health needs
Surveillance and assessment of the population's health and wellbeing	• Collect and structure data and information on the health and wellbeing of a defined population. • Develop and sustain relationships with groups and individuals with the aim of improving health and social wellbeing
Principle	**Domain:** Stimulation of awareness of health needs
Working with, and for, communities to improve health and wellbeing	• Communicate with individuals, groups and communities about promoting their health and wellbeing. • Raise awareness about the actions that groups and individuals can take to improve their health and social wellbeing.
Principle	**Domain:** Influence on policies affecting health

Developing health programmes and services and reducing inequalities	• Work with others to plan, implement and evaluate programmes and projects to improve health and wellbeing. • Identify and evaluate service provision and support networks for individuals, families and groups in the local area.
Principle	**Domain:** Facilitation of health-enhancing activities
Promoting and protecting the population's health and well-being	• Work in partnership with others to prevent the occurrence of needs and risks related to health and wellbeing. • Work in partnership with others to protect the public's health and well-being from specific risks.

Since publication of the first public health skills framework and the NMC Standards in 2004 there has been further refinement of the public health framework which was published in 2008 (Public Health Resource Unit and Skills for Health, 2008). The Public Health Skills and Career Framework has refined the ten areas of public health practice into four core areas and, in addition, identifies five defined areas of practice (see Box 3.2).

Box 3.2 Structure of the Public Health Skills and Career Framework

Core areas	Defined areas
1. Surveillance and assessment of the population's health and wellbeing	5. Health improvement
2. Assessing the evidence of effectiveness of interventions, programmes and services to improve population health and wellbeing	6. Health protection
3. Policy and strategy development and implementation for population health and wellbeing	7. Public health intelligence
4. Leadership and collaborative working for population health and wellbeing	8. Academic public health
	9. Health and social care quality

Source: Adapted from: Public Health Resource Unit/Skills for Health, 2008; Table 2.1, p. 8.

The Framework identifies competencies in each of the core areas and for practitioners in the defined areas at all nine of the NHS career framework levels. The Framework helps to identify the knowledge, the training and education, the requirements for regulation and the types of roles of public health practitioners in Bands 1-9. In Box 3.3 examples are provided of the competencies required for each of the core areas for a health visitor at Band 7.

Box 3.3   Examples of competencies in the core areas for Band 7 health visitors in relation to work with communities

Core areas	Competencies needed at Band 7 level
1. Surveillance and assessment of the population's health and wellbeing	Measure, analyse, compare and interpret the health and wellbeing and needs of various populations, communities and groups. (2) Advise others on the collection, analysis and reporting of surveillance and assessment data for your specific area of expertise. (5)
2. Assessing the evidence of effectiveness of interventions, programmes and services to improve population health and wellbeing	Formulate recommendations for change on the basis of critically appraised evidence. (2) Advise a range of audiences about evidence. (5) Review own area of work to ensure it is effective in achieving its aims. (6)
3. Policy and strategy development and implementation for population health and wellbeing	Work with a range of people and agencies to implement policies and strategies in interventions, programmes and services. (2) Contribute to the development of policies and strategies beyond own area of work. (3)
4. Leadership and collaborative working for population health and wellbeing	Engage and influence others in and beyond own organisation to improve population health and wellbeing. (2) Advocate for health and wellbeing and reducing inequalities. (5) Review the effectiveness of collaborative working and make the necessary improvements. (7)

For a health visitor team leader the framework provides a useful tool in identifying, supporting and monitoring the public health/community work of the skill mix team that she leads. Examples of competencies for staff at different bands are shown in Box 3.4. To explore the application of the public health core competencies to the work of your team with a community see Activity 3.3 (Appendix 3).

The NMC is reviewing the standards of education for preparation for health visitors in 2011/12 and it is to be hoped and anticipated that the new standards for preparation for health visitors will align explicitly with the principles of health visiting and the public health skills framework. This will enable health visitors to be clearly identified as key community/public health workers alongside colleagues in local government, public health departments and third sector community organisations.

As we celebrate the first 150 years of health visiting and look to the future, the importance of the work of health visitors with communities has been highlighted in the *Health Visitor Implementation Plan 2011-15. A Call to Action* (Department of Health, 2011). Health visiting services will provide four levels of provision: Community, Universal, Universal plus and Universal partnership plus (see Box 3.5). As illustrated in Box 3.5 health visitors need to make use of skills in community working in all four levels of provision. Working with communities they help to develop the skills and knowledge of communities to address local health issues; they need to have the ability to work with professional communities, for example with midwives and social workers in providing universal and universal plus services. To make appropriate referrals they need to know and understand local services and have relationships with people within those services.

Box 3.4   Examples of competencies in the core area of leadership and collaborative working for health visiting team members

Band level	Examples of competencies
2	Work effectively as a member of a team to improve population health and wellbeing. (1)
	Communicate effectively with people related to own work role to improve the population health and wellbeing. (2)
4	Be an effective member of various teams. (3)
	Communicate effectively for a range of purposes and with various Audiences. (5)
5	Lead on discrete areas of work. (2)
	Share knowledge to facilitate the development of others. (7)

Box 3.5   The new health visiting service: what it means for commissioners, providers and the profession

Community: Interactions at community level: *building capacity* and *using that capacity* to *improve health outcomes* and leading the Healthy Child Programme for a population.

Universal: Universal services for all families: *working with* midwives, *building strong relationships* in pregnancy and early weeks and planning future contacts with families. Leading the Healthy Child Programme for families with children under the age of 5.

Universal plus: Additional services that any family may need some of the time, for example care packages for maternal mental health, *parenting support* and baby/toddler sleep problems – where the health visitor *may provide, delegate or refer. Intervening early* to prevent problems developing or worsening.

Universal partnership plus: Additional services for vulnerable families requiring *ongoing support* for a range of special needs, for example families at *social disadvantage*, families with a child with a disability, teenage mothers, adult mental health problems or substance misuse.

Making sure the appropriate health visiting services form part of the high-intensity multi-agency services for families where there are safeguarding and child protection concerns.

Source: Adapted from: Department of Health, 2011: 10.

However, as identified by Cameron and Christie (2007) the low priority that has been given to public health/community skills in recent years has led to many health visitors feeling daunted by the prospect of re-engaging in community level work. This anxiety has been recognised in the roll out of the Health Visitor Implementation Plan 2011–15 (Department of Health, 2011) and health visitors will be able to access the new 'building community capacity' training module that has been commissioned from a team led by Professor Pauline Pearson (2011), University of Northumbria. This module will provide a combination of online and work-based facilitation support for health visitors to reinvigorate or develop new skills in community work through undertaking a community capacity building project in their area of practice (Pearson, 2011). Through redevelopment of these skills enabling health visitors to better connect with communities it is anticipated that health outcomes for children and their families will be improved (Lynch *et al.*, 2010).

As indicated above, one of the key aspects of the work of the health visitor with communities is the identification of the health needs and abilities of a community, the search for health needs, to inform planning of work with that community. The next section explores the process of health needs assessment (HNA).

Gaining an understanding of the health of your local community

There are a range of approaches to gaining a picture of the health of your local community or neighbourhood. Knowing the local community is fundamental to working in an area as Gilchrist (2007) comments:

> Learning about other people's cultures and histories is an important aspect of networking, enabling people to empathise with perspectives that are different from their own and to operate appropriately in different settings. (p. 146)

In this section we outline three approaches which help move from a general understanding of the needs of your community to a more detailed picture of the needs of a particular section of your community:

- windshield survey;
- developing a public health walk;
- health needs assessment.

There are a range of other approaches used by organisations to identify needs. A health impact assessment: 'is a systematic means of assessing health and measuring the health outcomes of policies and interventions on defined populations (Lock, 2000)' (cited in Naidoo and Wills, 2009: 44). A health impact assessment may be used both to measure the impact of health-related policies and the impact of other strategies which are not directly related to health but have consequences for health. Health equity audits are another way in which the health of populations is assessed, usually by organisations such as health trusts or local authorities. Health equity is different to health inequality but may contribute to it: 'health equity describes *differences in opportunity* for different population groups which result in different life chances, access to health services' (Hamer *et al.*, 2003: 11; emphasis in the original) which can lead to health inequalities. Hamer *et al.* (2003) describe a health equity audit as focusing on: '*how fairly resources are distributed in relation to the health needs of different groups*. (This may include resources such as services, facilities, and the determinants of health like employment and education.)' (p. 11, emphasis in the original). Local authorities and local health commissioners (formerly Primary Care Trusts) are required under the Local Government and Public Involvement in Health Act 2007 to undertake a Joint Strategic Needs Assessment to identify the health and wellbeing of their local population and plans to address health needs identified (Department of Health, 2007). In relation to health visiting the Health Visitor Implementation Plan (Department of Health, 2011) identifies the implementation of local Joint Strategic Needs

Assessments via Health and Wellbeing Boards as being key to the work of health visitors and other services working with young children and their families.

In the next section approaches which may be used by health visitors and health visiting teams will be discussed.

Windshield survey

The first activity of a health visitor in a new area will be to walk the patch or drive around the area, undertaking a 'windshield survey'. The purpose of this activity is to provide information about the obvious characteristics of the area and through this to identify strengths and challenges in the area. Hunt (2009) provides an overview of the type of information to be collected concerning the people, places and social systems evident in the community. Questions to be asked while undertaking the survey include: Who are the people in the streets, in the parks, shops and community centres? How are they dressed and what are they doing? What are the boundaries of the neighbourhood or area? What types and ages of buildings are there in the area? What condition are the houses in? Are there any open spaces and if so what are these used for? What types of shops are there? How many fast food outlets are there? What are the services available in the area? What health services are there? Is there a library and if so what types of health information does it provide? Are there schools, religious buildings or cinemas in the area? (Hunt, 2009: 147-148).

Doing a windshield survey at different times of day or on different days will yield different information, for example about the use of a park by older people on a health walk, younger people playing football or dog walkers exercising their dogs.

Public health walk

A key activity, as discussed above, for any health visitor working with and in a community is to get to know the area through walking around and experiencing the community. Doing this may lead to the identification of evidence of public health activities - for example, local reservoirs linked to water supply, buildings which were once local hospitals, old industrial waste indicating possible health risks or unemployment; as well as evidence of current public health issues - for example, the use made of parks, the number of fast food outlets in the area, children's centres and the number of people in a shopping centre during the day. Identification of these elements of the local area can help in understanding the health issues impacting on the current population as well as some of the attitudes of local people to healthcare provision.

Once these public health aspects have been identified they can be examined in more depth through exploring the history of the area, examining the local public health reports, reading novels and other books about the area and talking to local practitioners and residents. This exploration will help to provide information to help in understanding the relevance and impact of the different public health features identified in the area. The different public health

> **Box 3.6** A public health walk in Tower Hamlets, London
>
> | Evidence in the community | Relevance |
> | --- | --- |
> | The Women's Library | Previously the local wash house |
> | Tall Georgian houses with large windows on the top floor | Homes of the Huguenot weavers – providing light for their work; immigration to area |
> | A mosque | Previously a synagogue – evidence of immigration |
> | Signs on a building indicating a soup kitchen for Jewish immigrants | Immigration; poverty; community support |

features can then be woven together to form a walk tracing the public health history of a local area. In East London one such walk has been developed by lecturer and historian, John Eversley, and provides an introduction for student health visitors to the public health history in part of the borough of Tower Hamlets. Some of the elements included in this walk are shown in Box 3.6. Activity 3.4 (see Appendix 3) provides you with an opportunity to construct your own public health walk.

Health needs assessment

A health needs assessment involves the collection and analysis of information relevant to the health of a particular population. The Health Development Agency (HDA) (2004a) defines health needs assessment as:

> a systematic method for reviewing the health issues facing a population, leading to agreed priorities and resource allocation that will improve health and reduce inequalities. (p. 3)

Health needs assessment is therefore vital in terms of the commissioning of services as well as supporting the direction of the activities of a particular health visiting team. This definition is expanded by the HDA (2004b) identifying the key elements of health needs assessment (HNA):

> HNA is an approach that reviews systematically the health issues facing a given population. The starting point in HNA is a defined *population*. Health issues selected as priorities will usually be those that can help reduce *health inequalities*. The *primary outputs* are a *set of recommendations, an action strategy* based on the evidence gathered about that population, and the

identification of effective and acceptable interventions. These should be used to *influence policies and service delivery* in order to *improve health outcomes* [emphasis added, apart from 'population' which was bold in original]. (p. 5)

It can be seen from this description that HNA involves both the identification of need, plans to address that need and evaluation of the impact of the interventions put in place to meet the need. Hopper and Longworth (2002) state that there are three underpinning principles to HNA: Improvement; Integration and Involvement:

1. *Improvement* of health and inequalities by making changes that improve the most significant conditions or factors affecting health ...
2. *Integration* of this improvement in health into the planning processes ...
3. *Involvement* of:
   - people who know about the health issues in a community
   - people who care about those issues
   - people who can make changes happen. (p. 9)

These definitions focus on the identification of needs while Stewart *et al.* (2009) refer to the important identification of health assets in a community, alongside needs:

'The purpose of health needs assessment (HNA) is to identify the health assets and needs of a given population to inform decisions about service delivery to improve health and reduce health inequalities' (p. 133).

Understanding need

Before examining the process of HNA it is important to consider our understanding of need. Stewart *et al.* (2009) discuss a number of approaches to understanding need including Maslow's hierarchy of needs (Maslow, 1954). This considers the identification of need from the perspective of the individual with needs ranging from the fulfilment of basic physiological needs through to self-actualisation, the fulfilment by the individual of their potential. This approach to needs identification may be contrasted with that of Bradshaw (1972, 1994) who categorised need from 'the perspective of the person or organisation identifying the need' (Stewart *et al.*, 2009: 136). Although Bradshaw first proposed his taxonomy of need many years ago, as Scriven (2010) comments, it is still of great use in distinguishing levels of need. Bradshaw's fourfold classification of need is based on the derivation of the criteria adopted for recognising need, be it diagnostic or prescriptive. Bradshaw's taxonomy of need identifies four types of need:

1. Normative needs
2. Felt needs
3. Expressed needs
4. Comparative needs.

Normative needs

Normative needs are defined in accordance with some agreed standard. A desirable standard is laid down by the expert or professional and is compared with a standard which already exists. If an individual or group falls short of the desirable standard then they are identified as being in need. A normative definition of need is by no means absolute. It may not correspond with other definitions of need and, of course, different experts may have conflicting standards. It may be relatively easy to lay down standards for housing – where, for example, inside plumbing and electricity may be accepted as two standards of adequate housing – but it is more difficult to set standards in less tangible areas such as health without becoming involved in making value judgments. Thus normative definitions of need may be different according to the value judgments of differing experts. Furthermore, the idea of normative need demonstrates a particular view of service delivery in that it places the expert or professional at the centre of need assessment.

Felt needs

A felt need is a need expressed by an individual or community and is termed a want. Felt need alone may be an incomplete measure because it is limited by the perceptions and knowledge of the individual or community in that they may express a desire for a service without needing it, fail to recognise their own need, or assume that no solution exists which would be acceptable.

Expressed needs

Expressed need or demand is 'felt need' turned into action. Under this definition total need is defined as 'those people who demand a service'. Scriven (2010) comments that commercial classes for weight management provide an example of the response by industry to expressed needs or demands. There may be people, however, who do not turn felt need into demand or who are suffering from pre-symptomatic disease. Because of this, it is unsatisfactory to use, for example, waiting lists alone as a measure of unmet need. Other forms of information are also needed, for example, examination of the self-help groups in an area, the demands for well women clinics or fathers for parenting information, may all be seen as examples of expressed need.

Comparative needs

Comparative needs refer to the imputed needs of an individual or group not in receipt of services but similar in relevant characteristics to others receiving services. For example, if a person is in receipt of a service because of particular characteristics and another person also has these characteristics but is not receiving a service, then we can say that the second person is in need. This is an attempt to standardise provision, but provision may not correspond with need. In other words, even if area 'A' is receiving more resources than area 'B', area 'A' may still be in need.

Using the Bradshaw taxonomy of need the interrelations between the four definitions of need can be considered. For example, if we take the example of fluoridation of water supplies, this was accepted by public health experts, i.e. was a normative need, long before it was felt, demanded or supplied. The application of Bradshaw's taxonomy raises many issues for practice, not the least of which is the lack of clarity about what health visitors determine as normative need and what criteria we use in comparing provision in our areas with what is available in other parts of the district or country. As Naidoo and Wills (2009) conclude, 'needs are not objective and observable entities to which we must match our interventions. The concept of need is relative and is influenced by values and attitudes and by other agendas' (p. 257). Such other agendas will of course also include access to resources and finance to support services to meet the identified needs of the community. The process of HNA in partnership with community members and with reference to evidence such as that provided by Marmot *et al.* (2010) is one way of seeking to address these dilemmas.

Steps to undertaking health needs assessment

The HDA (which was joined with the National Institute of Clinical Excellence, forming the National Institute of Health and Clinical Excellence in 2005) has produced a guide (HDA, 2004a) and workbook (Hooper & Longworth, 2002) to support people in undertaking HNAs. A five-step process is described for undertaking an HNA as shown in Box 3.7. Activity 3.5 provides you with the opportunity to use these steps in undertaking an HNA in your locality.

A health needs assessment may be undertaken by a range of different people but involvement across different services and disciplines will enable collection and sharing of a wide range of information and will also ensure that those participating are ready to be involved in the planning and implementation of change. Hooper and Longworth (2002) suggest that some or all of the following might be involved in a HNA: members of the community affected by the issue; community leaders; religious leaders; shop owners; teachers and social workers; police, probation and community safety officers; GPs and members of the primary care team; local authority staff and elected members; service commissioners; members of community organisations, for example, allotment associations. They suggest that the following maxim is helpful in deciding who should be involved in the HNA:

- 'Who *knows* about the issue?
- Who *cares* about the issue?
- Who can *make change happen* related to the issue?'

(Hooper & Longworth, 2002: 29)

Box 3.7   Steps in undertaking a health needs assessment

Steps	Activities
Step 1: Getting started	What population? What are you trying to achieve? Who needs to be involved? What resources are required? What are the risks?
Step 2: Identifying health priorities	Population profiling Gathering data Perceptions of needs Identifying and assessing health conditions and determinant factors
Step 3: Assessing a health priority for action	Choosing health conditions and determinant factors with the most significant size and severity impact Determine effective and acceptable interventions and actions
Step 4: Planning for change	Clarifying aims of intervention Action planning Monitoring and evaluation strategy Risk-management strategy
Step 5: Moving on/review	Learning from the project Measuring the impact Choosing the next priority

Source: Health Development Agency, 2004a: 2

A HNA may therefore be undertaken by a cross-community team or a health visiting team may undertake a HNA of their practice population to help in planning the types of services to be provided by the team. In undertaking the HNA they may then engage with members of the wider community suggested above. A HNA may cover a whole population, for example in a neighbourhood, or may be focused on a particular part of the population, for example the needs of families with children over the age of two years. Such groups may or may not identify themselves as a community (for example, refer back to Figure 3.1, p. 89 in thinking about the community of interest). Once the focus of the HNA has been decided, the team undertaking the HNA needs to develop a realistic time plan for the HNA which will include the activities outlined in Box 3.7.

A major part of the HNA will involve the collection of information in relation to the health needs of the population. This information will be both quantitative and qualitative. It will involve accessing information from local, national and international sources, as well as undertaking local forms of qualitative data collection which might include interviews, focus groups or observation of use of services or spaces. Sources of information are shown in Box 3.8 and methods for identifying information with the local community are shown in Box 3.9 (other sources are provided in Chapter 6).

Box 3.8 Examples of sources of quantitative information on the health of a population

Source	Examples of types of information
The local public health report e.g. www.towerhamlets.nhs.uk/ publications	Local health needs and current priorities
The local joint community plan e.g. www.towerhamlets.gov.uk	Plan of action across local organisations to meet health and social needs
Association of Public Health Observatories www.apho.org.uk	• Health profiles • Health Impact Assessment Reports • Marmot Indicators for Local Authorities in England • APHO Tools Directory and Guide to Key Data Sources

UK National Statistics www.statistics.gov.uk	• Census information
	Theme areas including:
	  o Children, Education and Skills
	  o Health and Social Care
	  o People and places

NHS Evidence www.evidence.nhs.uk	• Clinical, non clinical evidence • Local, regional, national and international evidence • Government policy • To support high quality healthcare
NICE	• Clinical and cost effectiveness guidance • Appraisals of evidence • Tools to support implementation of evidence into practice
Child and Maternal Health Observatory www.chimat.org.uk	• Child Health Profiles • Information relating to the health of children, young people and maternal health • Tools to support needs assessment

Birth Cohort Studies, Centre for Longitudinal Studies www.cls.ioe.ac.uk	Evidence of impact of determinants of health on development and progress of children
PEGASUS (Professional Education for Genetic Assessment and Screening) www.pegasus.nhs/uk	• Antenatal and newborn screening statistics for local areas • Educational resources for health practitioners
Marmot Review www.marmotreview.org	• Marmot Report (2010) • Updated inequalities data • Evidence of initiatives to address inequalities in health
Joseph Rowntree Foundation ww.jrf.org.uk	Social policy research concerned with poverty, community development and empowerment
World Health Organisation www.who.org	• World health statistics • World guidelines • Annual world health report

---

Box 3.9   Examples of sources of qualitative information on the health of a population

Methods of gathering local information

- Observation in the local community of use of facilities and services
- Interviews with users of facilities and services
- Interviews with key informants, e.g. informal leaders of groups, shopkeepers, religious leaders
- Public meetings and forums
- Focus groups
- Using local media including radio phone-ins
- Reviewing local newspaper content
- Using internet sites e.g. a local community site, Facebook or Twitter groups
- Community health panels and citizens' juries

Research techniques including structured observation, rapid appraisal or ethnographic studies (Naidoo and Wills 2009: 264)

The information collected through these various methods may then be used to identify the extent of a health need in a particular population, the attitudes of people to the health need and the ability of that population to respond to the health need identified.

Box 3.10   Comparing health profile information

Health profile information, July 2010, Kingston-upon-Hull	Health profile information, July 2010, Surrey
The health of people in Hull is generally worse than the England average. Life expectancy for men and women, early deaths from cancer and from heart disease and stroke and deaths from smoking are all worse.	The health of people in Surrey is generally better than the England average. Levels of deprivation are low and life expectancy is higher than average.
In Hull *breastfeeding initiation, tooth decay in 5-year olds and teenage pregnancy are all worse than the England averages.* However, the percentage of physically active children is better than the England average.	While the proportion of children in Reception year classified as obese is below the England average, *physical activity levels are low.*

Source: Extracts from Health Profiles, Association of Health Observatories, 2010.

Starting with accessing information about your local area, the Health Profile, on the website of the Association of Public Health Observatories will provide a good starting point for identifying the health priorities in your area. Box 3.10 provides information from contrasting areas of England highlighting health needs in both areas which demonstrate the different focus of health visiting intervention needed in the two areas.

To explore the information in the Health Profile relevant to your area, complete Activity 3.6 (see Appendix 3).

Once the evidence of the extent of the health need has been compiled the HNA process then moves to development of interventions and an action plan to address the health need (see Box 3.7, p. 107). At this point it might be helpful to consider theory and skills that support work with communities.

Using health promotion models to support community working

There are a range of health promotion models that may be applicable to work with communities (Naidoo & Wills, 2009) but the model proposed by Beattie (1991/2003) has a particular focus on community development, as one aspect of the collective focus of an intervention. The model describes health promotion interventions being top-down or bottom up and focusing on the community or the individual. Where the focus is on the community and a bottom-up approach is being taken then community development activity will be supported. Naidoo and Wills (2009) identify the characteristics of community development based on Beattie's model to be:

> To *enfranchise* or *emancipate* groups or communities so they recognise what they have in common and how social factors influence their lives
> Practitioner is the role of 'advocate'
> Radical political ideology
> Activities include community development and action. (p. 78, emphasis in the original)

The health visitor using this model is working in partnership with community members supporting and acting as an advocate on their behalf and facilitating empowerment of individuals and the community. An important part of this process is the role that the health visitor has in strengthening networks and relationships between networks in the community thus enhancing the social capital in the community. Gilchrist (2007) discusses the literature which has demonstrated the importance of networks in providing support for health improvement and resilience of a community: 'While the physiological mechanisms for this resilience are unclear, it is probable that social networks provide a variety of forms of support and affirmation, including practical advice around health matters' (p. 142).

The work of the health visitor interfaces with very many people and organisations and this gives her the ability to provide a means of bridging and strengthening informal networks as well as professional and statutory network links. Joly (2009) in her PhD study demonstrates the existence of multiple overlapping and separate networks concerned with care of people who are homeless. The mapping of networks provides a means to locate gaps, poor or no communication between organisations working with the same community and thus means of developing and strengthening connections.

Identification of networks and work to strengthen networks to enable health needs to be addressed is essentially concerned with taking a strength-based approach to practice. One such approach is that of Appreciative Inquiry which takes a positive/strengths based stance and is based on the 4-D model which consists of four phases: discovery (the best of what is or has been), dreaming (what might be), designing (what should be) and destiny (what will be) (Reed, 2007; Radford, 2009). Using an Appreciative Inquiry approach requires participants to identify what has worked in the past and to draw on that experience to design solutions to address the current need. Various tools may be used to help in this process of identification of strengths and challenges one of which is Participatory Appraisal (PA) which makes use of visual tools. Pearson (2003) comments that PA, focuses on community level health and is an ideal approach for community based practitioners, such as health visitors, to use:

> PA takes a whole community approach to development rather than focusing on individuals, or individual groups of people in isolation. This has the effect of looking for rich, deep and broad community explanations for issues that would be missed if a narrower approach were used. Community practitioners who know and are part of communities are well placed to be involved in PA as facilitators, participants and users. (p. 176)

The above approaches may be helpful in engaging communities, particularly those that have long been disenfranchised. The term participation has many different meanings and efforts to engage people to participate may be met with both enthusiasm and resistance. Arnstein (1969) was the first to outline a ladder of participation describing the different levels of community participation:

- Citizen control
- Delegated power
- Partnership
- Placation
- Consultation
- Informing
- Therapy
- Manipulation

(Naidoo & Wills, 2009)

This ladder helps to demonstrate the limits of the transfer of power at the different levels of participation:

> [Arnstein] ranks the different degrees of citizen participation starting at the lowest rung of manipulation and ascending upwards to the highest level of participation, citizen control in which power is directly transferred from government to people.

(Draper *et al.*, 2010: 1103)

The application of this ladder to work with communities or the health visitors' experience in her team or work setting assists in the identification of barriers to the development of participant engagement in activities.

Another challenge in working with communities is the measurement both of the process and outcomes of community-based work (see Chapter 6). One aspect of this measurement is to gain an understanding of the level of participation of communities in health initiatives. Rifkin (1985) developed an approach to this measurement which examines participation on a continuum from little participation to wide participation (Draper *et al.*, 2010). Rifkin (1985) identified and defined a number of features of participation which are each measured on a scale and presented in the form of a spider diagram, with the legs of the spider comprising the measurement of: needs assessment, leadership, organisation, resource mobilisation, and management. By linking the scores for the five areas a spidergram is produced, showing the strength or weakness of each feature in a particular project. This approach has been widely used in community health projects with modification of the elements that form the spidergram in some cases, for example, in the application by Draper *et al.* (2010) to community-based child survival programmes in low income countries.

Summary

This chapter has considered some of the issues that need to be addressed by the health visitor and the health visitor team when working at the community level to support and enhance the experience of community health. Following an exploration of the meaning of community and the impact of community on health, the role of the health visitor and the skills and competencies underpinning current practice were explored. Working with a community requires the health visitor to develop an in-depth knowledge of the strengths and needs of that community. This may be achieved in a variety of ways, including one-to-one working. At the level of the community three approaches to developing such knowledge were outlined. The health visitor is supported in undertaking such assessments by a wealth of information and knowledge available via the internet. In fact one of the key skills in undertaking a health needs assessment is keeping focused and making use of relevant information and data to inform the process of need identification. Throughout the chapter skills and knowledge required by the health visitor to work successfully with communities have been referred to and the chapter concluded with reference to a number of such approaches.

References

Antonovsky, A. (1996) The salutogenic model as a theory to guide health promotion. *Health Promotion International*, **11**(1), 11-18.

Arnstein, S. (1969) A ladder of citizen participation. *American Institute of Planners Journal*, **35**(4), 216-224.

Association of Public Health Observatories (2010) Health Profiles. Available from: www.apho.org.uk (accessed 3 February, 2011).

Barrett, G., Naidoo, J. & Orme, J. (2007) *Capacity and capability in public health*. In: *Public Health for the 21st Century* (eds J. Orme, J. Powell, P. Taylor & M. Grey), 2nd ed, Ch. 5, pp. 83-97. Open University Press McGraw-Hill Education, Maidenhead.

Bauld, L. (2011) *The Impact of Smokefree Legislation in England: Evidence Review, March 2011*. Department of Health, London.

Beattie, A. (2003 (1991)) Knowledge and control in health promotion: a test case for social policy and social theory. In: *The Sociology of the Health Service* (eds J. Gabe, M. Calnan & M. Bury), Ch. 7, pp. 162-202. Routledge, London.

Bell, C. & Newby, H. (1971) *Community Studies*. Allen & Unwin, London.

Benson, J. (1976) The concept of community. In: *Talking about Welfare* (eds N. Timms & D. Watson). Routledge & Kegan Paul, London.

Bradshaw, J. (1972) The concept of social need. *New Society*, **30**, 640–643.

Bradshaw, J. (1994) The conceptualisation and measurement of need – a social policy perspective. In: *Researching the People's Health* (eds J. Popay & G. Williams), Ch. 3, pp. 45–57. Routledge, London.

Bryar, R. & Fisk, L. (1994) Setting up a community health house. *Community Practitioner*, **67**(6), 203–205.

Bryar, R., Kendall, S. & Mogotlane, S.M. (2011) *Reforming Primary Health: A Nursing Perspective: Contributing to Health Care Reform, Issues and Challenges.* ICHRN, ICN, Geneva (in press).

Cameron, S. & Christie, G. (2007) Exploring health visitors' perceptions of the public health nursing role. *Primary Health Care Research and Development*, **8**(1), 80–90.

Campbell, A., Converse, P. & Rodgers, W. (1976) *The Quality of American Life: Perceptions, Evaluations and Satisfaction.* Russell Sage Foundation, New York.

Change4Life (undated) Home Page. Available from: www.nhs.uk/Change4Life/Pages/change-for-life.aspx (accessed 12 March, 2011).

Council for the Education and Training of Health Visitors (1965) *Syllabus Examination for Health Visitors in the United Kingdom.* Council for the Education and Training of Health Visitors, London; cited in J. Robinson & R. Elkan (1996) *Health Needs Assessment. Theory and Practice.* Churchill Livingstone, Edinburgh.

Council for the Education and Training of Health Visitors (1967) *The Function of the Health Visitor.* Council for the Education and Training of Health Visitors, London, cited in J. Robinson & R. Elkan (1996) *Health Needs Assessment. Theory and Practice.* Churchill Livingstone, Edinburgh.

Cowley, S. & Frost, M. (2006) *The Principles of Health Visiting: Opening the Door to Public Health Practice in the 21st Century.* Community Practitioners' and Health Visitors' Association, London.

Craig, P.M. (1995) *A Different Role: Health Visiting in a Community Project.* Glasgow City Health Project, Glasgow.

Craig, P.M. & Lindsay, G.M. (eds) (2000) *Nursing for Public Health. Population-based Care.* Churchill Livingstone, London.

Crow, G. (2002) Community Studies: Fifty Years of Theorization. *Sociological Research Online*, **7**(3), 1–13, Available from: www.socresonline.org.uk/7/3/crow.html (accessed 23 March, 2011).

Dahlgren, G. & Whitehead, M. (1991) *Policies and Strategies to Promote Social Equity in Health.* Institute for Futures Studies, Stockholm.

Dench, G., Gavron, K. & Young, M. (2006) *The New East End: Kinship, Race and Conflict.* The Young Foundation, London.

Department of Health (2007) *Guidance on Joint Strategic Needs Assessment.* Department of Health, London.

Department of Health (2011) *The Health Visitor Implementation Plan 2011–15. A Call to Action.* Department of Health, London.

Draper, A.K., Hewitt, G. & Rifkin, S. (2010) Chasing the dragon: Developing indicators for assessment of community participation in health programmes. *Social Science & Medicine*, **71**(6), 1102–1109.

Drennan, V. (ed.) (1988) *Health Visitors and Groups. Politics and Practice.* Heinemann Professional Publishing Ltd, Oxford.

Gilchrist, A. (2007) *Community Development and Networking for Health.* In: *Public Health for the 21st Century* (eds J. Orme, J. Powell, P. Taylor & M. Grey), 2nd edn, Ch. 8, pp. 135–152. Open University Press McGraw-Hill Education, Maidenhead.

Greer, S. & Minar, D. (1969) *The Concept of Community.* Aldine Press, Chicago.

Hall, D.M.B. & Elliman, D. (2006) *Health for All Children*, 4th edn, revised. Oxford University Press, Oxford.

Hamer, J., Jacobson, B., Flowers, J. & Johnstone, F. (2003) *Health Equity Audit Made Simple: A briefing for Primary Care Trusts and Local Strategic Partnerships. Working Document January 2003.* NICE, London.

Hart, J.T. (1971) The Inverse Care Law. *The Lancet,* **I**, 405–412.

Health Development Agency (2004a) *Health Needs Assessment.* HDA, NICE, London.

Health Development Agency (2004b) *Clarifying Health Impact Assessment, Integrated Impact Assessment and Health Needs Assessment.* HDA, NICE, London.

Hillery, G.A. (1955) Definition of community – areas of agreement. *Rural Sociology,* **20** (June), 111–123.

Hillery, G.A. (1982) *Developing and Testing a Community Theory. A Research Odyssey.* Transaction Inc., New Brunswick.

Hooper, J. & Longworth, P. (2002) *Health Needs Assessment Workbook.* HDA, NICE, London.

Hunt, R. (2009) *Introduction to Community-Based Nursing,* 4th edn. Walters Kluwer, Lippincott Williams & Wilkins, Philadelphia.

Joly, L.M.A. (2009) *A mixed method study to explore interagency working to support the health of people who are homeless.* PhD thesis. University College London, London.

Knight, B. & Hayes, R. (1981) *Self Help in the Inner City.* Voluntary Services Council, London.

Konig, R. (1968) *The Community.* Allen & Unwin, London.

Krupat, E. & Guild, W. (1980) Defining the city: The use of objective and subjective measures for community description. *Journal of Social Issues,* **36**(3), 9–28.

Layard, R. & Dunne, J. (2009) *A Good Childhood inquiry: Searching for Values in a Competitive Age.* Penguin Group, London, cited in Y. Roberts, M. Brophy & N. Bacon (2009) *Parenting and Wellbeing: Knitting Families Together.* The Young Foundation, London.

Lock, K. (2000) Health impact assessment. *BMJ,* **320**, 1395–1398, cited in: J. Naidoo & J. Wills (2009) *Foundations for Health Promotion.* 3rd edn. Bailliere Tindall Elsevier, Edinburgh.

Luker, K. & Orr, J. (eds) (1992) *Health Visiting: Towards Community Health Nursing.* Blackwell Science, Oxford.

Lynch, J.W., Law, C., Brinkman, S., Chittleborough, C. & Sawyer, M (2010) Inequalities in child health development: Some challenges for effective implementation. *Social Science & Medicine,* **71**(4), 1244–1248.

MacIver, R.M. & Page, C.H. (1962) *Society. An Introductory Analysis.* Macmillan, London.

McNaught, A. (2009) *Leadership in Community Development,* Chapter 12, pp. 165–176. In: *Professional Practice in Public Health* (eds J. Stewart & Y. Cornish). Reflect Press Ltd, Exeter.

Marmot, M., Atkinson, T., Bell, J., *et al.* (2010) *Fair Society, Healthy Lives. The Marmot Review,* Marmot Review Team, University College London.

Maslow, A. (1954) *Motivation and Personality.* Harper, New York.

Mguni, N. & Bacon, N. (2010) *Taking the Temperature of Local Communities. The Wellbeing and Resilience Measure (WARM).* The Young Foundation, London.

Midwinter, E. (1973) *Patterns of Community Education.* Ward Lock Publications, London.

Moos, R.H. (1976) *The Human Context; Environmental Determinants of Behaviour.* John Wiley & Sons, Inc., New York.

Moos, R.H. (2002) The mystery of human context and coping: an unravelling of clues. *American Journal of Community Psychology,* **30**(1), 67–88.

Mulgan, G. (2010) *Investing in Social Growth. Can the Big Society be More than a Slogan?* The Young Foundation, London.

Naidoo, J. & Wills, J. (2009) *Foundations for Health Promotion,* 3rd edn. Bailliere Tindall Elsevier, Edinburgh.

National Institute for Health & Clinical Excellence (2008) *Community Engagement*. NICE, London.

Nursing and Midwifery Council (2004) *Standards of Proficiency for Specialist Community Public Health Nurses*. Nursing and Midwifery Council, London.

O'Dwyer, L.A., Baum, F., Kavanagh, A. & Macdougall, C. (2007) Do area-based interventions to reduce health inequalities work? A systematic review of the evidence. *Critical Public Health*, **17**(4), 317-335, cited in A.K. Draper, G. Hewitt & S. Rifkin (2010) Chasing the dragon: Developing indicators for assessment of community participation in health programmes. *Social Science & Medicine*, **71**(6), 1102-1109.

Orr, J. (1992) The community dimension. In: *Health Visiting: Towards Community Health Nursing* (eds K. Luker & J. Orr), Ch. 2, pp. 43-72. Blackwell Science, Oxford.

Pearson, L. (2003) Capturing client voices for community development using participatory appraisal. In: *Practice Development in Community Nursing. Principles and Processes* (eds R.M. Bryar & J.M. Griffiths), Ch. 9 pp. 175-193. Arnold, London.

Pearson, P. (2011) Personal communication.

Public Health Resource Unit & Skills for Health (2008) *Public Health Skills and Career Framework. Multidisciplinary/Multi-agency/Multi-professional April 2008*. Available from Solutions for Public Health Website*: http://www.sph.nhs.uk/what-we-do/public-health-workforce/outcomes/public-health-skills-and-career-framework/* (accessed 16 March, 2011).

Radford, A. (2009) *Reflections on AI and Their Implications for Sustaining AI as a Way of Life*. www.aradford.co.uk (accessed 23 March, 2011).

Reed, J. (2007) *Appreciative Inquiry - Research for Change*. Sage, London.

Rifkin, S.B. (1985) *Health Planning and Community Participation: Case Studies in South-east Asia*. Croom Helm Ltd, Beckenham.

Roberts, Y., Brophy, M., Bacon, N. (2009) *Parenting and Wellbeing: Knitting Families Together*. The Young Foundation, London.

Robinson, J. & Elkan, R. (1996) *Health Needs Assessment. Theory and Practice*. Churchill Livingstone, Edinburgh.

Scriven, A. (2010) *Promoting Health. A Practical Guide*. Balliere Tindall Elsevier, Edinburgh.

Starfield, B. (1996) Public health and primary care: A framework for proposed linkages. *American Journal of Public Health*, **86**(10), 1365-1369.

Stewart, J., Cornish, Y., Patel, S. (2009) Health needs assessment. In: *Professional Practice in Public Health* (eds J. Stewart & Y. Cornish), Ch. 10, pp. 133-147. Reflect Press Ltd, Exeter.

Swann, B. & Brocklehurst, N. (2004) Three in one: the Stockport model of health visiting. *Community Practitioner*, **77**(7), 251-256.

Tönnies, F. (1955; first published 1887) *Community and Association*. Routledge & Kegan Paul, London.

Tucker, W.H. (1979) The nature of a community. In: *Community Health Care and the Nursing Process* (ed. M.J. Fromer). C.V. Mosby, St Louis.

Watt, G. (2002) The inverse care law today. *The Lancet*, **360**(9328), 252-254.

Weaver, B.R. (1977) Conceptual basis for nursing intervention with human systems: communities and societies. In: *Distributive Nursing Practice: a Systems Approach to Community Health* (eds J.E. Hall. & B.R. Weaver), J.B. Lippincott Co., Philadelphia.

Weiner, R. (1975) *The Rape and Plunder of the Shankhill*. Notarms Press, Belfast.

World Health Organization/UNICEF (1978) *Declaration of Alma Ata*. WHO, Geneva. Available from: www.who.int/NPH/docs/declaration_almaata.pdf (accessed 10 October, 2010).

World Health Organization (2008) *Primary Health Care: Now More than Ever*. WHO, Geneva.

Young, M. & Willmott, P. (2007 (1957)) *Family and Kinship in East London*. Penguin Modern Classics, London.

Young Foundation (2010) *How Can Neighbourhoods Be Understood and Defined?* The Young Foundation, London.

Young Foundation (2011) *Community Action Toolkit*. Available from: www.youngfoundation.org/community-action-tool-kit (accessed 13 March, 2011).

Appendix 3   Activities for Chapter 3

Working with communities is essentially about participation so in this chapter we want you to participate. It may be that you will undertake these activities on your own or working with other team members or people in your local community.

Activity 3.1

Your definition of community and your communities

Write down your definition of community and discuss this with a colleague. Do you share the same understanding? What are the differences in your definitions?

Think about the different communities that you belong to. Write down all these communities and group them under relevant headings.

Activity 3.2

Public health practice

Consider the ten areas of public health practice from Barrett *et al.*, 2007 and identify an example from your practice with a community which illustrates your application of one or more of the areas of public health practice.

Areas of public health practice	Example(s) from your practice
Surveillance and assessment of the population's health and wellbeing;	
Promoting and protecting the population's health and wellbeing;	

(Continued)

Activity 3.3

Setting up a new service

With reference to Box 3.4 consider how the members of your health visiting skill mix team might respond to setting up a service to meet the need of fathers for support in developing their parenting role.

Activity 3.4

Developing a public health walk

Explore your local area on foot, talk to local health visitors and public health colleagues, consult the local librarian and library services and talk to local residents to identify the historical and contemporary public health issues in your area. Construct a walk to illustrate the impact of these issues in your area. Invite colleagues and local residents to participate in and develop the walk.

Activity 3.5

Undertaking a health needs assessment

Identify a neighbourhood in which you are working and use the HDA 5 Step model (HAD, 2004a) to undertake a health needs assessment of the neighbourhood. In doing this identify one health need and develop an implementation plan and evaluation process to address that need

Steps	Activities	Your neighbourhood
Step 1: Getting started	• What population? • What are you trying to achieve? • Who needs to be involved? • What resources are required? • What are the risks?	
Step 2: Identifying health priorities	• Population profiling • Gathering data • Perceptions of needs • Identifying and assessing health conditions and determinant factors	
Step 3: Assessing a health priority for action	• Choosing health conditions and determinant factors with the most significant size and severity impact • Determine effective and acceptable interventions and actions	
Step 4: Planning for change	• Clarifying aims of intervention • Action planning • Monitoring and evaluation strategy • Risk-management strategy	
Step 5: Moving on/ review	• Learning from the project • Measuring the impact • Choosing the next priority	

Activity 3.6

Accessing health profile information

Access the health profile for your area on the APHO website (www.apho. org.uk) and compare the information in the profile with a contrasting area in another part of Britain. What are the key priorities for health visiting that you can identify from this information? How does the comparison affect your assessment of health issues in your area?

4

Approaches to Supporting Families

Karen I. Chalmers
The University of Manchester, Manchester, UK

Introduction

Health visitors are well positioned to contribute to the proposed changes to the public health system and improve the health of the nation (Department of Health, 2010). Improving the social determinants of health is critical if health inequalities are to be reduced across social groups (Marmot *et al.*, 2010). The Social Exclusion Task Force estimates that about 2% of families with children in Britain experience five or more disadvantages and that, for many, these persist into adulthood (Cabinet Office, 2006, 2007). Disadvantages include no parent in the family in work, living in poverty or overcrowded housing, no parent with educational qualifications, mother with mental health problems, low income and other disadvantages. Children living in deprived areas are 8% more likely to be obese, 9% more likely to be of low birth weight and 12% more likely to have an accident than those living in the rest of England (Audit Commission, 2010). As well, there is increasing evidence of the impact of the home environment on the neurological development and physical and psychosocial health of infants and young children and that these impacts can have a long-lasting effect on the children's health and development. Building resilience and wellbeing of young children across the social gradient is critical for improvement in health of the population (Marmot *et al.*, 2010). Supporting families with young children is seen as one important approach to improve the social determinants of these families and improve their current and future health (Marmot *et al.*, 2010).

Supporting families to improve health and to prevent ill health, particularly families with young children, has been the cornerstone of health visiting practice since the inception of the service. This chapter explores approaches and programmes in which health visitors support

Health Visiting: A Rediscovery, Third Edition. Edited by Karen A. Luker, Jean Orr and Gretl A. McHugh.

families with young children with a goal of improving family health. The specific objectives of the chapter are to:

- assess some models of intervention in family life and their application to health visiting practice;
- explore the role of policies influencing health visitors' work in supporting families;
- examine programmes to support families with young children, including the Family Nurse Partnership Programme;
- examine the role of the health visitor-client relationship when providing supportive care to young families;
- reflect on the challenges when planning services for and working with families.

Models of intervention in family life

The 'family' is one institution in our society which is viewed as being important, not only for individual welfare but for the overall good of society. The family is used as a symbol in all discussions of social life and social welfare and it is seen as a necessary function of the state to intervene in family life through the provision of services and benefits as well as controlling behaviours through policies and laws (e.g. the use of infant and child car seats). Health visitors are, more than most other health workers, involved in visiting families in their homes and in providing a unique service by working with families across all social classes and during periods of family transitions and crises. To work with families in this way gives health visitors considerable experience of family life and the tensions which are a normal part of living, thus placing health visitors in a privileged position to monitor social and economic policies affecting health. It is also a responsibility to work with individuals and families in this personal and important sphere of their lives.

The notion of intervening in family life to assess need is complex and has within it tensions based on the relationships between the state and the family. On the one hand, the family is seen as being a private and personal unit especially when there are no children and the dominant values of society are being upheld. On the other hand, due to the importance of the family, particularly in relation to the wellbeing of children, intervention with the family is seen by many as a legitimate action of the state. Wasoff and Hill (2002) argue that parenting is now a designated area of policy intervention, not only to support parents but to tackle social inclusion for the sake of the wider community. The state first intervenes in the family often when a woman becomes pregnant and almost always when the child is born. Pregnancy and childbirth result in the private family being scrutinised by professionals. Doctors often legitimise when a woman is pregnant and decide on the availability of abortion, if that is requested. The medical profession tends also to control contraception, at least in part. Social workers, and more recently health visitors, have a major role in deciding if children are being adequately cared for and when, or if, they should be taken into care, and parents may perceive that they have to 'measure up' to professionals' expectations. The focus on child-rearing skills objectifies parenting as caring labour and hides the fact that it has a gendered status and is largely undertaken by women in the family. Also, it is women who usually find themselves on the interface with social and health services, particularly if they are caring for children or aged or disabled family members. The economic need means more women in the workforce, which has led to seeing full-time mothering as a problem, particularly in the case of lone parents. The State gives token acknowledgment to the role of women as mothers and caregivers and emphasises these roles in order to support the policy shift in community care (House of Commons, 1990; Department of Health (DH), 2006, 2008a, 2009b). While there is increasing recognition of the social costs imposed on carers (which most commonly means women) and increasingly carers' needs are being identified by governments (e.g. OPSI, 2004; Carers UK, 2008), there is little real help coming from government.

Three models relevant to health visiting practice in families with young children

Historically, the focus of health visitors' work was on families, specifically families with infants and pre-school children. Although individuals, social groups and 'the community' were also cited in health visitor texts and position statements, in practice, the dominant focus was usually children and women in the mothering role. Although there is a call over the past decade for more involvement of health visitors in wider public health roles (Department of Health, 2001, 2010, 2011b), there remains a dominant emphasis in the heath visiting role of working to support young families.

Articulating the theoretical underpinnings of practice may assist practitioners in clarifying what actually or potentially influences day to day practice. Below, three models or approaches of health visitors' work in supporting young families are outlined. These models have not been gener- ated strictly from empirical research although there is some research which supports how health visitors work with young families (see below). Rather, these models have been synthesised from the health visitor literature. The models include the child-centred model, the family-centred model and the ecological model.

1.   The child-centred model

This model was the dominant model of health visiting practice for many years. Within the child focused model, the proper focus of services is seen to be the wellbeing of the young child, with other family members, especially fathers, playing secondary roles. Fathers, and their role in promoting and supporting the health of families, received little attention. Health visitors worked primarily with mothers in their homes and clinics with the goal of promoting the healthy development of children. They had contact at designated times to carry out development assessments (as advocated in the Hall Report (Hall & Elliman,

2006) and health teaching at each age milestone. All families received the home visiting service. The universality of the service is seen as eliminating the stigma of professionally perceived needs or problems permitting intervention 'upstream' (Marmot *et al.*, 2010: 155) to prevent health and behavioural problems (primary prevention) or to detect these problems early before they become entrenched (secondary prevention).

Health visitors have no statutory right of access to the home, but negotiate their entry to the home based on the 'normality' of the service ('everyone receives it'). Because the focus was on the child, the wellbeing of other family members was perceived to be secondary or was minimally considered. There is currently strong research evidence of the importance of prenatal and early childhood development, including neurological development, as a determinant of health and health equalities (Irwin *et al.*, 2007). Interventions to promote healthy child development are critical. While health teaching to parents related to child development remains important., the means to promote healthy child development are also now seen as entailing a wider focus than just the child within the family.

2. The family-centred model

The family-centred model also recognises the importance of children's health; however, the means of securing enhanced child health is viewed within a holistic 'family lens'. This approach has the satisfactory health and functioning of the family as its main aim. This model tends to be more concerned with resolving difficulties and conflicts within the family and thus improving the overall functioning and wellbeing of the family as a whole, as well as its members. The underpinnings of this model are influenced by family theories, primarily family systems theory, as well as other family theories such as structural-functioning theory and family development theory (Wright & Leahy, 1994). These theories were developed in social science disciplines and adapted by some applied disciplines, such as clinical psychology and specialty fields within social work. Aspects of these models and theories are now taught in nursing and health visiting courses. For example, genograms of families (see Figure 4.1) are used in practice as a pictorial means of viewing the family holistically (e.g. Haringey NHS Teaching Primary Care Trust, 2004; Birmingham Primary Care Trusts, 2007; McGoldrick *et al.*, 2008). Activity 4.1 (see Appendix 4 at the end of the chapter) provides an opportunity to create a genogram and provides further information about genogram symbols.

It is important, though, that theories developed and applied by other disciplines are not 'imported' into health visiting without careful consideration of the practice context. These theories, though, may assist health visitors to view families holistically, expand their 'lens' of practice from 'child' to 'family' and direct them to view the influences on the child's health from a broader perspective.

3. Ecological model

This model has its origins in Bronfenbrenner's (1979) 'person in context' framework. This is an integrated framework which recognises the interrelationship and interdependence of all aspects and levels in society. For example, the young

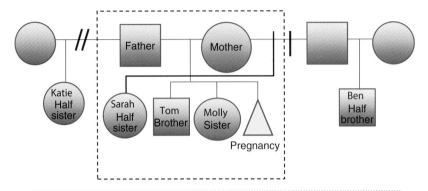

Figure 4.1 Family genogram.

child can be viewed as nestled within a family which is viewed within the neighbourhood and community and the larger sociopolitical and cultural environments. The model outlines four distinct levels: the microsystem, mesosystem, exosystem and macrosystem. Viewing children's health through this approach acknowledges the various immediate and more distant environments as major impacts on children's health and development. It also provides additional 'targets' for legitimate health visitors' interventions. This might involve meeting with extended family members as well as parents to discuss the child's health needs (i.e. mesosystem) or developing groups in the community to support young families in the community (i.e. exosystem) or influencing governments to implement child health promotive policies (macrosystem).

This model recognises the transitions of families and communities and helps to provide a means of viewing today's families within the context of the many influences on their lives. For example, this model would direct the health visitor to recognise the diversity of family units such as sole parent, same sex parents, adoptive families and others to assess the strengths, resources and stressors coming from the different systems which influence individual and family health. This model also resonates with the call for health visitors to work within a family centred public health role (Department of Health, 2001). However, the ecological model more clearly articulates the interrelationship and interconnectedness of the individual to the external environments than is outlined in the public health perspective. It has been advocated as a promising approach for the health visiting service while needing further research to test directly the utility of the framework in practice (Bryans *et al.*, 2009: 564). Bronfenbrenner's (1979) ecological model is also one of the theoretical underpinnings of the Family Nurse Partnership Programme and elements are present in the Starting Well Project (see p. 132, 137).

Application of models in practice

Although the above models are presented separately, there is little empirical evidence that, in actual practice, health visitors in the past or currently function solely within one conceptual perspective. Also, there are many other models or perspectives which health visitors may be using purposefully or informally in their work with young families such as strengths based interventions (DH/Unite/CPHVA, 2009). Health visitors' practice with young families is also influenced by many other factors such as the numbers of health visitors in communities and other available resources. One of the most important factors is the policy initiative under which the service is offered. For example, policies may direct health visitors' service provision to all of the under fives or to a targeted group of young children who are deemed to be at particular risk for poor health and development. (The influence of policy on health practice is outlined in more detail in the section below.)

There is some evidence, however, that, even within existing policies which direct service provision, health visitors operate within conceptual models which place more or less emphasis on particular aspects of their work. Understanding how practice is actually delivered is gleaned from empirical research on practice. Research studies which gather information through observation and interviews with health visitors and clients are particularly helpful.

For example, in an early study of health visiting practice in the north of England, health visitors were interviewed about aspects of their practice (Chalmers, 1992b). At this time, all health visitors in the study were carrying out universal home visiting to families with children from the early post natal period to age five. Although the focus of the study was not directly on how health visitors worked with fathers, this became evident from the analysis of their descriptions of practice. The particular approach that the health visitors used was influenced by their conceptualisation of men/fathers as important (or not) in promoting the family's health, including the health of young children and also factors in the actual client–health visitor situation which enhanced or restricted their work with the fathers. There was considerable variation in the approach to promoting the health of the children and health visitors' involvement with the fathers in these households. Some health visitors, for example, did not appear to conceptualise men as particularly important in their work with the families but did seek them out (i.e. worked with them) when they assessed the mother as incompetent in some way in the mothering role. Some health visitors were clearly working from a child centred model while others were more family focused.

In a more recent research example on health visiting practice in central Scotland carried out in 2003–2004 (Bryans et al., 2009), the actions of the health visitors in their day-to-day work with families were analysed using an ecological perspective. The study used a mixed method design involving audio-recorded interviews with health visitors and clients, observations of home visits of health visitor–client interaction and a review of documents and workshops with health visitor participants. The findings illustrated considerable work by the health visitors at the micro, meso and exosystems. The researchers articulated that Bronfenbrenner's (1979) framework captured how health visitors worked with individuals and families in a culturally sensitive, person-focused and context specific way (p. 571).

Thus, research on actual practice can help to uncover what 'informal' models may be influencing health visiting practice, regardless of the policies operating at the time.

Policies

As noted above, health visitors' practice with young families is highly influenced by government policies. Governments attempt to direct social change by various policy instruments such as programmes to benefit specific groups such as children. It is governments which develop, implement, revise and retire polices. In addition, other nongovernmental organisations such as professional associations, unions and voluntary associations attempt to influence government policies by lobbying, making presentations at government committee meetings and producing position statements or other reports on topics of interest to their agendas.

Several government policies in the past decade have been directed to improving children's health. In the report, *Every Child Matters* (HM Government, 2003), the development of a national Common Assessment Framework (CAF), was proposed. Five key outcomes for children were articulated – be healthy; stay safe; enjoy and achieve; make a positive contribution; and achieve economic wellbeing (Department for Education and Skills, 2004). The Common Assessment Framework (CAF) (discussed further in Chapter 5) has been implemented widely in a most organisations and boroughs; however, the process of completing a CAF may be a barrier for being used as originally intended. The detailed document is reported to be time-consuming and requires written consent prior to sharing with other organisations. The e-CAF (electronic) system may be a great asset to staff, as it aids information sharing and all professionals involved with children and their families can see what information has been collected and likely will reduce duplication in assessment. Increasingly, services are recognising that the CAF can meet both required assessment and referral information (Personal communication, S. Stewart, 29 June 2010).

The *Every Child Matters* report was followed shortly by the *National Service Framework for Children, Young People and Maternity Services* report (Department of Health, 2004). An outcome of this report was the initiation of the *Child Health Promotion Programme* (Department of Health, 2008b), now the *Healthy Child Programme* (Department of Health, 2009) to provide preventative services tailored to the individual needs of children and families (Audit Commission, 2010).

Health visiting is increasingly seen at the forefront of the Government's plans to deal with health inequalities and improve public health (Hoskins, 2009; Department of Health, Social Services and Public Safety, 2009). Chapter 2 discusses this further. However, the numbers of health visitors has declined and there is little agreement on the focus of their role throughout the United Kingdom (Audit Commission, 2010). This has now been recognised and a plan is in place to increase the number of health visitors by 4200 by the year 2015. One early approach advocated by the Department of Health (2001), as noted above, is the family-centred public health role. This role aims to strengthen the community-based, population approach of public health and integrate this with individual and family work. The focus of the health visitor role moves away from surveillance of children's health and towards a public health framework with a focus on groups, communities and populations. Health visitors would still work with young families but work more in partnerships with the families and base their services according to identified needs. The emphasis would be on universality, meaning that all families would have access to a range of services provided by a team of people, but not all families would receive the same service from the same person (p. 15). Through community assessments, the needs of other groups in the community would be identified and services developed to address these needs (e.g. homeless people). This perspective has resonance with the Council of Education and Training of Health Visitors' (CETHV) original principles of health visiting which addressed searching for health needs; stimulating an awareness of health needs; influencing policies which affect health needs and facilitating health enhancing activities (CETHV, 1977).

Many similar policy changes affecting health visiting practice with families are occurring in Northern Ireland. The Department of Health, Social Services and Public Safety (DHSSPS) published a new strategy for health visiting and school nursing, *Healthy Futures: The Contribution of Health Visitors and School Nurses in Northern Ireland* (DHSSPS, 2010). One of the key aims of this strategy is to support families using a model of progressive universalism (p. 25). This means that a universal team delivers child health promotion programmes and identifies children, young people and families in need. The team is made up of a skill mix which enables those with the most skill to work with those with the most needs. This approach is based on the UNOCINI (Understanding the Needs of Children in Northern Ireland) Threshold of Needs model (DHSSPS, 2006) which divides need into four levels. The first level is universal need which is seen as families who enjoy wellbeing and require no additional support. Level 2 is called 'additional needs' where there is increased vulnerability. Level 3 is complex needs requiring targeted preventive services and level 4 is specialist needs with those in need of protection (looked after children or with serious enduring health problems). The input of health visitors will vary according to needs assessment and they will be working as part of an integrated child health service. Families who are deemed to be most challenging and complex will receive additional support which follows a rigid programme of intervention, such as the Family Nurse Partnership. It is proposed that this will be the future provision in England (UNOCINI, 2008).

Nongovernmental organisations have responded to the changes made or proposed by governments and advocate for particular future health visitor roles. The Health Visitor Review Group (Department of Health, 2007) proposed the future role as a public health nursing role focusing on early intervention, prevention and health promotion for young children and families including home visiting. The concept of proportionate universalism (Department of Health, 2010; Marmot *et al.*, 2010) (earlier referred to as progressive universalism) is now stressed in which services are planned and delivered to provide support according to needs at the neighbourhood and individual levels. Working with vulnerable families with high needs is an important component of the work including readiness to provide health protection services. Also, the health visitor would deliver the *Healthy Child Programme* during pregnancy and the first year of life using a family focused public health approach (Department of Health, 2009a). This includes knowing the community, working across organisational boundaries and an emphasis on teamwork and partnership. Additional areas of practice include the delivery of wider public health packages to other risk groups in the community (i.e. homeless people) and primary care nursing services for children and families.

The United Kingdom Public Health Association (UKPHA) has responded to the concerns about the future role of the health visitor (UKPHA, 2009). Many of the same issues and recommendations are highlighted in this report. Health visitors are seen as key professionals in delivering the public health agenda to promote health and reduce health inequities particularly through the services to families with young children. The principles of progressive universalism are recommended based on an assessment at the area/population level and the individual/family level.

Clearly, from the review of current policy documents, the wellbeing of children is an increasing concern and health visitors are seen as contributing to the support of families with young children. In the sections below, the evidence for family support programmes is explored.

Evidence for interventions to support families

Over the years, several home visiting and other child health programmes have been developed to address the needs of families with young children. These programmes build on a long tradition of child health services delivered by health visitors (in the United Kingdom) and public health nurses (in the United States, Canada and other countries). With the growing number of well-designed longitudinal studies, there is increasing evidence, primarily from North America, that home visiting programmes contribute to several improved outcomes in mothers and children. Many of these studies have been critiqued and reported in several systematic reviews and meta-analyses (e.g. Elkan *et al.*, 2000). In a 'review of reviews' by the National Health Service (NHS Health Development Agency, 2004), nine systematic reviews were included in the analysis of studies on antenatal, postnatal and child health visiting. While the focus of programmes and the variables used to assess outcomes may vary, all of the studies are designed to gather evidence as to 'what works' in supporting young families. From this review, the evidence suggests that home visiting programmes are associated with improved parenting, improvements in some child behaviours, improved cognitive development particularly in some subgroups such as low birth or premature infants, reduction in accidental child injuries and improved detection and management of postnatal depression. There is little or inconclusive evidence on other variables such as incidents of child abuse, immunisation uptake, reduced hospitalisation or maternal employment (NHS Health Development Agency, 2004: 4). Other reviews have examined parent training programmes and found benefit to maternal mental health (Barlow *et al.*, 2002, 2003).

Despite the promising findings from the evaluation studies and reviews, the variation in studies (the design, sample characteristics, time periods of data collection and many other factors) makes it difficult to 'tease out' the critical features of the home visiting programme which may be contributing to the study outcomes. In a meta-analysis of 60 home visiting programmes, no one characteristic of the programmes was found to be a significant influence across outcomes (Sweet & Applebaum, 2004).

Characteristics of programmes to support families with young children

Programmes to support young families may vary on many important characteristics. Important questions that need consideration when examining and evaluating programmes are outlined in Box 4.1. While this list of questions is not exhaustive, it may assist in thinking about the number of factors which will

---

Box 4.1 Questions to consider when assessing child health programmes

- Is the service offered to all infants/children (universal) or to a particular group (targeted)?
- If the latter, what criteria are used to identify the target group?
- Is the programme designed to enrol women during the prenatal or postnatal period or either time period?
- What are the conceptual underpinnings of the programme, if known (e.g. strengths based, learning theory, support based on interpersonal/therapeutic relationships between parent and nurse, etc.)?
- Who delivers the programme (the professional – health visitor or public health nurse – or an assistant – a home visitor, community 'mothers', etc.)?
- What is the programme's age cut off for the child (i.e. two years, school enrolment, etc.)?
- What services does the family receive and how often do they receive services?
- What are the services (if any) that the family receives once they complete the programme? If services are provided, what are these services?

influence the development, implementation and evaluation of programmes to support families. Think about the child health programmes which are delivered in your area and begin to complete Activity 4.2 (see Appendix 4).

In the next sections, several programmes delivered in the United Kingdom are presented and the available evidence to evaluate outcomes is discussed. Similarities and differences in the conceptual underpinnings of programmes are identified, where possible, as well as how the programme was operationalised or put into actual practice. Also outlined are the key elements of the programme and what variables or criteria are/were used to evaluate the programme. Where possible, information is provided on the evaluated findings of the programme and additional recommendations for changes or future development. It is not intended that this be an exhaustive list of all programmes; rather examples of current and/or seminal programmes indicating what intervention appear to 'work' or not work in supporting young families. Of particular interest is the Family Nurse Partnership Programme (FNP) which is currently undergoing a wide-scale evaluation in many sites throughout England. Although the characteristics of programmes outlined below vary, all have the goal of improving the health and wellbeing of children.

Early home visiting programmes

The first and major structured home visiting programme in the United Kingdom was the Child Development Programme (also called First Parent Health Visiting Programme). It originated from Bristol University under the leadership of Professor Walter Barker and was supported by the Bernard Van Leer Foundation of The Hague (Barker, 1984; Barker & Anderson, 1988). It was a large-scale programme intervention and evaluation project which focused on altering the human environment surrounding the disadvantaged child during the earliest years of life and supporting the parents to make positive changes.

The First Parent health visitor visited antenatally and postnatally at monthly intervals by appointment (or more frequently if necessary in the early months). The home visits focused on seven fields of child development, namely: language, social development, cognitive development, pre-school educational development, nutrition, health, general development. The health visitors' work was specialised in that they did not engage in other health visiting duties. The programme stressed the importance of working with the parents in partnership and recognised that the parents are the 'experts' of their own children. Parents were encouraged to seek their own solutions to the problems of child rearing with help and advice with the health visitor who acted more as a guide rather than the authority on child care.

The programme was evaluated during 1986-92 (retrospective data on 2113 families) and 1993-98 (prospective data from 459 families) as part of the National Health Service provision (Emond *et al.*, 2002: 150). Outcomes were assessed when the children were one and two years of age. Overall, there were few differences between the group receiving first parent services and comparison mothers and children. Breast feeding was higher in the first parent group but there were no differences on measures of self-esteem, locus of control or depression rates (mothers) or measures of development at ages one and two (children). Also, no differences were found on measures of health service utilisation including immunisation rates, uptake of child health surveillance or use of hospital services. At the time of this programme implementation, there was universal home visiting to all new infants and children. The authors conclude that the comparison health visitors may have adapted their practice to be more in keeping with the approach used in the study programme, thus masking any potential differences between the services.

Despite the (somewhat) disappointing outcomes from the evaluation, this remains a seminal programme on health visiting. The concepts introduced – targeting the disadvantaged child, structured home visiting, the emphasis on positive parenting and parents as experts, respectful relationships between the health visitor and parent, and the importance of support – are the cornerstones of most home visiting programmes which followed.

As part of the development of the First Parent Programme, the concept of a 'Community Mothers' Programme (CMP) was developed in Dublin in 1983 in response to limitations in resource provision for high needs families. Community mothers visit families with first (and sometimes) second children monthly. Women are selected on the basis of being experienced and competent mothers with the ability to empathise with and empower others. The mothers are volunteers although they are given nominal expenses for each visit. The emphasis is on support, encouragement and guidance rather than direct advice. The programme is run in the Republic of Ireland by the Health Service Executive (Prevention Action, 2008). Modified versions of this programme were initiated in some other communities in the United Kingdom.

Evaluations completed to date indicate some successes likely attributed to the CMP. Children receiving this service were more likely to have received all of their primary immunisations, to be read to daily, played more cognitive games and were exposed to more nursery rhymes. They were less likely to begin drinking cows' milk before 26 weeks and to receive inappropriate foods related to their age. Mothers in the intervention group also had a better diet than controls. At the end of the study they were less likely to report being tired and miserable and reported more positive feelings. The researchers concluded that nonprofessionals can deliver a health promotion programme on child development effectively but whether they can do so as effectively as professionals required further study (Johnson et al., 1993). Similar positive results for mothers and infants were found in a group of travellers in Ireland (Fitzpatrick et al., 1997).

A follow-up study of participants in the original randomised controlled trial (RCT) (see above) when the children were age eight years old focused on child health, nutrition, cognitive stimulation, parenting skills, and maternal self-esteem. The study found that the benefit to the children and mothers continued. The researchers concluded that the CMP had sustained beneficial effects on parenting skills and maternal self-esteem seven years later with benefit extending to subsequent children (Johnson et al., 2000).

The CMP did not widely diffuse throughout the United Kingdom although there are reports that a few areas continue to provide this service. The use of volunteers and paraprofessionals to deliver child development programmes is under debate in other locations. It is influenced by the discussion on skill mix and also the notion that 'like-minded' persons who have experienced particular life events can have a positive influence on others experiencing similar situations. The question remains as to the use of replacements for health visitors with disadvantaged families. There is some evidence from the United States that paraprofessionals as home visitors are less effective than professional practitioners. In a randomised controlled trial in the USA, Olds et al. (2002) concluded that public health nurse home visitors were more effective than the nonprofessional home visitors on a number of maternal and child health outcomes two years after the programme ended, such as reduced lower birth weight in subsequent pregnancies and greater responsiveness of mothers toward their children. However, there were some benefits for mothers and children who received care from paraprofessionals compared with controls (Olds et al., 2004). In a programme in one Canadian province, paraprofessional home visitors appear to be meeting the programme objectives (Heaman et al., 2006). It is not clear what all the critical factors are that influence the success of programmes using nonprofessionals or volunteers although guidance for the home visitors is considered to be critical (Heaman et al., 2007).

Current home visiting programmes

Family Nurse Partnership Programme

Background

United States Model

The Family Nurse Partnership (FNP) (sometimes referred to as the Nurse Family Partnership Programme) is a joint Department of Health/Department for Children, Schools and Families (DCSF) project that is testing a model of intensive, nurse-led home visiting for vulnerable, first time, young parents in the UK. The NFP concept was developed in 1977 by psychologist David Olds, who worked with nurses in Elmira, New York, to test the idea of home visiting with disadvantaged mothers who had at least one of the following risk factors: being a teenager, unmarried, or of low socioeconomic status (Olds et al., 1986). It was further tested in randomised trials in Memphis, Tennessee, beginning in 1988, and in Denver, beginning in 1994 (Dawley et al., 2007).

The intent of the programme is to provide support to the new mother as she learns to parent her infant often in a very stressful environment. The nurses receive extensive training for the role including building therapeutic relationships. Nurses work with approximately 25 families during hour-long visits beginning prior to the 29th week of pregnancy. Visits take place every two weeks. The mother's participation in the programme is voluntary. The focus of the visits is on six domains: personal health, environmental health, friends and family, the maternal role, use of healthcare and human services, and 'maternal life course development' (which encompasses planning for future pregnancies, education, and employment) (Dawley et al., 2007).

Evidence from the three large controlled trials carried out on participants in Elmira, Memphis and Denver USA have shown that the programme provides significant and consistent improvements in the health and wellbeing of the most disadvantaged children and their families in both the short and long term. Benefits include: improved school readiness; fewer subsequent pregnancies; better prenatal health; improvement in women's antenatal health, fewer subsequent pregnancies, greater interval between births, reductions of between 50 and 70% in child injuries, neglect and abuse; increases in employment, increases in father's involvement, reduction in welfare dependency, reduced substance use initiation (Kitzman et al., 1997; Olds et al., 1997, 1998, 2007). There are over 23 States delivering the programme to approximately 13 000 at-risk, first-time mothers. Also, the model is being tested in other countries such as the Netherlands and Germany as well as England (Dawley et al., 2007).

The Family Nurse Partnership (FNP) Programme

The FNP programme was introduced in September 2006 in England as part of the government's *Social Exclusion Action Plan* (Cabinet Office, 2009). The government pledged in the *New Opportunities White Paper* to roll out one-to-one support to all vulnerable pregnant women through the FNP over the next decade.

Family Nurse Partnership nurses (mainly health visitors and usually called family nurses in this programme) visit parents from early pregnancy until the child is 24 months old, building a close, supportive relationship with the whole family and guiding mothers to adopt healthier lifestyles, improve their parenting skills, and become self-sufficient (Cabinet Office, 2009). Families are referred to the FNP through Midwifery Services and Specialised Midwifery and other partner agencies such as Leaving Care, Teenage Pregnancy Services, GP, Health Visitors, Education Re-integration Officer, Probation, Social Services and in some cases self-referral. The enrolment criteria are: age under 20 years; vulnerable / hard to reach; NEET – meaning no education, employment or training; first time mother; gestation 14–28 weeks; and not newly delivered (i.e. must be pregnant) (personal communication, S. Stewart, 29 June, 2010).

The programme is voluntary and has been taken up by 90% of the families who have been offered it. Highly trained nurses and midwives backed by a partnership between Primary Care Trusts and local authorities provide the intensive one-to-one maternity and paediatric care for the mothers in their homes (Cabinet Office, 2009).

Initially the programme was piloted at ten sites (Blackpool, Calderdale, Hastings and Rotherham, Islington, Milton Keyes, Nottingham, Plymouth, Southhampton, Stockport, Stoke). In March 2008, after initial positive feed-back, with an additional £30 million, the initiative was expanded to 20 new sites throughout the country.

Characteristics of the programme

While the FNP Programme is modelled after the US programme, it has been customised to the UK context. The programme entails weekly or fortnightly structured home visits. The programme is theoretically driven based on ecological (Bronfenbrenner, 1979), attachment (Bowlby, 1969) and self-efficacy (Bandura, 1977) theories. Ecological theory stresses social context and interactions among individuals and the environments in which they are situated (see above). Attachment theory highlights the importance of the mother-infant relationship and self-efficacy theory focuses on the importance of individuals' beliefs in achieving and directing behaviours (Department for Children, Schools and Families and Department of Health, 2008). Self-efficacy in the parent role is encouraged by the strengths based focus (i.e. focus on the parents' strengths not limitations).

The curriculum is specific and detailed with a plan for the number, timing and the content of the visits. The visit content is divided into five domains with the proportion of time specified (personal health 35-40%; maternal role 23-25%; life course development 10-15%; family and friends 10-15%; environmental health 5-7%). There is ongoing supervision of the practitioner and detailed records are kept. The core of the programme is the formation of a strong, therapeutic, empathetic relationship with the mother (Department for Children, Schools and Families and Department of Health, 2008).

At each pilot site a supervisor leads a team of up to six family nurses, each with a caseload of approximately 25 families. Family nurses receive relevant training to deliver the programme. They are also linked to Sure Start Children's Centres (see below), and encourage families to make active use of local community resources, including activities such as parenting groups and educational activities. On most sites the scheme is offered to mothers under the age of 20, though some sites are now offering FNP to mothers up to the age of 24 (Cabinet Office, 2009).

The programme focuses on improved outcomes across three areas:

- improving antenatal health;
- enhancing child development and school readiness;
- linking the family to wider social networks and employment. (Cabinet Office, 12 January 2009)

Evaluation and outcomes

First year evaluation

The aim of the initial (first year) evaluation was to determine if the FNP programme could be delivered effectively in England in a variety of sites. It addressed the pregnancy and post partum period. The evaluation used multiple methods with multiple informants from three domains – the families, the workforce and the wider organisation of services. A mix of qualitative and quantitative methods was used to gather data. The project was directed by Professor Jacqueline Barnes from the Institute for the Study of Children,

Families and Social Issues at Birkbeck, University of London (Department for Children, Schools and Families and the Department of Health, 2008).

Although the findings were positive, not all sites were able to meet recruitment and retention targets. Also, the number of visits to women was just over half (53%) of the targeted number. The programme was acceptable to the first time mothers and also seemed acceptable to the fathers who participated. Participating practitioners valued the programme although they found the work to be demanding. The evaluation was helpful in identifying best practice and barriers to working effectively with the women including how to strengthen the delivery of the service (Department for Children, Schools and Families and the Department of Health, 2008).

Second year evaluation – pilot sites

This evaluation reports on the second year of a four year evaluation study that is assessing the feasibility of delivering the Family FNP Programme in England. The evaluation is focused on the 10 initial test sites. The report focuses on the infancy phase of the programme (ages birth to 12 months) addressing how it can be delivered with consistency and fidelity to the programme model (i.e. David Olds, see above) and how well the programme is meeting the stated objectives. This includes the extent of involvement of the fathers, the acceptability to families and practitioners, factors influencing families' engagement and retention as well as views of the family nurses, supervisors, and children's services commissioners concerning the programme (including costs) (Department for Children, Schools and Families and Department of Health, 2009).

The evaluation involved analysing the data collected from service delivery forms, case studies, structured face to face (n=154) and telephone (n=98) interviews with a sample of families receiving the programme (and some who had left the programme n=42). Questionnaires and interviews were implemented with professionals delivering the programme and local commissioners of services for young children, Children's Centre managers and FNP project leads (Department for Children, Schools and Families and Department of Health, 2009).

Overall, the findings are quite positive and the programme is close to meeting the objectives although there were considerable differences between study sites. The evaluation found that the majority (87%) of clients received at least half of the expected visits during pregnancy and early infancy. Although retention issues were identified, clients who left the programme were generally positive about it. The programme was well received by the families, particularly their relationship with their family nurse. Fathers were present in over 20% of the pregnancy visits and almost one-quarter of the infancy visits. Overall, family nurses and supervisors were satisfied with the programme. Commissioners were variable in their support of the programme citing costs (about £3000 per client per year) and problems with infrastructure and delivery issues (Department for Children, Schools and Families and Department of Health, 2009).

Third year evaluation

The third year evaluation follows the first wave of enrolled families to age 24 months (the usual programme leaving time). The aims of this evaluation were to determine if the programme was implemented as expected in the toddler age group; assess if the programme was acceptable to mothers, partners and family nurses; explore the nature of the experience of completing the programme from the perspective of mothers and nurses; and finally to determine the likelihood that the programme is providing benefit to children, women and families (Department of Health, 2011a: 10). The evaluation used data from the nurses' completed work data forms, interviews with and diaries completed by nurses and interviews with mothers. The findings suggest that the aims are being met. Some selective findings include a low attrition rate during the toddler period (7%); continued involvement of many fathers in the home visits; and mothers' positive attitudes and interactions with their toddlers and, for many, a move to taking up education or paid work.

Evaluation of outcomes (2009–2013)

The Department of Health in England has commissioned an evaluation to generate evidence about the benefits and costs of the FNP. Although the evidence from the initial three evaluations (outlined above) is positive, this study will allow an assessment of the effectiveness of the programme. The South East Wales Trials Unit (SEWTU) at Cardiff University and other collaborators are conducting a randomised controlled trial to compare the outcomes of the programme compared to usual services. The study is being carried out in 18 centres, eight of which have already participated in the earlier evaluation (see above). Half of the women will be randomised to receive routine care from maternity services plus the FNP and half will be randomised to receive routine care from maternity and child health services. The study aims to recruit 2400 pregnant first-time mothers and began in April 2009. Women are recruited to the study ideally within the first 15 weeks of pregnancy but no later than 24 weeks. All participants are to be followed up until their child's second birthday with final results expected in early 2013. Outcomes will be assessed in three domains: pregnancy and birth, the health and wellbeing of the child and the life course and economic self-sufficiency of the mother (The South East Wales Trials Unit (SEWTU), undated).

The 18 participating centres (Local Authority and Primary Care Trusts) throughout England are: Barnsley, Cornwall, Coventry, Cumbria, Derby City, Berkshire East, Hull, Lambeth, Leeds, Liverpool, Manchester, Northamptonshire, South Birmingham, Southwark, Sunderland, South East Essex, Tower Hamlets and Walsall. These sites were selected by the Department of Health.

Flying Start – Wales

Background

Flying Start is an initiative of the Welsh Assembly Government. The Flying Start Health Visiting Core Programme is one component of the initiative with a focus on partnership with parents and other professionals to provide support to families from the antenatal period through school age (Welsh Assembly Government, undated). The programme includes midwives, health visitors, registered nurses and nursery nurses working in Flying Start areas across five boroughs.

Characteristics of the programme

All mothers receive a detailed assessment in the antenatal period and a detailed care plan is developed. The intensity of the follow-up is based on the level of need that is identified (low, medium or high). In addition, all families are invited to antenatal groups. Postnatally, all families receive home visits until the infant is six weeks old and then visits are made according to assessed need. The assessments included structured measures on the infant and mother, including the mental health of the mother. Groups are offered to all mothers on topics including infant care, massage and maternal depression (Flying Start Health Core Visiting Programme (Welsh Assembling Government, undated)). The goal is to provide all families with the level of care they need and reflects the notion of progressive universalism (discussed above).

Evaluation and outcomes

No formal evaluation of this initative was identified. An annual audit is to be undertaken and a report submitted to the Clinical Governance Forum (Flying Start Health Core Visiting Programme (Welsh Assembling Government, undated)).

Starting Well – Scotland

Background

The Starting Well programme began as a demonstration project in 2000 in recognition of the need to improve the health of the Scottish population (McIntosh, 2006). The aim of the project was to demonstrate improved health for children through measures to support families and access to community resources. Similar to other programmes noted above, the programme attempted to address problems of social exclusion through supportive, empowering interventions, delivered by health visitors with an enhanced public health role. The project was established in two areas of Glasgow and funded for a three-year period by the Scottish Executive. The project uses conceptual elements of the Triple P – Programme (also discussed in this chapter), developed in Australia such as empowering parents through interventions to increase their knowledge, skills and confidence (The Starting Well Demonstration Project, undated). It was also influenced by David Old's work in the United States on home visiting (discussed earlier). However, the project differed from Old's model: deprived communities were targeted rather than vulnerable high-risk families; the programme was universally delivered to all infants not just targeted to high-risk and first parents; contact with the health visitors began largely after birth; the programme was integrated with other existing services, e.g. the midwifery services; paraprofessionals were employed for aspects of the service delivery as well as professional health visitors (McKenzie *et al.*, 2004).

Characteristics of the programme

The home visiting component, delivered by health visitors, is structured and intensive (weekly for two months, fortnightly from two to six months, then monthly) (McIntosh, 2006). The families receive visits until the child is age three. The project is not limited to first-time parents. Evidence-based guidelines are in place to ensure consistent information is provided and detailed records are kept. The community component includes funding for local projects to improve children's health. Examples of funded projects include: toy libraries, a fathers' breakfast programme, a play at home programme to assist parents develop skills in helping children learn through creative play, and many others (Starting Well Demonstration Project, undated). Unlike some programmes, health visitors are not exclusively working with this project.

Evaluation and outcomes

The Department of Public Health of the University of Glasgow conducted the independent evaluation. The aims of the evaluation were to: measure the impact of the project on children and families; understand the theory, processes and context of the Starting Well intervention; and analyse the policy implications of the project (Scottish Government, 2004). Early evaluation of Starting Well suggests some benefits for the involved families. Using a quasi-experimental design, outcomes at age six months were examined in 213 (intervention) and 146 comparison families (Shute & Judge, 2005). In the intervention group there were improved outcomes in maternal depression and childrens' dental registration. When follow-up data of the children were collected at 18 months, however, there were no differences in maternal depression although there was a small but positive effect on the quality of the home environment; higher levels of client satisfaction with levels of health visitor support; and continued higher levels of dental registration (Scottish Government, 2004).

Other aspects of the evaluation focused on the implementation processes within the Scottish healthcare system (McIntosh, 2006). A qualitative longitudinal study of 20 mothers and their health visitors using tape-recorded interviews sought feedback on the programme when the infants were three to four months and nine to 10 months of age (McIntosh, 2006). Health visitors in one of the areas found it difficult to maintain the intensive home visiting schedule during the early months and had to cut back on the scheduled number of visits. Health visitors highlighted the importance of building trust as the relationship was developed and mothers reported feeling helped and supported by their health visitors. Health visitors considered that the mothers over time gained confidence and knowledge in infant care and using community resources and reduced their anxiety around parenting. Semi-structured interviews with staff involved in developing and implementing the programme (n=44) identified complexities in implementing a public health focused programme (Mackenzie, 2008).

The findings of these evaluations are providing guidance for the development of Phase II of the Starting Well programme (Scottish Government, 2005).

The Triple – P Programme – Positive Parenting Programme

Background

There are many additional parent support programmes which have been developed and implemented in full or in part in the United Kingdom. The Triple P - Positive Parenting Programme is a prevention and treatment programme from birth to 16 years developed in Australia and widely implemented throughout the world including North America, Australia, New Zealand, parts of Europe and Asia, as well as some locations in England, Ireland and Scotland (Sanders, 1999, 2008). It is a programme targeting all families with young children (universal) incorporating five levels of interventions of increasing intensity. The rationale for the levels of intervention is based on the recognition of different levels of dysfunction and behavioural problems in children and parents' differing needs and approaches for receiving assistance (Sanders, 1999).

The first level of intervention is a universal information media campaign directed to all parents and focusing on common parenting problems. Interventions include electronic and print media, radio, etc. on general parenting topics (Sanders, 2008). Level 2 targets parents interested in parenting education or having specific concerns about their child's behaviour. Their need may be addressed through a group seminar or telephone or short face to face brief intervention. In Level 3, parents require more information and support. The final two levels provide intensive parent and family programmes for children at risk for more severe behavioural problems (Sanders, 2008).

Characteristics of the programme

The programme targets five different developmental periods from infancy to adolescence. Within each level are very broad interventions directed to the whole population and focused interventions targeted only to high-risk children (Sanders, 2008). The characteristics of the programme are its flexible approach to parenting and family support. The central goal of the programme is to develop self-regulation in all involved (parents, children and practitioners). Five core principles of positive parenting are encouraged to promote social competence and emotional self-regulation in children: These include providing a safe engaging environment, a positive learning environment, reasonable expectations, assertive discipline and taking care of oneself as a parent (Prinz et al., 2009).

The programme is evidence-based with an emphasis on prevention and early intervention as well as treatment. It is multidisciplinary in delivery and theory based with a particular focus on social learning theories (Sanders, 2008). The flexibility and the focus on prevention and early intervention means that health visitors, with additional training/education can utilise components in their day to day work with families.

Evaluation and outcomes

The overall programme has been evaluated in over 43 controlled trials and 22 field evaluations with positive findings including reduced instances of child abuse (ages birth to age eight) in a population trial involving 18 countries (Prinz et al., 2009). Level 4 interventions have been critiqued through a meta-analysis with a report of short- and long-term improvements in childrens' behaviour problems (de Graaf et al., 2008). Level 3 is currently being evaluated in the Netherlands (Spijkers et al., 2010). Aspects of the Triple P Programme are being used in several locations in the United Kingdom including Glasgow, Birmingham, Liverpool and other areas. However, there are few reports of evaluated projects. There is some evidence of positive outcomes in programmes carried out by health visitors including a reduction in maternal anxiety and depression and negative interactions with their children (Long et al., 2001) and a randomised controlled trial on children with conduct disorders is currently underway in Birmingham (ISRCTN Trial registration, 2009).

Sure Start Programmes

Background

While not a home visiting programme, Sure Start is a family support resource which works in conjunction with home visiting programmes. For this reason, as well as its widespread dissemination in England, it is included with this section on home visiting programmes. Sure Start Local Programmes (SSLPs) were developed in 1999 to work with parents and expectant parents to promote physical and intellectual development of children initially under four years but later extended to under age five years with the move to Sure Start Children's Centres programmes. Social Services funding initially concentrated on the most deprived localities but now has extended funding to provide universal access for families. The Centres have been implemented in three phases with the aim of having 3400 children's centres in place by 2010 – one for every community. All SSPLs have now become Children's Centres. Between 1998/99 and 2010/11 an estimated £7.2 billion pounds has been spent on Sure Start (Audit Commission, 2010). Sure Start covers a wide range of programmes, both universal and those targeted to particular local areas or disadvantaged groups within England (Department for Children, Schools and Families, 2010).

Characteristics of the programme

Services include play and early education learning experiences, child care, primary and community healthcare, support for children with special needs, and parenting and family support through area based programmes (Audit Commission, 2010). There is an emphasis on coordination of services, outreach and community development to improve the services which families receive. All three- and four-year-old children are guaranteed an early learning placement (12 1/2 hours per week) Department for Children, Schools and Families, 2010).

Family and parenting support is a strong emphasis in Sure Start Local Programmes. This may include therapeutic services such as counselling (cognitive behavioural therapy, family therapy, art therapy), adult learning services and general support. Support is provided either directly by staff or through coordination and referral (Barlow *et al.*, 2007).

Evaluation and outcome

The National Evaluation of Sure Start is being led by Professor Edward Melhuish and colleagues at the Institute for the Study of Children, Families and Social Issues, Birkbeck, University of London. This is an extensive evaluation addressing implementation, impact, local context analysis, cost effectiveness and support to local programmes. Findings to date suggest benefits to children and families who participate in Sure Start programmes. The impact of Sure Start local programmes on three year olds and their families was assessed through evaluation of 14 outcomes including language development, social and emotional development and physical health. Accidental injury decreased and immunisation rates increased, although improvements were slight (Melhuish & Belsky, 2008). In another study of children at age three, differences in implementation of SSLPs were examined in relation to effectiveness using a quasi-experimental study (Belsky *et al.*, 2006). The outcomes assessed were mothers' reports of community services, family functioning and parenting skills, child health and development, and children's verbal ability at age 36 months. The results suggested that SSLPs had beneficial effects on nonteenage mothers (i.e. better parenting, better social functioning in children). Also, programmes which were led by health services appeared to result in better outcomes than those led by other agencies. Benefits have also been found in other studies which examined children at risk of conduct disorders (Hutching *et al.*, 2007).

Another programme of Sure Start aims to improve outcomes for young parents under 18 years. Sure Start Plus is a pilot programme launched in 2001 in participating Local Authorities. The pregnancy strategy aims to reduce by half the conception rate of under 18 year olds and to increase the participation of teenage parents in education, training or employment (Malin & Morrow, 2009). The key service was provided by advisors; this one-on-one support entailed advice, practical help and in-depth emotional support as well as advocacy with other agencies. The evaluation found that the supportive services provided by the Sure Start Plus advisors were successful in addressing the crisis needs and helping the young women to develop skills for parenting and further opportunities (Wiggins *et al.*, 2005). The programme increased support for emotional needs, improved the young woman's family relationships; reduced the incidence of domestic violence, improved accommodation and increased participation in education for teenagers under 16 years. The programme was less successful, though, in changing specific heath behaviours (i.e. reducing smoking, increasing breast feeding) or participation in education for those over age 16 years. Also, there was less success in supporting young fathers, in part due to lack of available resources to work with the young men (Wiggins *et al.*, 2005).

The conclusion, to-date, is that the Sure Start along with the direct funding from Primary Care Trusts has resulted in 'modest' health improvements (Audit Commission, 2010: 40). The national evaluation of Sure Start addressing effectiveness (i.e. outcomes) of Sure Start Programmes is currently underway and will continue until 2012 (National Evaluation of Sure Start, 2009) with the report expected by 2014 (Audit Commission, 2010).

Table 4.1 provides an overview of the programmes already discussed.

Table 4.1   Child health promotion programmes.

Programme name, location, dates	Key elements of the programme	Key findings	Recommendations and comments
Community Mothers' Programme (CMP) (Northern Ireland) developed in Dublin in 1983.	• Community mothers (volunteers) visit monthly first born (and sometimes) second children; emphasis on support, encouragement and guidance rather than direct advice.	• Several positive findings: For children – primary immunisations; read to daily; nutrition. • For mothers – better diet than controls; less likely to report being tired and miserable and reported more positive feelings. • Benefits to children and mothers continued to age 8.	Programme did not widely diffuse throughout the United Kingdom The use of volunteers and paraprofessionals to deliver child development programmes is under debate in other jurisdictions.

(Continued)

Table 4.1 (Continued)

Programme name, location, dates	Key elements of the programme	Key findings	Recommendations and comments
Family Nurse Partnership (FNP) (England) - based on David Old's (US) programme; introduced in 2006.	• Based on ecological, attachment and self efficacy theories; • Targeted to vulnerable families from antenatal to age 24 months; • Structured intensive home visits to build close, supportive relationships and guide parents to adopt healthier lifestyles, improve their parenting skills, and become self-sufficient	• Initially piloted at ten sites and in 2008, after initial positive feedback, expanded to 20 new sites throughout the country.	A randomised controlled trial is ongoing with results expected in 2013.
First Parent Health Visiting Programme (Child Development Programme) (UK) - developed by Professor Walter Barker of Bristol University in early 1980s; implemented in the UK.	• Ante and post natal home visits at monthly intervals by appointment; • Targeted to disadvantaged children; • Structured home visiting with focus on child development; • HVs work in partnership with families; parents are the 'experts' of their own children	• Outcomes assessed at ages one and two years. Few differences between the group receiving first parent services and comparison mothers and children.	Evaluation may have been influenced by 'control' health visitors using principles from the programme.
Flying Start (Wales) - developed and implemented in five boroughs	• The programme includes midwives, health visitors, registered nurses and nursery nurses;	• No evaluation was identified. An annual audit is carried out.	

(Continued)

Table 4.1 (*Continued*)

Programme name, location, dates	Key elements of the programme	Key findings	Recommendations and comments
	• Visits are based on assessment of need (low, medium, high), i.e. progressive universalism.		
Starting Well Phase I Demonstration Project (Scotland) – implemented in two areas in Glasgow in 2000 & funded for a three-year period.	• Uses elements of the Triple P Programme (Australia) and David Old's programme (USA); • Structured and intensive home visiting; • Universally delivered to all infants largely after birth; • Programme integrated with other existing services, e.g. the midwifery services; has a community component which funds local projects to improve children's health. • Paraprofessionals as well as health visitors employed.	• Early evaluation suggests there may be some benefits to mothers and children (i.e. reduction in maternal depression).	Information on Phase II was not available.
Sure Start programmes including Sure Start Centres (United Kingdom) – developed in 1999.	• Promote physical and intellectual development of children up to age 5 including play and learning experiences, support for parents, primary	• Extensive evaluation underway addressing implementation, impact, local context analysis, cost effectiveness	• Specialised supports may also be available to parents including therapeutic services such as counselling (cognitive behavioural,

(Continued)

Table 4.1 *(Continued)*

Programme name, location, dates	Key elements of the programme	Key findings	Recommendations and comments
	and community healthcare, coordination of services, outreach and community development. • Initially centres targeted to deprived areas but not service is universal.	and support to local programmes. • To-date Sure Start along with the direct funding from Primary Care Trusts resulted in 'modest' health improvements.	family therapy) adult learning and general support.
Triple P – Positive Parenting Programme (some locations in the United Kingdom) – developed in Australia	• Preventive and treatment programme for children from infancy to age 16 years; • Five levels of intervention of increasing intensity; • Core principles of promoting competence and self-regulation; evidence-based interventions.	• Well evaluated in over 43 trials; • Some research available with positive benefits of health visitors carrying out components of the programme.	• Aspects of the programme can be delivered by many disciplines.

Working with families

While detailed evaluations are not yet fully available to date for all of the programmes reviewed above, there appears to be recognition of the importance of practitioners developing supportive, trusting relationships with parents and the need to work in partnership with families. These concepts are clearly articulated in some of the programmes, particularly in the FNP Programme, and form part of the conceptual underpinnings of this programme. These concepts, though, are not particularly 'new' in professional-client relationships, nor, many would argue, are they 'new' to health visiting practice. However, the importance of developing supportive relationships when working with young, vulnerable families is now clearly articulated (Hall & Hall, 2007).

What, though, is meant by supportive relationships? The current perspective would suggest that within supportive relationships there is respect for different values and the uniqueness and strengths of each individual is observed and recognised. This perspective is in contrast to the 'traditional' view of the professional as one with expert knowledge; this view recognises that parents are 'expert' in their knowledge of their own children. This perspective of 'parents as experts' was clearly articulated in the early Child Development Programme (see above) (Barker & Anderson, 1988). Within this approach, the health visitor acts not as the authority on child rearing but as an 'advisor' or 'guide' to assist the parent to move forward with their parenting goals.

However, I would suggest that the 'traditional' perspective of the relationship and the current view have many similarities. The professional still holds considerable power in structuring and directing the interaction (i.e. interview, home visit). The fluidity of the interaction may mask the agenda which the professional holds. It is largely the professional's concept of the client's needs and problems which shape who is recruited into programmes and what will be discussed. This is likely the case regardless of the type of interviewing/home visit (i.e. within structured or other programmes). In fact, many child visiting programmes have a type of 'curriculum' (i.e. Baby First Programme, Woodgate et al., 2007) and some, such as the FNP Programme even designate the percentage of the visit which is allocated to different topics (see above). While it remains to be determined if this is the 'best way' to assist high needs families, it may be helpful to ponder the response of the parent to the interaction. If parents do not feel that their needs are being addressed, they may withdraw from the interaction and the relationship between the health visitor and client may be impaired. As a result, critical life events which are affecting their health and parenting capacity may not be acknowledged and appropriate interventions, including referrals not made. It is interesting to reflect on reports of child abuse, spousal abuse and incest which have come to light months or years after professionals have 'worked with' people but did not uncover the core problems affecting the wellbeing of these families.

What, then, is the nature of the health visitor-parent relationship when working with young families? The health visitor-client relationship is seen to be a therapeutic one (Department for Children, Schools and Families and Department of Health, 2009) facilitating the feeling of trust between the health visitor and client and assisting in the movement towards the achievement of the goals of the programme. Trust is defined as 'confidence in or reliance on some quality or attribute of a person or thing' (Shorter Oxford English Dictionary, 1973: 2374). Trust is the foundation upon which effective practice is built, and it is a necessary part of the relationship if health visitors and parents are to work together. It is the therapeutic relationship that facilitates the growth and strengthens the trust between health visitor and client.

But what is the interaction from the parent's perspective? The very nature of the visit from the health visitor must appear to the client to have some of the characteristics of any other visit by a friend or relative. There are, of course, differences which are apparent, such as the health visitor being the one to initiate the visit, determine its length and define its purpose. In addition, the client is aware that the health visitor has information of a personal nature relating to the family and has some power over the fate of the family. The interaction, despite this, may be perceived by the client to be similar to any conversation in which she is at liberty to ask questions in order to establish who the health visitor is and what type of person she is. There is no doubt that the health visitor is being observed and judgments are being made as to her attitudes, trustworthiness, friendliness, knowledge and personal appearance. At some point the client realises that this is more than a normal type of social visit and may at that stage become concerned as to her role and appropriate conduct.

As health visitors, we are aware of the social skills which are used in an interaction and the difficulties of employing such skills as listening or questioning. Yet we do not seem to recognise the efforts of the client in listening and the emotional labouring it takes to reflect on feelings or discuss emotive issues. How often do we recognise that a visit may be tiring for the client as well as for us and that the client may be expending considerable energy in hosting the visit?

The health visitor also has to recognise that she may impose her reality on the visit. We may see what we want to see, or what we have been taught to expect. How do we identify what is the case and what we think is the case? As health visitors, our knowledge comes from our own education and experiences; however, there is no guarantee that the subjects we study fully describe the reality of people's lives. In recent years, qualitative research approaches, such as phenomenology, have been employed which acknowledge and validate the lived experience of people as they carry out their lives.

There is an increasing body of knowledge on family health which can provide health visitors with an understanding of the impacts of many social determinants on the life and health of their clients. Featherstone and Trinder (2001), for example, see a lack of recognition of the gendered and generational power dynamics within families where men may be a potential risk to the mother and child. This knowledge can sensitise health visitors to the types of stressors which the family may be facing, while not dismissing that there are also strengths. Most health visitors may have little direct personal experience with the impacts of poverty, relationship breakdown, partner abandonment, beatings, negative cultural views of women in society, low literacy, severe stresses of motherhood (e.g. post partum depression) and many others. It is helpful, and I would argue necessary, to acknowledge these potential impacts as the health visitor begins his/her work with young vulnerable families.

Empirical evidence on relationship development

There is evidence that parents value supportive relationships with their health visitors. In a qualitative study, mothers have reported on the importance of a supportive relationship with their health visitor (Worth & Hogg, 2000).

In a large survey (n = 4775) of parents of under fives, 76% of respondents wanted parenting support and advice on child health and development. Parents reported valuing health visitors' knowledge of health and having a relationship with them (Family and Parenting Institute, 2009: 6). In another survey through *Netmums*, a website run by local mothers, mothers reported valuing the health visitors' expertise on child development and parenting and the time and support they received from their health visitor (Russell & Drennan, 2007).

Despite the importance of developing supportive relationships between parents and health visitors, there is little empirical literature which documents just how relationships are developed and the outcomes of this process (Heaman *et al.*, 2007). Some early work on home visiting interactions using observation (videotaping) and follow-up interviews with clients and public health nurses suggests the importance of a friendly, relaxed affect when connecting with community clients and attention to both verbal and nonverbal cues during the interactions (Kristjanson & Chalmers, 1990). Trust has been identified as important enabling the disclosure of sensitive topics (Jack *et al.*, 2002; McIntosh, 2006).

In an early study on health visiting practice, several issues influenced building and maintaining the health visitor–mother relationship (Chalmers & Luker, 1991; Chalmers, 1992b). Both health visitors and parents (usually mothers) controlled what they offered and accepted from each other. What was 'given' and 'received' and acted upon was a complex process involving many factors related to the health visitor, the client and the context in which the interaction took place. The 'offer' had to be something of value to the client and this varied from client to client. This might include timely and helpful information, support for the care the mother was providing to the child, material supports, etc. When the health visitor was seen as 'giving' something helpful, the relationship was able to develop and flourish. When this happened, the health visitor was often able to progress in her work with the family and uncover other concerns with the child or the family which needed attention.

Relationship development, though, is not always easy or straightforward. In a study of a Canadian home visiting programme for families with high-risk young children, developing supportive relationships was seen as an important goal of the service by public health nurses and clients (Heaman *et al.*, 2006, 2007). However, public health nurses also expressed that establishing professional–client boundaries was important but sometimes difficult when young parents saw the relationship as a 'friendship' with the expectation of social activities such as attendance at birthday parties. Also, child safety issues are real concerns in some contexts and this influences the process of developing helping relationships (Woodgate *et al.* 2007). The health visitor–client interaction is further explored in Activity 4.3 (see Appendix 4).

Working in partnership with parents may be more of a concern to health visitors than parents. Heaman and colleagues (2007) in their study of home visiting note that parents did not talk about partnerships with their home visitor although public health nurses and home visitors (paraprofessionals) reported they valued working in partnership. Other research on participation using tape recordings of health visitor–parent interactions suggests that client participation is rarely initiated by clients or health visitors (Kendall, 1993). However, more recent research suggests that when participation is viewed as consensus in relation to the needs identified and satisfaction with the level of participation, the views of public health nurses and parents were more similar than different (Mulcahy & McCarthy, 2008). It may be that parents' views of participation and working in partnership do not always mirror professionals' perspectives.

With the move away from universal home visiting to visiting targeted families, successful recruitment of families (usually mothers) into programmes is crucial if the family is to receive the potential benefit of the programme. For example, the FNP is voluntary and eligible pregnant young women can refuse the service. It is recommended that health visitors working in the FNP programme meet women during pregnancy (even if they are not providing services during this time) in order to foster a connection with the woman (Hall & Hall, 2007). Engaging with the woman at this early stage is a crucial skill if the programme is to meet its targets and women are to receive ongoing services.

Much more understanding is needed, not only about how to develop supportive relationships and work in partnership with families, but also about the role these relationships play in achieving the programme outcomes. Relationships, though, are not the only challenges when attempting to support families. Several additional challenges may affect the capacity of the health visitor to develop supportive relationships and influence the overall outcomes of the programme. In the next section, these challenges are examined when planning services for and delivering services to young families.

Challenges

Working with young families who have high needs can often be challenging regardless of the programme framework within which the health visitor works. In this section, we examine some of those challenges and possible underlying reasons for these difficulties.

Public health agenda

The public health approach to supporting families is a population health approach focusing the identification of community wide needs using various assessment frameworks and statistical data. Targets or goals are then established to 'benchmark' changes that are needed and programmes are introduced to improve health indices. The health indices may include such health behaviours as breastfeeding rates in the population, smoking rates in pregnant women, school completion for teenage mothers and so on. These indices and goals are very important for governments and health and social care planners to see the 'big picture'. While the goals and targets are evidence-based, the public health agenda is programme driven rather than client driven. The health visitor working within this framework needs to ensure that the stated 'targets' are met. This, at times, may conflict with the clients' stated needs and wants from the offered service and influence the capacity of the health visitor to work in partnership with the family. For example, if a programme goal is to reduce prenatal smoking rates, the health visitor who addresses this issue enthusiastically and repeatedly (with accurate but unwanted information on the hazards of smoking) may hinder the development of the relationship with the client, resulting in little engagement around this or other health issues or even client withdrawal from the programme. A skilled health visitor has to learn when and how to raise the programme identified goals in a way that keeps the client engaged.

Level of evidence

To date the available evidence to support positive outcomes of many programmes for young families is mixed. This may be due to a number of factors: poorly designed evaluation studies; overly ambitious 'unreachable' targets in the original programme plan; conceptualisations of service delivery that are difficult to implement fully; 'importing' programmes from other jurisdictions which appeared promising (but did not deliver); and many other reasons. Also, programmes may suit some clients more that others and this may affect findings. It is not always clear why some programmes do not deliver the outcomes which were expected (or hoped for). Also, as noted above, health visitors deliver programmes through themselves as 'agents' or, in some cases, through leading skill mix teams. The capacity to develop supportive and helpful relationships within the context of particular programmes is a critical skill that health visitors must learn and practise. It is also important that we continue to learn through qualitative research and process evaluations, how to deliver programmes that address the complex and varied needs of parents.

Adhering to the programme criteria

Most programmes in the current healthcare context are to be delivered according to structured criteria over specific time periods. In the FNP programme, for example, the visit is divided into specific focal areas with a time allotment for each area. Whether this approach is the 'best practice' for all families in a programme will need further assessment through feedback (research based) from parents and practitioners. In the process evaluation of the Baby First Home Visiting Programme delivered in one Canadian province, public health nurses raised the issue of the suitability of the structured use of the curriculum (programme content and delivery) for all the families and that deviation from the structured format may be needed to allow for flexibility in delivering the service (Woodgate et al., 2007). Also, the child health visiting programme literature concludes that many families do not receive the programme according to the stated objectives. For example, families receive only about half of the intended visits and 20-67% of families leave the programme prior to the intended termination date (Gomby, 1999). The evaluations to-date of the FNP Programme found that 87% of clients received at least half of the expected visits during pregnancy and early infancy (Department for Children, Schools and Families & Department of Health, 2009). If families are not receiving the full complement of the visits or the visits do not conform to the programme standards, this creates difficulty in evaluating if the outcomes to families are related to potential deficiencies in the programme or difficulty adhering to the programme criteria. It is important that programme evaluations build in, if possible, interviews with clients who do not complete the programme (or otherwise do not adhere to the stated objectives) to provide helpful information on issues related to retention and programme delivery.

High needs families

A question which receives little attention in the literature is whether there are some high needs families who are not suitable for health visiting programmes and additional exclusion criteria for enrolment of these families are needed. The FNP, for example, attempts to enrol all consenting parents who meet the age, gestation and NEET criteria described earlier in the participating areas. It may be that some families are not appropriate for the home visiting programme and might benefit more from other services such as family therapy, child protection supports, addiction supports, direct assistance (i.e. live-in home helps) or other types of services (Woodgate et al., 2007). At the time of recruitment and enrolment, however, it may not always be known if women are experiencing problems with addictions, mental health and other major problems. Research which permits an analysis of those families participating in programmes who achieve the desired outcomes and those who do not may shed more light on the question of excluding some families from these visiting programmes.

On the other hand, many high needs families may potentially benefit from home visiting programmes but, for a variety of reasons, may not be recruited into the programme. They may have had negative experiences with persons perceived to be 'in authority', be fearful of exposing their parenting to professional criticism or overwhelmed with general living concerns. The experience of parent support programmes such as Sure Start, Head Start (in the United States) and other programmes suggests that the most 'needy' parents are the least likely to participate; this has been called the 'inverse-care law' (Hall & Hall, 2007). In an evaluation of the Starting Well Programme in Glasgow (Wright et al., 2009), only 47% of families (of 302) rated as 'high need' were identified by age four months (the programme standard). The initial recruitment contact is crucial if these families are to engage with the programme.

Practice specialisation

Does a specialised approach (i.e. working in one programme only such as the FNP) provide the best outcomes for families? This appears to be an assumption underlying the structuring of this and other programmes in which the health visitors/nurses work solely in one programme. The FNP Programme (and others) are reported to be intensive and demanding on the staff and supervisors (Department for Children, Schools and Families & Department of Health, 2009). Little is known to-date about provider burn-out and retention of staff in these programmes. Other models for health visiting practice, such as the family-centred public health role (Audit Commission, 2010) may entail working across various 'levels' such as groups and the community (e.g. community development) as well as families. However, this more 'generic' approach raises questions as to the skill set which health visitors need to work effectively at all levels, including the 'community level' (Chalmers & Bramadat, 1996). It is likely that many skills, such as in-depth community assessments and community development, entail advanced knowledge and practice that are gained through specialised education and opportunities to learn these skills in the community. Also, when practitioners work across several areas, the child support programme may take a 'back seat' to other public health priorities such as mandated communicable diseases control (Woodgate *et al.*, 2007). However, working in only one programme may contribute to the concern of service 'silos' in which many practitioners from different agencies are providing services to the same family. As the Common Assessment Framework (see above and Chapter 5) becomes more widely available, this problem may be reduced.

Concerns about child safety

Despite the importance accorded to building relationships based on partnerships, this is not always easy to do. Child safety as well as client denial and blocking of problems have been reported as particularly stressful for home visitors (Chalmers, 1994; Woodgate *et al.*, 2007). Health visitors attempting to work 'in partnership' with clients may encounter instances when they are concerned that the parent is not providing adequate care or is not moving forward in learning appropriate caregiving behaviours. The health visitor needs skills to communicate expectations clearly to parents concerning the level of care expected while doing this in as supportive a context as possible. There is little in the 'partnership' literature as to how this process is best learned and managed.

Adequate resources

Programmes to support parenting of young children need sufficient resources to deliver the programme as outlined. This includes a manageable ratio of families per health visitor. The FNP has set this at 25 families per family nurse. In addition, there needs to be other community supports available where families can access peer support from other families, resources for children's play (such as Sure Start children's centres programmes). Supports from supervisors are also critical (Woodgate *et al.*, 2007) and both the practitioners and supervisors need adequate in-service training to carry out their roles well.

It is important that there is sufficient and ongoing in-service education to ensure that health visitors' skills match the needs of vulnerable families. This includes skills in assessments. Recent evidence based on direct observation of parent–child interactions (interactions were videotaped and subjected to rigorous analysis) suggests considerable variation by health visitors in identi-fication of problems in the parent–child interactions (Wilson *et al.*, 2010). This study points to the need for the adequacy of resources (both amount and type) to uncover the learning needs of health visitors, regardless of the type of programme within which they work. This is a particular issue for health visitors given that most of their work takes place in the home with little opportunity for their assessments to be 'validated' by a supervisor or peers. Also, with the implementation of progressive (now referred to as proportion-ate) universalism in some jurisdictions, it is imperative that practitioners assess the level of need in families in order to allocate ongoing resources (Wilson *et al.*, 2010).

Summary

In this chapter, approaches and programmes to support families with young children were examined. Currently, there appears to be political support to invest in programmes which lead to improved outcomes for children and par-ents. Details of the outcomes of FNP Programme, once available, will provide important data which can be used for wide spread implementation or adjust-ment of the programme.

Improving the social determinants of health for young families is critical if the long term impacts on high needs children and parents are to be amelio-rated. However, programmes, are just one component of measures to enhance the wellbeing of vulnerable families. Social support, social cohesion and social involvement (i.e. social capital) (Moore *et al.*, 2006) are increasingly seen as key approaches to help mitigate the effects of social determinants of health and improve health outcomes to the most disadvantaged members of society (Marmot, 2006). Health visitors can have a role to play at this broader com-munity level as well as the family and make a substantial contribution to improving the nation's health.

Note

* Some parts of this chapter were adapted from Orr. (1992).

References

Audit Commission (2010) *Giving Children a Healthy Start: Health Report*. Available at: www.audit-commission.gov.uk (accessed 9 March, 2011).

Bandura, A. (1977) Self-efficacy: towards a unifying theory of behavioural change. *Psychological Review*, **84**, 191–215.

Barker, W. (1984) *Child Development Programme,* Early Childhood Development Unit, Senate House, University of Bristol, Bristol.

Barker, W. & Anderson, R. (1988) *Child Development Programme: An Evaluation of Process and Outcomes.* Early Child Development Unit, University of Bristol.

Barlow, J., Coren, E. & Stewart-Brown, S. (2002) Meta-analysis of the effectiveness of parenting programmes in improving maternal psychosocial health. *British Journal of General Practice,* **52**(476), 223-233.

Barlow, J., Coren, E. & Stewart-Brown, S. (2003) Parent-training programmes for improving maternal psychosocial health (Review). *Cochrane Database of Systematic Reviews,* **76**, 223-233.

Barlow, J., Kirkpatrick, S., Wood, D., Ball, M., & Stewart-Brown, S. (2007) *Sure Start National Evaluation Summary: Family and Parenting Support in Sure Start Local Programmes.* Available from: http://www.education.gov.uk/research/data/uploadfiles/NESS2007SF023.pdf (accessed 9 March, 2011).

Barrett, G., Naidoo, J. & Orme, J. (2007) Capacity and capability in public health. In: *Public Health for the 21st Century* (eds J. Orme, J. Powell, P. Taylor & M. Grey), 2nd ed, Ch. 5, pp. 83-97. Open University Press McGraw-Hill Education, Maidenhead.

Belsky, J., Melhuish, E., Barnes, J., Leyland, A.H. & Romaniuk, H. (2006) The National Evaluation of Sure Start Research Team Effects of Sure Start local programmes on children and families: early findings from a quasi-experimental, cross sectional study. *British Medical Journal,* **332**, 1476. doi:10.1136/bmj.38853.451748.2F (published 16 June, 2006).

Birmingham Primary Care Trusts (2007) *Health Visitor and School Health Record Keeping Guidelines.* Available from: www.bpcssa.nhs.uk/policies/_south%5Cpolicies%5C764.pdf (accessed 9 March, 2011).

Bowlby, J. (1969) *Attachment and Loss. Volume 1. Attachment.* Basic Books, New York.

Bronfenbrenner, U. (1979) *The Ecology of Human Development: Experiments by Nature and Design.* Harvard University Press, London.

Bryans, A., Cornich, E. & McIntosh, J. (2009) The potential of the ecological theory for building an integrated framework to develop the public health contribution of health visiting. *Health and Social Care in the Community,* **17**(6), 564-572.

Cabinet Office (2006) *Reaching Out: An Action Plan on Social Exclusion Publication.* Stationery Office, London.

Cabinet Office (2007) *Families at Risk: Background on Families with Multiple Disadvantages.* Stationery Office, London.

Cabinet Office (2009) *Social Exclusion Task Force, Family Nurse Partnership.* Available from: http://webarchive.nationalarchives.gov.uk/+/http://www.cabinet-office.gov.uk/social_exclusion_task_force/family_nurse_partnership.aspx (accessed 9 March, 2011).

Carers UK (2008) 2008 Carers UK: National Carers' Strategy. Available from: http://www.carersuk.org/Aboutus/MoreaboutCarersUK/StrategyAnnualReportAccounts (accessed 18 March, 2011).

Chalmers, K.I. (1992a) Giving and receiving: an empirically derived theory of health visiting practice. *Journal of Advanced Nursing,* **17**(11), 1317-1325.

Chalmers, K.I. (1992b) Working with men: an analysis of health visiting practice in families with young children. *International Journal of Nursing Studies,* **29**(1), 3-16.

Chalmers, K.I. (1994) Difficult work: health visitors' work with clients in the community. *International Journal of Nursing Studies,* **31**(2), 168-182.

Chalmers, K.I & Luker, K. (1991) The development of the health visitor-client relationship. *Scandinavian Journal of Caring Sciences,* **5**(1), 33-41.

Chalmers, K.I. & Bramadat, I. (1996) Community development: analysis of the role for community health nurses. *Journal of Advanced Nursing*, **24**, 719-726.

Council for the Education and Training of Health Visitors (CETHV) (1977) *An Investigation into the Principles of Health Visiting*. CETHV, London.

Dawley, K., Loch, J. & Bindrich, I. (2007) The Nurse Family Partnership. *American Journal of Nursing*, **107**(11), 60-67.

Department for Children, Schools and Families & Department of Health (2008) *Nurse-Family Partnership Programme: First Year Pilot Sites, Implementation in England. Pregnancy and the Post Partum Period*. Research Report DCSF-RW051 (authors: L. Barnes, M. Ball, P. Meadows, J. McLeish, J. Belsky and the FNP Implementation Research Team, Institute for the Study of Children, Families and Social Issues, University of London Birkbeck). Department for Children, Schools and Families, London.

Department for Children, Schools and Families & Department of Health (2009) *Nurse-Family Partnership Programme: Second Year Pilot Sites, Implementation in England. The Infancy Period*. Research Report DCSF-RR166 (authors L. Barnes, M. Ball, P. Meadows, J. McLeish, J. Belsky and the FNP implementation team, Institute for the Study of Children, Families and Social Issues, Birkbeck, University of London). Department for Children, Schools and Families, London.

Department for Children, Schools and Families (2010) *Home Page: Sure Start Children's Centres*. Available from: http://www.dcsf.gov.uk/everychildmatters/earlyyears/surestart/whatsurestartdoes/ (accessed 9 March, 2011).

Department for Education and Skills (2004) *Common Assessment Framework*. Available from: http://www.education.gov.uk/consultations/downloadableDocs/ACFA006.pdf (accessed 15 February, 2011).

Department of Health (2001) *The Health Visitor and School Nurse Development Programme: Health Visitor Practice Development Resource Pack*. Department of Health, London.

Department of Health (2004) *National Service Framework for Children, Young People and Maternity Services*. Department of Health, London.

Department of Health (2006) *Our Health, Our Care, Our Say: A New Direction for Community Services*. The Stationery Office, London.

Department of Health (2007) *Facing the Future: A Review of the Role of Health Visitors*. Department of Health, London. Available from: http://www.phru.net/phn/healthvisitingreview/Literature%20Review%20and%20Evidence/health%20visitor%20review.pdf (accessed 9 March, 2011).

Department of Health (2008a) *NHS Next Stage Review: Our Vision for Primary Care and Community Care (Darzi Report)*. Department of Health, London.

Department of Health (2008b) *Healthy Child Programme*. Department of Health, London.

Department of Health (2009a) *Healthy Child Programme: Pregnancy and the First Five Years of Life*. Department of Health, London.

Department of Health (2009b) *Transforming Community Services: Enabling New Patterns of Provision*. Department of Health, London.

Department of Health (2010) *White Paper – Healthy Lives, Healthy People: Our Strategy for Public Health in England*. Department of Health, London.

Department of Health (2011a) *The Family-Nurse Partnership Programme in England: Wave 1 Implementation in Toddlerhood & a Comparison between Waves 1 and 2a of Implementation in Pregnancy and Infancy*. Institute for Study of Children, Families and Social Issues, Birbeck, University of London.

Department of Health (2011b) *Health Visitor Implementation Plan 2011-15: A Call to Action February 2011*. London, Department of Health.

Department of Health, Social Services and Public Safety (2006) *UNOCINI and the Comprehensive Assessment of Children in Need*. DHSSPS, Northern Ireland.

Department of Health, Social Services and Public Safety (2009) *Review of Health Visiting and School Nursing in Northern Ireland 2009-2011/12*. DHSSPS, Belfast.

Department of Health, Social Services and Public Safety (2010) Redesign of community nursing - *Healthy Futures: The Contribution of Health Visitors and School Nurses in Northern Ireland*. DHSSPS, Belfast. Available from: http://www.dhsspsni.gov.uk/microsoft_word_-_hvsn_review_-_main_report_-_june_2009.pdf (accessed 23 August, 2010).

Department of Health/Unite/CPHVA (2009) *Getting it Right for Children and Families. Maximising the Contribution of the Health Visiting Team. 'Ambition, Action, Achievement'*. Department of Health, London.

Elkan, R., Kendrick, D., Hewitt, M., *et al.* (2000) The effectiveness of domiciliary health visiting: a systematic review of international studies and a selective review of British literature. *Health Technology Assessment*, **4**(13), i-v, 1-339.

Emond, A., Pollock, J., Deave, T., Bonnell, S., Peters, T.J. & Harvey, I. (2002) An evaluation of the First Parent Health Visiting Scheme. *Archives of Disease in Childhood*, **86**, 150-157. doi:10.1136/adc.86.3.150.

Family & Parenting Institute (2009) *Health Visitors: A Progress Report*. National Family & Parenting Institute, London. Available from: http://www.familyandparenting.org/Filestore//Documents/Our_work/Campaigns/HealthVisitors_a_progress_report.pdf (accessed 10 March, 2011).

Featherstone, B. & Trinder, L. (2001) New Labour, families and fathers. *Critical Social Policy*, **21**(4), 534-536.

Fitzpatrick, P., Molloy, B. & Johnson, Z. (1997) Community mothers' programme: extension to the travelling community in Ireland. *Journal of Epidemiology and Community Health*, **51**(3), 299-303.

Gomby, D.S. (1999) Understanding evaluations of home visiting programmes. *Future Child*, **9**, 27-43.

de Graaf, I., Speetjens, P., Smit, F., de Wolff, M. & Tavacchio, L. (2008) Effectiveness of the Triple P- Positive ParentingProgram on behavioural problems in children: meta-analysis. *Behaviour Modification*, **32**(5), 714-35. doi: 10.1177/0145445508317134. Available from: www.triplep.net/cicms/assets/pdfs/pg1as100gr5so142.pdf (accessed 9 March, 2011).

Hall, D.M.B. & Elliman, D. (2006) *Health for All Children*, 4th edn. Oxford University Press, Oxford.

Hall, D.M.B. & Hall, S. (2007) *The 'Family-Nurse Partnership': Developing an Instrument for Identification, Assessment and Recruitment of Clients*. Department for Children, Schools and Families. Ref: DCSF-RW022. Available from: http://www.education.gov.uk/research/data/uploadfiles/DCSF-RW022.pdf (accessed 9 March, 2011).

Haringey NHS Teaching Primary Care Trust (2004) *Guidelines for Use of New Health Visiting and School Nursing across Haringey TPCT* (authors: J Grant & D Cole). Available from: www.haringey.nhs.uk/.../1789_clinical_records_system_health_visitors_and_school_nurses_1_.pdf (accessed 9 March, 2011).

Heaman, M.I., Chalmers, K.I., Woodgate, L. & Brown, J. (2006) Early childhood home visiting programme: factors contributing to success. *Journal of Advanced Nursing*, **55**(3), 291-300.

Heaman, M.I., Chalmers, K.I., Woodgate, R. & Brown, J. (2007) Relationship work in an early childhood home visiting program. *Journal of Paediatric Nursing*, **22**(4), 319-330.

HM Government (2003) *Every Child Matters*. Presented to Parliament by the Chief Secretary to the Treasury by Command of Her Majesty, September 2003 (Cm 5860). The Stationery Office, London. Available from: http://www.education.gov.uk/consultations/downloadableDocs/EveryChildMatters.pdf (accessed 18 March, 2011).

Hoskins, R.A.J (2009) Health visiting – the end of a UK service? *Health Policy*, **93**, 93–101.

House of Commons (1990) *The National Health Service and Community Care Act*. HMSO, London.

Hutching, J., Bywater, T., Daley, D., Gardner, F., Whitaker, C., Jones, K., Eames, C. & Edwards, R.T. (2007) Parenting intervention in Sure Start services for children at risk of developing conduct disorder: pragmatic randomised controlled trial. *British Medical Journal*, **7**(334), 678 doi:10.1136/bmj.39126.620799.55 (published 9 March, 2007).

Irwin, L., Siddiqi, A., Hertzman, C. (2007) Early child development: a powerful equalizer. *Final Report for the World Health Organization Commission on the Social Determinants of Health*. Available from: http://www.who.int/social_determinants/resources/ecd_kn_report_07_2007.pdf (accessed 10 March, 2011).

ISRCTN Trial registration (2009) *An Evaluation of the Triple P Parent Programme in Birmingham: Support for Parents of 5-11 Year Old Children Displaying Problem Behaviour*. Available from: www.controlled-trials.com/ISRCTN10429692 (accessed 10 March, 2011).

Jack, S.M., DiCenso, A., Lohfeld, L. (2002) A theory of maternal engagement with public health nurses and family visitors. *Journal of Advanced Nursing*, **49**(2), 182–190.

Johnson, Z., Howell, F., Molloy, B. (1993) Community mothers' programme: randomised controlled trial of non-professional intervention in parenting. *British Medical Journal*, **29**(306), 1449–1452.

Johnson, Z., Molloy, B., Scallan, E., *et al.* (2000) Community Mothers Programme – seven year follow-up of a randomized controlled trial of non-professional intervention in parenting. *Journal of Public Health Medicine*, **22**(3), 337–342.

Kendall, S. (1993) Do health visitors promote client participation? An analysis of the health visitor–client interaction. *Journal of Clinical Nursing*, **2**(2), 103–109.

Kitzman, H., Olds, D.L., Henderson, C.R Jr. *et al.* (1997) Effect of prenatal and infancy home visitation by nurses on pregnancy outcomes, childhood injuries, and repeated childbearing. A randomized controlled trial. *Journal of the American Association*, **278**(8), 644–652.

Kristjanson, L. & Chalmers, K.I. (1990) Nurse-client interactions in community based practice: Creating common meaning. *Public Health Nursing*, **7**(4), 215–223.

Long, A., McCarney, S., Smyth, G., Magorrian, N., Dillon, A. (2001) The effectiveness of parenting programmes facilitated by health visitors. *Journal of Advanced Nursing*, **34**(5), 611–620.

McGoldrick, M., Gerson, R., Petry, S.S. (2008) Genograms: Assessment and intervention (3rd ed.), W.W. Norton & Co., New York.

McIntosh, J. (2006) The process of health visiting and its contribution to parental support in the Starting Well demonstration project. *Health and Social Care in the Community*, **15**(1), 77–85.

Mackenzie, M. (2008) 'Doing' public health and 'making' public health practitioners: putting policy into practice in 'Starting Well'. *Social Science & Medicine*, **67**(6), 1028–1037. doi:10.1016/j.socscimed.2008.05.021.

McKenzie, M., Shute, J., Berzns, K. & Judge, K. (2004) *The Independent Evaluation of 'Starting Well': Final Report.* Health Promotion Policy Unit, University of Glasgow, Glasgow.

Malin, N. & Morrow, G. (2009) Evaluating the role of the Sure Start Plus Advisor in providing integrated support for pregnant teenagers and young parents. *Journal of Health and Social Care in the Community,* **17**(5), 495–503.

Marmot, M. (2006) Status syndrome: a challenge to medicine. *Journal of the American Association,* **295**(11), 1304–1307.

Marmot, M., Atkinson, T., Bell, J. *et al.* (2010) *Fair Society, Healthy Lives. The Marmot Review.* Marmot Review Team, University College London.

Melhuish, T. & Belsky, J., The National Evaluation of Sure Start Research Team (2008) *The Impact of Sure Start Local Programmes on Three Year Olds and Their Families.* Institute for the Study of Children, Families and Social Issues. University of London, Birkbeck.

Moore, S., Haines, V., Hawe, P. & Shiell, A. (2006) Lost in translation: a genealogy of the 'social capital' concept in public health. *Journal of Epidemiology and Community Health,* **60**, 729–734.

Mulcahy, H. & McCarthy, G. (2008) Participatory nurse/client relationships: perceptions of public health nurses and mothers of vulnerable families. *Applied Nursing Research,* **21**(3), 169–172.

National Evaluation of Sure Start (NESS) (2009) *BBK NESS Site Home Page.* Available from: www.ness.bbk.ac.uk (accessed 9 March, 2011).

NHS Health Development Agency (2004) *Ante-natal and Post-natal Home Visiting Programmes: A Review of Reviews. EVIDENCE BRIEFING* (authors: J. Bull, G. McCormick, C. Swann & C. Mulvihill); available from: http://www.hda.nhs.uk/ evidence or https://www.nice.org.uk/niceMedia/documents/home_visiting.pdf (accessed 9 March, 2011).

Office of Public Sector Information, OPSI (2004) *Carers (Equal Opportunities) Act.* Available from: www.opsi.gov.uk/acts/acts2004/ukpga_20040015_en_1 (accessed 10 March, 2011).

Olds, D.L., Eckenrode, J., Henderson C.R.,Jr. *et al.* (1997) Long-term effects of home visitation on maternal life course and child abuse and neglect. Fifteen year follow-up of a randomized trial. *Journal of the American Association,* **278**(8), 637–643.

Olds, D.L., Henderson, C.R., Jr, Cole, R. *et al.* (1998) Long-term effects of nurse home visitation on children's criminal and antisocial behavior: 15-year follow-up of a randomized controlled trial. *Journal of the American Association,* **280**(14), 1238–1244.

Olds, D.L., Henderson C.R., Jr, Tatelbaum, R. and Chamberlin, R. (1986) Improving the delivery of prenatal care and outcomes of pregnancy: a randomized trial of nurse home visitation. *Pediatrics,* **77**(1):16–28.

Olds, D.L, Kitzman, H., Hanks, C. *et al.* (2007) Effects of nurse home visiting on maternal and child functioning: age-9 follow-up of a randomized trial. *Pediatrics,* **120**(4), e832–845.

Olds, D.L., Robinson, J., O'Brien, R. *et al.* (2002) Home visiting by paraprofessionals and by nurses: a randomized controlled trial. *Pediatrics,* **110**(3), 486–496.

Olds, D.L., Robinson, J., Pettitt, L. *et al.* (2004) Effects of home visits by paraprofessionals and by nurses: age 4 follow-up results of a randomized trial. *Pediatrics,* **114**(6), 1560–1568.

Orr, J. (1992) Assessing individual and family health needs. In: *Health Visiting: Towards Community Health Nursing* (eds K. Luker & J. Orr), pp. 107–158. Blackwell Science, Oxford.

Prevention Action (2008) *Ireland's Community Mothers Take the Pressure off Family Life*. Available from: http://www.preventionaction.org/what-works/ire-lands-community-mothers-take-pressure-family-life (accessed 18 August, 2010).

Prinz, R.J., Sanders, M.R, Shapiro, C.J., Whitaker, D.J. & Lutzker, J.R. (2009) Population-based prevention of child maltreatment: the U.S. Triple P system population trial. *Prevention Science*, **10**, 1–12.

Russell, S. and Drennan, V. (2007) Mothers' views of the health visiting service in the UK: a web-based survey. *Community Practitioner*, **80**(8), 22–26.

Sanders, M.R. (1999) Triple P-Positive Parenting Program: towards an empirically validated multilevel parenting and family support strategy for the prevention of behavior and emotional problems in children. *Clinical Child Family Psychology Review*, **2**(2), 71–90.

Sanders, M.R. (2008) Triple P-Positive Parenting Programme as a public health approach to strengthening parenting. *Journal of Family Psychology*, **22**(3), 506–517.

Scottish Government (2004) *Independent Evaluation of 'Starting Well' Final Report* (authors: M. Mackenzie, J. Shute, K. Berzins, K. Judge). Available from: www.scot-land.gov.uk/Publications/2005/04/20890/55054 (accessed 26 August, 2010).

Scottish Government (2005) *Detailed Plan for Phase Two of the National Health Demonstration Project Starting Well*. Available from: www.scotland.gov.uk (accessed 26 August, 2010).

Shorter Oxford English Dictionary (1973) Clarendon Press, Oxford.

Shute, J.L. & Judge, K. (2005) Evaluating 'Starting Well', the Scottish national demonstration project for child health: outcomes at six months. *Journal of Primary Prevention*, **26**(3), 221–240.

South East Wales Trials Units (SEWTU) (undated website) *Evaluating the Family Nurse Partnership in England: A Randomised Controlled Trial (Building Blocks Study)*. Dr Mike Robling Chief Investigator, Cardiff_University. Available from: http://medic.cardiff.ac.uk/archive_subsites/_/_/medic/subsites/buildingblocks/index.html (accessed 26 July, 2010).

Spijkers, W., Jansen, D., de Meer, G. & Reijneveld, S.A. (2010) Effectiveness of a parenting programme in a public health setting: a randomised controlled trial of the positive parenting programme (Triple P) level 3 versus care as usual provided by the preventive child healthcare (PCH). *BMC Public Health*, **10**, 131 (published online 15 March 2010), doi: 10.1186/1471-2458-10-131.

Starting Well Demonstration Project (undated) Available from: www.gorbalslive.org.uk/data/community/.../startingwell.htm (accessed 26 August, 2010).

Stewart, S. (2010) Personal communication, 29 June.

Sweet, M.A. & Applebaum, M.I. (2004) Is home visiting an effective strategy? A meta-analytic review of home visiting programs for families with young children. *Child Development*, **75**(5), 1435–1456. doi: 10.1111/j.1467-8624.2004.00750.

United Kingdom Public Health Association (UKPHA) (2009) *Health Visiting Matters: Re-establishing Health Visiting*. Available from: www.ukpha.org.uk (accessed 10 March, 2011).

UNOCINI (2008) *Guidance*. Understanding the Needs of Children in Northern Ireland. Available from: http://www.welbni.org/index.cfm/go/publications/key/6832628E-09E1-D43F-4F0E0109B9D314BD:1 (accessed 10 March, 2011).

Wasoff, F. & Hill, M. (2002) Family Policy in Scotland. *Social Policy and Society*, **1**(3), 171–182.

Welsh Assembly Government (undated) *Flying Start Health Visiting Core Programme – Play, Learn, Grow*. Available from: http://www.wales.nhs.uk/site-splus/866/opendoc/140318/&47125823-1143-E756-5C54492FA3987A90 (accessed 10 March, 2011).

Wiggins, M., Rosata, M., Ausaterberry, H., Sawtell, M. & Olicwe, S. (2005) *Supporting Teenagers Who Are Pregnant or Parents: Sure Start Plus National Evaluation: Final Report*. Social Science Research Unit, Institute of Education, University of London, London. Available from: www.ioe.ac.uk/ssru/reports/ssplusevaluation-finalreport.pdf (accessed 10 March, 2011).

Wilson, P., Thompson, L., Puckering, C., *et al.* (2010) Parent-child relationships: are health visitors' judgements reliable? *Community Practitioner*, **83**(5), 22-25.

Woodgate, R.L., Heaman, M.I., Chalmers, K.I. & Brown, J. (2007) Issues related to delivering an early childhood home visiting program. *American Journal of Maternal and Child Health Nursing*, **32**(2), 95-101.

Worth, A. & Hogg, R. (2000) A qualitative evaluation of the effectiveness of health visiting practice. *British Journal of Community Nursing*, **221**(5), 224-228.

Wright, C.M., Jeffrey, S.K., Ross, M.K., Wallis, L. & Wood, R. (2009) Targeting health visitors: lessons from Starting Well. *Archives of Disease in Childhood*, **94**(1) 23-27.

Wright, L.M. & Leahy, M. (1994) *Nurses and Families: A Guide to Family Assessment and Intervention*. FA Davis, Philadelphia.

Appendix 4   Activities for Chapter 4

Activity 4.1   Using genograms in health visiting

To gain some practice using genograms within health visiting, draw a genogram relating to your own family or a family you are currently visiting.

Genogram symbols
These are just some of the symbols which can be used when compiling a genogram.

A dotted line is drawn around the people who currently live in the same house.

(Continued)

Activity 4.1 (Continued)

Symbols representing examples of children and birth

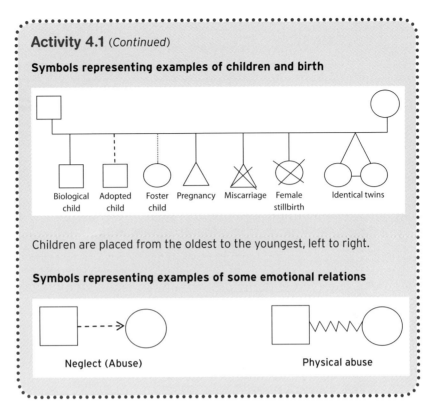

Children are placed from the oldest to the youngest, left to right.

Symbols representing examples of some emotional relations

Neglect (Abuse)   Physical abuse

Activity 4.2 Assessing child health programmes

Think about the child programmes which the health visiting service in your area offers. Answer the following questions:

Questions to consider	Assessment of child health programme
Is the service offered to all infants/ children (universal) or to a particular group (targeted)?	
If a particular group, what criteria are used to identity the target group?	
Is the programme designed to enrol women during the prenatal or postnatal period or either time period?	

(Continued)

Activity 4.2 *(Continued)*

Questions to consider	Assessment of child health programme
What are the conceptual underpinnings of the programme, if known (e.g. strengths based, learning theory, support based on interpersonal/therapeutic relationships between parent and nurse, etc.)?	
Who delivers the programme (the professional – health visitor or public health nurse – or an assistant – a home visitor, community 'mothers', etc.)?	
What is the programme's age cut-off for the child (i.e. two years, school enrolment, etc.)?	
What services does the family receive and how often do they receive services?	
What are the services (if any) that the family receives once they complete the programme? If services are provided, what are these services?	
Has the programme undergone a rigorous evaluation? If this has been done, what are the outcomes and the recommendations (if any) for changes?	

Activity 4.3 Health visitor–client interaction

- Reflect on a recent visit with a family.
- Do you feel this was a good interaction? If so, why was this? If not why not?
- In either situation, is there anything you would do differently during your next contact?

5

Safeguarding Children: Debates and Dilemmas for Health Visitors

Julianne Harlow

University of Bolton, Bolton, UK

Martin Smith

Mersey Deanery School of Public Health, Liverpool, UK

Introduction

The first decade of the new millennium has seen an increase in political and societal demands to tackle various forms of child abuse in order to safeguard children. It is widely acknowledged that for all practitioners involved in working with vulnerable children and their families, safeguarding children can be both difficult and challenging on the one hand, and yet intensely rewarding on the other. A plethora of policies relevant to safeguarding children underpinned by the United Nations Convention on the Rights of the Child (UNICEF, 1989) exists at all levels of society. Such policy charts the growing emphasis on safeguarding work and has refocused the roles of numerous professionals and practitioners. For those health visitors who work with children and families, the increased emphasis on safeguarding children has led to both tensions within and a reinforcement of the value of their (public health) role in practice. This chapter will address these tensions to contextualise the contemporary role of health visitors as public health practitioners in safeguarding. It will recognise the importance of leadership in health visiting practice to ensure the safety and wellbeing of children. Although this chapter will focus on health visiting from the perspective of specialist community public health nursing, it will also be relevant to other key practitioners working in the field of safeguarding children.

Given the emphasis on leadership within specialist community public health nursing (NMC, 2004) it is important that health visitors understand how to work with ambiguity and ethical decision-making in complex situations where

Health Visiting: A Rediscovery, Third Edition. Edited by Karen A. Luker, Jean Orr and Gretl A. McHugh.
© 2012 Blackwell Publishing Ltd. Published 2012 by Blackwell Publishing Ltd.

there may be competing interests and needs amongst family members. In order to reach these understandings, this chapter will begin with an exploration of some of the key concepts surrounding child abuse and safeguarding children. Initially, consideration of how UK society currently defines a 'child' will be given as understanding the concept of 'child' has ramifications for health visitors as they seek to practice within a society and legislative and policy framework, that presents inconsistencies and tensions. The meaning of child abuse will be explored as a social construct and from a temporal perspective, along with other associated terms. This will highlight how society has come to respond to various forms of child abuse which constitute a continually evolving phenomenon. In the UK, this response is currently expressed in terms of safeguarding children; the concept of safeguarding and its relationship with child protection will be explored.

Health visiting has had to respond to the changing nature of child abuse, safeguarding and child protection in contemporary society whilst having been subject to a range of political changes as a profession. Such changes have had an impact upon how the health visiting role has been interpreted at both national and local levels. In terms of the evidence base there have been a number of descriptive studies undertaken that highlight different aspects of health visitor's work with child abuse by Elkan *et al.* (2000). However, the evidence base for demonstrating the effectiveness of health visiting in dealing with child abuse was noted to be somewhat limited (Elkan *et al.*, 2000). Indeed, more recently, the evidence relating to the cost effectiveness of early years' services as a whole is also said to be limited (Health Select Committee, 2009). These issues are not unusual across services such as health visiting, as the nature of the roles make it difficult to distinguish cause and effect relationships.

Nevertheless, there are clear policy drivers that demonstrate an unequivocal recognition that health visitors have an important role in safeguarding children. This role aligns itself with a public health approach which recognises the wider determinants of heath and the impact upon not only the children but also the parents and carers of children. Consequently, this challenges perceptions that working with individuals and families in a safeguarding context are separate in some way to a public health role for health visitors.

This chapter places an emphasis on the fact that good leaders are role models for ethical safeguarding practice. Health visitors are required to be accountable for their practice and fit for professional standing. These are statements which underpin the Nursing and Midwifery Council (NMC) standards for safe and effective practice (NMC, 2004). However, accepting them at face value risks minimising the importance of a clear understanding of why accountability and safe practice are essential in safeguarding work. Health visitors therefore need to develop and maintain skills of critical thinking and reflection in order to fulfil their role not only as effective practitioners in a multidisciplinary arena but also as leaders within the health visiting team and in engaging with other partners. The value of supervision for enabling a reflective, critical approach has been increasingly recognised as essential for safe and effective practice (DCSF, 2008). However, as supervision becomes increasingly established in practice it is equally important to recognise how the quality of supervision impacts upon the quality of both leadership and practice.

Overall, this chapter takes a considered approach to safeguarding children through an analysis of health visiting practice emphasising the significance of leadership. This is not a reference piece or step-by-step account of how to safeguard, as this information is readily available through existing texts and up-to-date policy. For example, the process is explained with a series of very useful flow charts by the Department for Education and Skills (DfES, 2006) and is readily available on the internet. This chapter is an analytical contribution designed to underpin contemporary health visiting practice and demonstrate:

- how an understanding of policy and legislation is relevant to safeguarding practice;
- the evidence associated with the impact of child abuse;
- the utilisation of supervision to support critical reflection and thinking.

All of these contribute to the development of leadership in practitioners working in the safeguarding arena.

Throughout the chapter consideration will be given to examples of published inquiries into child deaths and serious case reviews that are particularly relevant for health visiting. The reader will also have the opportunity to undertake activities as they progress through the text. The chapter draws from relevant legislation and policy. Whilst health visitors are not required to be legal experts, they need an understanding of the legislative framework as it relates to their safeguarding role. This understanding helps to ensure safe, effective and accountable safeguarding practice and the tailoring of health promotion activities. The movement towards integrated services and closer working with other professionals such as social workers, reinforces this as legislation forms the basis of joint discussions and decision-making regarding vulnerable children and their families. A health visitor's knowledge and confidence in respect of relevant safeguarding and child protection law requires constant updating on policies and practices.

The key concepts

Defining child

Throughout its history, health visiting has been associated with the health and wellbeing of children as the main group and focus for professional practice. This is not without reason, as the promotion of health and the prevention of ill health (CETHV, 1977) is dependent upon the roots for a long and healthy life being established at an early age. It has been argued (e.g. Symonds, 1991) that if health visitors focus on children and families this detracts from the broader, whole population approach. It is important to recognise, however, that children form a distinct population within the general population. A population of children has its own distinct health characteristics and health needs that vary according to age, developmental stage and a range of genetic, social and environmental factors. Furthermore, as most children live within families, focusing on the health of families with young children means that not only is the health of the current population of children enhanced, but so too is the health of the future adult population.

Current legislation such as the Children Act 1989 and the Children Act 2004 is informed by the United Nations Convention on the Rights of the Child (UNICEF, 1989) and defines a child as 'anyone who has not yet reached their 18th birthday'. However, within the UK, tensions exist within law and policy on how chronological age and developmental capacity vary as a marker for childhood. Take as an example the unborn child. Policy sets out procedures and timescales for addressing safeguarding concerns regarding unborn children For example, 560 unborn children were the subject of child protection plans in the year ending March 2009 (NSPCC, 2009). Such plans only come into place at birth as the fetus has no legal rights to protection in respect of even the most extreme of circumstances. In utero, however, the foetus may be subjected to a range of harmful behaviours and abuses such as domestic abuse, tobacco smoke, alcohol and drugs, all of which are known to cause potential harm to the health and development of the fetus. Just as the beginning of childhood is an ambiguous and contested concept, so too is the point at which childhood ends.

Although in law a child is a child until they are 18, in the UK 16 year olds can legally have a sexual relationship with a member of the same or opposite sex of the same age or older. Sixteen year olds may marry or enter a civil partnership with their parents' consent; however, they cannot purchase alcohol or cigarettes, learn to drive or vote. Further tensions exist within specific pieces of legislation and policy. The Sexual Offences Act 2003 for example, deems that sex for children and young people under 16 years of age is illegal. However, young people under the age of 16 may request and be prescribed contraception if they are deemed competent to do so in line with Department of Health guidance (DH, 2004a).

Similarly, in respect of decision-making for medical treatment, children may give or withhold their consent to medical treatment if they are deemed as competent. Increasing importance is given to the child's wishes in accordance with age and evolving capacity for understanding. Courts can and do, however, override these wishes when they are deemed not to be in the best interests of children and young people. Other tensions in respect of service provision and the chronological age of children exist. For example, young people aged 16 or above requiring hospital admission may be considered too old for admission to a paediatric ward and consequently may be exposed to adult environments and services which may not cater appropriately for their needs and which may potentially be harmful. Whilst analysis of society's use of chronological age in determining when particular behaviours (healthy or not) may be considered legal falls outside this chapter, the discussion reflects the ambiguities and contentious nature of society's attempts to determine the age at which childhood begins and ends. Activity 5.1 (see Appendix 5 at the end of the chapter) may be useful in helping you to explore the concept of 'child' further.

Defining childhood

Difficulties in reaching a consensus in respect of defining childhood are evidenced by contested concepts within the literature. Different forms and sources of literature offer various perspectives on what constitutes a 'child' and are influenced by political, temporal, spatial and cultural factors. Smith (2010) presents an analysis of the concept of childhood in contemporary society and suggests that perspectives on childhood are subject to disparate positions with little to support childhood as a 'clear and coherent entity' (Smith, 2010: 194). He suggests that there may be certain universal features of childhood that act as determinants of children's lives which are:

- physical growth;
- increasing competencies;
- inexperience;
- vulnerability.

He further argues that these features should be considered as principles in relation to the variations of experiences and the child's context, which may be heavily influenced by such factors as history, culture and genetics. Nevertheless these features expose the extent to which childhood is commonly viewed in adult terms; that is as a deficit in preparation for adulthood and as Smith (2010: 5) suggests 'a means to an end'. In contrast to these features, Smith considers other perspectives on childhood that recognise the importance of the child's view; the need to understand the child's lived experience as well as a perspective on how the child formulates their own sense of the world in their own terms. Children draw from the source material of the adult world around them; however, their behaviour through play and interaction with others helps them to create their own roles and identities and develop their relationships.

These different perspectives on childhood present dilemmas for health visitors who are often required to draw on their own professional and personal values, as adults, to make judgements based on a biopsychosocial model reflecting the immaturity of children with limited rights and interests. In addition, health visitors need to develop an understanding of the world through the child's eyes and ensure they give a clear priority to the views of children in families and rely less upon traditional perspectives of childhood which view children as Prout (2005, cited in Smith, 2010) sees it, from a standpoint of immaturity and incompleteness (in relation to children and adulthood). For health visitors to be successful in working with children and understanding their needs and experiences they need to be able to see them and utilise their higher level communication skills through observation and active listening and engage more fully, more directly and more empathically with children. This will enable health visitors to develop more robust assessments of children's needs and the extent to which they feel safe from harm.

A recent tighter focus of early intervention and practice with those families and children deemed particularly vulnerable has become known as *progressive universalism* (or it is referred to by Marmot *et al.* (2010 as *proportionate universalism*). This is thought to make a more significant impact on the reduction of health inequalities affecting the lives of children. Progressive universalism has been defined as a 'universal service that is systematically planned and delivered to give a continuum of support according to need at neighbourhood and individual level in order to achieve greater equity of outcomes for all children' (DH, 2007: 8). However, a consultation with CPHVA members found that the concept has not been easily embraced by some health visitors (CPHVA, 2007). It was suggested that the term *'regressive' universalism* could be more appropriate to reflect the fact that not everyone would get an adequate standard of service. If health visitors were denied the opportunity to build a relationship with all families they would feel it impossible to provide a service based on a progressive universalism. Indeed other major charitable organisations have suggested that the term progressive universalism is just another means to justify the cutting of health visitor numbers (FPI, 2007). Whilst the concept of progressive universalism assists health visitors in focusing services on those with the most recognised need, in the context of safeguarding children, it presents a challenge as child abuse does occur across all social classes. It involves children of all ages and is most likely to be hidden and not easily recognised. Focusing health visiting practice only on those perceived as vulnerable at neighbourhood or individual level means that opportunities for identifying and responding to abuse across the population will be reduced. Indeed, Lord Laming in his report to the House of Commons (Laming, 2009) highlighted the tensions between health visitors supporting families with complex needs and the health visitor's role in offering a universal service to all. He makes the point that large numbers of children in the population do not have a child protection plan and therefore sees the universal role of health visitors as crucially important in being able to develop strong relationships with all families and that there is a value in all children being seen in their home environment.

Defining safeguarding

Before reading on, it may be useful to consider your own perceptions of the meaning of *safeguarding* and begin to complete Activity 5.2 (see Appendix 5). Over recent years the term *safeguarding children*, coined in Section 17 of the Children Act 1989 has increasingly replaced that of *child protection*. Whilst *safeguarding,* as a term, is now widely represented in the mainstream language of policy and practice, it represents a multifaceted concept that may be open to interpretation by many different groups, agencies, professionals and individuals. Whilst literature offers various perspectives of *safeguarding children* the importance of professionals sharing an agreed definition of what constitutes safeguarding cannot be overstated. Agreed definitions are vital in terms of understanding the aims that should be achieved in respect of safeguarding practice whilst simultaneously forming a basis for more specific procedural policy that details how safeguarding practice should be carried out. A current definition of safeguarding and promoting the welfare of children is:

> Protecting children from maltreatment; preventing impairment of children's health or development; ensuring that children are growing up in circumstances consistent with the provision of safe and effective care; and undertaking that role so as to enable those children to have optimum life chances and to enter adulthood successfully.
>
> (DCSF, 2010: 34)

Whilst this definition does not offer any detail of the activities associated with the safeguarding role, or how effective safeguarding practice might be achieved, it does have a number of strengths. One of the most significant is it reflects the five outcomes identified as being most important to children and young people in the consultation of *Every Child Matters* (HM Government, 2003). These are:

- Be healthy.
- Stay safe.
- Enjoy and achieve.
- Make a positive contribution.
- Achieve economic wellbeing.

The process of consulting with children and young people and allowing them to express their views is compliant with articles 12 and 13 of the United Nations Convention on the Rights of the Child. In addition to the process being respectful of children's rights, the content of the five outcomes is also compliant with the rights of children.

In incorporating the five outcomes, the broad definition of safeguarding above represents a current and holistic view that safeguarding children is much more than protecting children from abuse. Defining safeguarding, in a holistic way, effectively widens the scope of practice increasing the opportunities for health visitors and school nurses to work proactively in partnership with children and families to safeguard and promote children's welfare. However, as indicated by the placement of the term *protecting children from maltreatment*, child protection is nevertheless a very important part of safeguarding work. Equally, protecting children from harm demands much more than just having systems in place to manage child maltreatment. Recent suggestions highlighted by Puffett (2010) of a replacement of the term safeguarding with the term child protection would be a retrograde step. Political attempts to manipulate the discourse and subsequent direction of policy detract from the fact that for children, the issue of preventing child maltreatment remains. Therefore, whilst child protection per se refers to the activities undertaken to protect those children who are suffering or likely to suffer significant harm (DCSF, 2010), the concept of safeguarding enables a wider, more holistic understanding of the need to protect children from harm and subsequently aim to reduce the need for child protection activities. A proactive, preventative approach such as this reflects many aspects of the health protecting, health promoting public health role of the health visitor.

A robust legislative and policy framework underpins the role of the health visitor in safeguarding children and incorporates a range of global, national, professional and local policies and procedures. This reflects society's recognition of the seriousness of child abuse and neglect as public health issues and also the value that health visitors bring to a safeguarding role.

According to the World Health Organisation, the maltreatment of children is a major global issue. Each year, millions of children worldwide are the victims of and witnesses to physical, sexual and emotional violence. In 2002 for example, there were 31 000 child deaths attributed to homicide with infants and very young children at greatest risk (WHO & ISPCAN, 2006). For all these children there are health consequences as a result of their exposure to abuse that impact physically and emotionally on their wellbeing and development, not only through childhood. but sometimes into adulthood too.

Safeguarding children requires a global political response. The development of policy at a national and international level for protecting children against abuse has, in recent decades become increasingly child-centred with a growing recognition of the rights of children. Global safeguarding policy is underpinned by The United Nations Convention on the Rights of the Child (UNICEF, 1989). The UNCRC has become the world's most ratified convention with only two UN member States, the USA and Somalia having declined (Somalia did state its intention to ratify in 2009). This international treaty consists of 41 substantive articles that detail a range of children's civil, political, economic, social and cultural rights which every child is deemed to require to live a safe, happy and fulfilled childhood. The convention was clearly a significant undertaking by the UN which challenged its member states to recognise the importance of the state in supporting children, meeting their health and development needs and if necessary intervening to protect them from harm. However, without any significant level of accountability the UK Government has ratified the Convention but not incorporated it into UK law in the form of a specific Act of Parliament.

Consequently there may be some difficulty in enforcing children's convention rights. Whilst the UNCRC places emphasis on the rights and needs of children and the aim of ensuring an optimum state of child wellbeing, UK policy has continued to wrestle with the rights of children and the rights and wishes of parents. Health visitors therefore find themselves working within a policy framework that on the one hand espouses the rights and interests of children and on the other sees parental choice as key to how children are parented. A health visitor's access to a child is through the parent who is the gatekeeper to observation and communication with the child. Although the fact that the UNCRC has not been incorporated into English law by an Act of Parliament may be considered a limitation of the value placed on children's rights in

England, there is other evidence concerning the extent to which the seriousness of children's rights are taken. The Government for example, is bound to making regular reports to the Committee on the Rights of the Child, a UN monitoring body. In court settings children's Convention rights are referred to and used in legal arguments and decision-making, whilst in policy in respect of children, reference is often made to the fact that such policy and guidance reflects the principles of the United Nations Convention on the Rights of the Child. An example of this may be seen on page 24 of *Working Together to Safeguard Children: A Guide to Inter-agency Working to Safeguard and Promote the Welfare of Children* (DCSF, 2010).

The UNCRC is clearly a very important document that holds great relevance for health visitors and can be explored further in Activity 5.3 (see Appendix 5). Of particular significance to the health visitors' role is Article 19, which requires that States Parties take appropriate measures to protect children from all forms of physical and mental violence, injury, abuse and neglect. Article 19 therefore acts as a mandate for national safeguarding legislation and policy, which encompass the roles of public sector employees and professionals such as health visitors. Other articles found within the UNCRC may also be considered directly relevant to the health visitor's role in safeguarding children.

Newell (cited in Martell, 1999: 121) stated that health visitors need to see themselves as part of a new 'movement to build a human rights culture for children'. In respect of health visiting practice and children's rights per se this is a laudable goal and one which health visitors should strive for. However, in the context of the health visitor's role in safeguarding and protecting the most vulnerable children it becomes an urgent element of essential practice. Health visitors therefore need a fundamental awareness and working knowledge of the Convention Rights that underpin their work with children, families and the communities in which they live as well as the ability to act as advocates for children in spite of the challenges they face within everyday practice. Current challenges in health visiting include those brought to light by the Unite/CPHVA's (2008) Omnibus survey and subsequently emphasised by Lord Laming (2009). These include; large and complex caseloads, staff shortages and resultant time pressures which may reduce the effectiveness of child and family interactions and assessment.

In addition to these challenges, health visitors also face other issues within the context of health visiting practice and safeguarding children, for example the problem of balancing the needs and rights of children with the competing rights of parents. The European Convention on Human Rights (ECHR) was incorporated into English law through the Human Rights Act 1998. This important piece of legislation confers a range of human rights on all UK citizens and requires all public authorities, including health authorities and therefore health visitors to perform their duties and enact their role in accordance with these rights. Again, health visitors need to embed their safeguarding practice within their knowledge and understanding of this legislation which is relevant to the professional context of their safeguarding and child protection roles. Of particular relevance to and sometimes causing tension within child protection activity is Article 8 of the ECHR, the right to respect for private and family life, home and correspondence. Whilst it is unlawful for public authorities to behave in a way that is incompatible with this right, there are a number of exceptions. Exceptions include activity which is: in the interests of public safety, for the prevention of crime, for the protection of health or morals and the protection of the rights and freedoms of others. All the exceptions specified are relevant to professionals' roles in protecting children. The challenge for health visitors and other professionals, however, is to ensure that the degree of interference with families' rights under Article 8 is proportionate. It is important to recognise that the rights conferred by the ECHR and Human Rights Act extend not only to adults but children too. They therefore add impetus to the Convention on the rights of the child and the requirements of health visitors as public servants.

The recent emphasis on safeguarding children within contemporary society justifies, underpins and guides the health visitor's role in safeguarding children. Major shifts in national child protection and safeguarding policy generally occur reactively, precipitated by high profile child deaths or scandals involving children and subsequent inquiries. For example, the death of Dennis O'Neill, beaten and starved to death aged 12 whilst in foster care in Shropshire, precipitated the Monckton Inquiry (Home Office, 1945) and the Children Act 1948. Later, the 1987 crisis in Cleveland where 121 children were removed from their families following dubious diagnoses of sexual abuse was detailed in the Cleveland Report (Butler-Sloss, 1988) and gave impetus to the Children Act 1989. The Children Act 1989 is described as having radically affected all aspects of legal practice concerning children (White *et al.*, 2002), consequently the practice of all professionals working with children, especially those defined by the Act as being 'in need' of support and/or protection was also affected.

The death of Victoria Climbié in 2000 from severe physical abuse and neglect at the hands of her great-aunt and partner led to an inquiry (Laming, 2003) and a range of policy and organisational changes, including *Every Child Matters: Change for Children* (DfES, 2004) and its legislative spine, the Children Act 2004. More recently, the death of baby Peter Connelly in 2007 (known initially as 'Baby P') precipitated the commissioning of a report by Lord Laming (2009) on the recent progress made to implement effective arrangements for safeguarding children and subsequently a revision of *Working Together to Safeguard Children*. Such policy changes impact on and present a challenge to the professional practice of health visitors when considered alongside a raft of other policy initiatives being introduced at regular intervals. Activity 5.4 (see Appendix 5) enables this to be explored further taking into account local policy initiatives. Keeping an up-to-date working knowledge of policy changes presents a challenge to health visitors who need to be able to identify new learning needs on a regular basis and access the knowledge and support needed to fulfil their safeguarding role.

National policy also informs professional policy. The *Standards of Proficiency for Specialist Community Public Health Nurses* (NMC, 2004: 12) feature safeguarding children and specify that Specialist Community Public Health Nurses need 'in depth knowledge of child protection' (NMC, 2004: 15). Furthermore, the Chief Nursing Officer (DH, 2004b) has emphasised that it is the responsibility of all nurses to improve outcomes for vulnerable children and identified child protection learning as a priority. Driven from a high level from both the NMC as professional regulator and central government departments, there is no shortage of professional policy and guidance around safeguarding children. Clearly, professional practice and the policy that guides that practice should reflect the principles contained within the NMC Code of Conduct (NMC, 2008). Whilst the Code is not explicit in respect of safeguarding and child protection activity per se, it is an extremely valuable form of professional policy that provides a broad foundation of ethical guidance and contains core professional values that may be applied to health visitors' safeguarding practice. Furthermore it is the minimum standard against which professionals are measured in relation to the NMC's function of protecting the public. Thus it is vital that health visitors have a working knowledge of the Code and its application within a safeguarding and child protection context.

Defining child abuse

Although children have been exposed to harmful acts and behaviours from the beginning of time, an understanding of what society considers as child abuse today only began to emerge during the nineteenth century. At that time children were seen as the property of adults and not as individuals in their own right. They were often subjected to all manner and types of abuse and neglect. Indeed, a measure of society's value of children was their utility as small individuals who could perform dangerous roles by virtue of their size as factory and mill workers, coalminers and chimney sweeps. During this time there was growing political pressure to tackle this and other forms of exploitation of children for economic gain. Legislative change ensued with a series of Factory Acts that increasingly excluded younger children from working and limited the hours that older children could work.

A number of Education Acts gradually introduced compulsory education whilst legislation such as the Infant Life Protection Act 1872 was enacted, designed to tackle the barbaric practice of *baby farming*. This was the term used to describe the taking in of children for a commercial fee, many of whom subsequently lived in overcrowded conditions, were subjected to abuse and neglect and frequently murdered. Although baby farming as such no longer exists in contemporary English society, informal, private arrangements between parents and other family members or friends are sometimes still made and may put children at risk. Whilst this practice is not confined to any one ethnic group, in today's multicultural society it is important to acknowledge that in some countries entrusting children to relatives in Europe who can offer educational and other opportunities, not available to them in their home country is not uncommon (Laming, 2003). Where private unregulated care arrangements are made in an abusive context, children may be used primarily as a mechanism to gain access to financial support, housing and other benefits, may not have their needs met and may be at risk of harm. Health visitors need to be alert to the above possibilities, and be prepared to share their concerns in a procedurally appropriate manner. The accounts of relevant nineteenth-century legislation such as those outlined earlier are relevant to society in the twenty-first century. They show a clear marker for the birth of law and other forms of policy that we would now consider reflects the ethos of safeguarding children in a holistic sense, that is, taking account of the wider socio-environmental factors that impact upon the lives of children. They also illustrate the fact that despite legislation and policy, abuse and neglect for financial gain still occur.

Despite an acknowledgement of society's role in addressing the welfare of children there are also accounts during the nineteenth century of the serious injuries sustained by children as a result of acts of physical abuse (Kempe & Kempe, 1978). In contrast to the broader understandings of child welfare above, accounts of physical abuse and neglect were predominantly recognised and interpreted within a medical discourse through autopsy findings and epidemiological analysis of population data on injuries sustained by children. Such data presented a picture of the extent to which children were abused and neglected. The first UK Act of Parliament to recognise the need to address the extent of physical abuse was the Prevention of Cruelty to Children Act 1889 which for the first time allowed the state to intervene between parents and children. This Act was later amended in 1894 to acknowledge mental cruelty, create an offence where a sick child was denied medical attention and allow children to give evidence in court. This could be interpreted as the beginnings of society's recognition of the rights of children to voicing their thoughts and opinions as well as their right to protection from emotional abuse and neglect. It would be many years from the beginning of the twentieth century before the rights and interests of children would be considered more fully with firmer legislation and stronger penalties for the perpetrators of abuse.

The association of health visiting with child protection arose during the mid-late nineteenth century as it became aligned with the maternal and child welfare movement as a result of appalling poverty and insanitary conditions (Robinson, 1982). Indeed, Robinson notes that in 1867 the Ladies Sanitary Reform Association set out the duties of its visitors to include: 'teaching' hygiene, child welfare, mental and moral health and providing social support. These activities clearly align health visiting with an interest in the welfare of children. However, caution does need to be applied in interpreting the drivers for this 'teaching'. Smith (2004) challenges the altruistic and romanticised perception of the origins of health visiting with reference to middle-class fears over the spread of epidemics (Wohl, 1986), concerns over the fitness of the workforce and army recruits (Caraher & McNab, 1997) and as a source of occupation for middle-class women (Cowley, 1996). Whatever the drivers were, health visiting became increasingly aligned with maternal and child welfare and the basis for what we would now consider as a 'safeguarding' role was recognised in legislative terms through the Children Act 1908 where health visitors were appointed as Infant Life Protection Visitors.

According to Robinson (1982) the development of health visiting in the twentieth century was influenced both by the development of the NHS and its relation with other occupational groups. The Children Act 1948 was heavily influenced by the Monckton Inquiry (Home Office, 1945) into the death of Dennis O'Neill which highlighted how divided administrative responsibilities across departments increased the risk of errors (Robinson, 1982). Robinson presents an analysis of the influence of the Children Act 1948 with the development of new children's services and the NHS Act of 1946 for health visiting and highlights the degree of ambiguity over its development and the parallel development of the social work profession, both of which were based within local authorities but with an overlapping set of skills and functions. The point here for health visitors is that to this day we continue to see a blurring of the interface between the preventative and reactive roles of both professions. This is borne out by Lord Laming (2009) who highlights how social workers' caseloads have risen and how, as a result, health visitors have increasingly carried child protection issues that would previously have been referred on to children's social care services. This demonstrates that the threshold for accepting referrals of children at risk of suffering abuse is not consistent and is dependent in part on resourcing. Whilst Lord Laming acknowledges that this situation is both inappropriate and unmanageable for health visitors, it remains a challenge to be addressed. The situation also serves to illustrate the impact that the under-resourcing of one professional group has on another.

The term that first articulated the concept of child abuse in modern society was that of the 'Battered-Baby Syndrome' which emerged in 1961 having been coined by Kempe (Kempe & Helfer, 1972). The term was emotive and deliberatively provocative, designed to shock paediatricians and society in general out of complacency. Although the term succeeded in its aim, the limitations were acknowledged as being open to interpretation, lacking clarity and causing confusion. For some, the term represented a narrow interpretation of only the severest forms of physical abuse whereas for the authors it encompassed the total spectrum of abuse. Whilst the term syndrome was used in the context of referring to a set of symptoms, it also presents connotations of a disease process which may detract from the often premeditated and deliberate nature of child abuse. Clearly, however, the early recognition of the phenomenon of child abuse was not confined to one particular person, place or time. Recognising the issue and naming it took a number of intellectuals and professionals from a variety of countries just short of a century.

Different sources of literature offer various terms, definitions and perspectives that relate to what constitutes child abuse. It is important that health visitors work to definitions of child abuse that are agreed across professional groups so that a common consensus is reached in working together to prevent, identify and respond to behaviours, contexts, situations and settings that may be abusive. The current definition of child abuse aimed at the inter-agency workforce and offered by recent statutory guidance is:

> Abuse and neglect are forms of maltreatment of a child. Somebody may abuse or neglect a child by inflicting harm, or by failing to act to prevent harm. Children may be abused in a family or in an institutional or community setting, by those known to them or, more rarely, by a stranger for example, via the internet. They may be abused by an adult or adults, or another child or children.
>
> (DCSF, 2010: 38)

This is a contemporary definition, key for practitioners working with and coming into contact with children. Although neglect is recognised as one of the forms of child maltreatment it is clearly differentiated in the definition above from other forms of abuse which may be further categorised as physical, emotional and sexual. Highlighting and giving prominence to neglect in this way reflects its significance both in terms of it being the most reported form of abuse (DCSF, 2009) as well as increasing recognition of the deleterious impact of neglect on the health and wellbeing of children. Indeed, neglect is considered as separate from abuse as it relates to acts of omission rather than commission, i.e. it is based on shortfalls in meeting the needs of children rather than specific acts they are subjected to. This can be seen in the DCSF definition of neglect which refers to a 'persistent failure to meet a child's physical and/or psychological needs likely to result in the serious impairment of the child's health and development' (DCSF, 2010: 39). Highlighting neglect in this way may counteract the problem that neglect may not be perceived as abuse or maltreatment by some. That said, it is important to also acknowledge that whilst neglect may be referred to as a passive form of maltreatment by some authors, this does not reflect cases where neglect appears to have been premeditated and actively pursued as a form of child abuse, for example as in the recent case of Khyra Ishaq (Radford, 2010). Health visitors need to be mindful that differentiating neglect from physical, emotional and sexual abuse does not diminish its significance and, indeed, it could be argued that is likely to have the greatest impact on a health visitor's workload.

Defining child abuse and neglect is only the first step for health visitors in applying these concepts to real situations in practice and can be explored further in Activity 5.5 (see Appendix 5). However, there is a broader context here that relates to the formative nature of child abuse and neglect that practitioners need to consider. The concept of child abuse becomes problematic when trying to determine whether an action (or omission) should be considered abusive or not; given that how child abuse is defined and refined is subject to change over time and across different societies in different parts of the world. By attempting to define child abuse and neglect, we do so at a given point in time and within a broader context of what society considers constitutes satisfactory parenting and what behaviours towards children are considered acceptable or not.

Different forms of child abuse receive heightened prominence in various forms of literature such as policy, research and the media at different times, often as a result of specific child abuse cases that are highlighted due to various aspects of their shocking nature. These cases lie within a broader context of an ever-increasing knowledge and evidence base of child abuse theory, safeguarding and child protection practice and greater improvements in techniques for investigation by authorities. Technological advances, in particular, have paradoxically influenced how child abuse is defined. On the one hand, improvements in forensic techniques have underpinned a pathologisation of child abuse by providing a medium for more sophisticated diagnosis and intervention. On the other hand, twenty-first-century technology in the form of the internet and mobile phones has been increasingly used as a vehicle for accessing children, to abuse them directly but also as a means of sharing information relating to the abuse of children in the form of still or moving images or the written word. Thirty years ago such technology did not exist, and such activity could not have been imagined as a form of child abuse. These examples illustrate an ever-expanding societal and technological context where forms and understandings of child abuse continue to evolve. It is important that health visitors remain alert as to what constitutes both existing and newly emerging forms and definitions of child abuse as they seek to interpret behaviours and practices within families and communities. Some increasingly accepted behaviours and practices, such as allowing children access to social networking sites for example, may on face value appear harmless yet pose known risks in respect of adults accessing and grooming children for the purposes of abuse. Indeed, the recent case of a man convicted for eight and a half years for abusing hundreds of children through social networking sites (BBC News, 2010) is evidence of this growing phenomenon. Furthermore, social networking sites and mobile phones also afford children a mechanism through which they may abuse other children in the form of cyber-bullying.

It is important also to recognise that incidents of abuse, whatever the form do not occur in a vacuum within the lives of children; but that survival from abuse has its lifelong impacts upon the health and wellbeing of its victims (see Box 5.1).

Box 5.1 The health impacts of child abuse: examples from research

Symptoms of post-traumatic stress disorder (PTSD) common among adult survivors of childhood abuse with victims of past traumatic events more vulnerable to current life stressors (Kendall-Tackett, 2000).

PTSD associated with:

- significant impact on brain function (Van der Kolk, 1984);
- parental lack of support (Pine & Cohen, 2002);
- witnessing threats to caregiver (Scheeringa et al., 2006).

Chronic hyper-arousal associated with abnormal levels of stress hormones and alteration of certain brain structures (Bremner, 1999).

(Continued)

Box 5.1 (*Continued*)

An association between neglect and:

- adverse effects on the development of a child's brain (Glaser, 2000);
- mal-development of neural systems associated with social and emotional functioning (Perry, 2002);
- reduced brain mass (Perry, 2002).

Adults with four or more Adverse Childhood Experiences (ACE Study):

- had higher rates of ischemic heart disease, cancer, stroke, chronic bronchitis, emphysema, diabetes, skeletal fractures, and hepatitis (Felitti *et al.*, 1998);
- were more likely to have had 50 or more sexual partners, and to have had a sexually transmitted disease (Felitti *et al.*, 2001);
- were more likely to consider themselves as alcoholics, have used illegal drugs, and have injected drugs (Felitti *et al.*, 2001).

Survivors of childhood abuse are more likely to:

- smoke (Felitti *et al.*, 2001);
- have higher rates of obesity (Felitti, 1991);
- develop Irritable Bowel Syndrome (Talley *et al.*, 1995; Kendall-Tackett, 2000);
- report diabetes or three or more symptoms of diabetes (Kendall-Tackett & Marshall, 1999);
- experience sleeping difficulties, including repetitive nightmares (Teegan, 1999);
- have twice the physical symptom reported in primary care; more primary care visits, and twice as much surgery (Hulme, 2000);
- consider themselves as alcoholics, have used illegal drugs, and have injected drugs, and have an increased risk of attempted suicide (Felitti *et al.*, 2001);
- have a greater risk of developing major depression compared with people who do not have an abuse history (Briere & Elliot, 1994);
- suffer from conduct disorders, depression and suicide (Fergusson *et al.*, 1996);
- have children with hyperactivity, conduct problems, peer or emotional problems (Roberts *et al.*, 2004).

Female survivors of child sexual abuse:

- are ten times more likely to have a history of drug addiction and two times more likely to have been alcoholics than members of the control group (Briere & Runtz, 1987);
- have a higher risk of sexual activities than non-abused females with: earlier age of first intercourse; two or more partners; unprotected intercourse and STIs (Kendall-Tackett, 2002).

Whilst the quality of these studies may vary there is a clear and consistent pattern of messages that makes the association between child abuse and its impact on health explicit. This is more so with some forms of abuse that have been easier to measure/observe e.g. physical abuse and less so with sexual abuse, neglect and emotional maltreatment that may be more challenging to research. Despite the variance across the studies, the wealth of evidence to date suggests an association between child abuse and poor health that could be readily applied to Bradford Hill's criteria for causation (Bradford Hill, 1965).

This evidence demonstrates that the health visitor's role in safeguarding is not only to seek to protect a child from harm in the short term, but also to optimise and promote the child's future trajectory for health into adulthood. It is also important to consider that when working with parents/adults experiencing the health problems mentioned above, they may have been exposed to adverse childhood experiences or indeed be survivors of child abuse themselves.

Defining significant harm

The concept of significant harm represents a legal definition of child abuse, and was first introduced in Section 31(9) of the Children Act 1989. The concept reflects a threshold that legitimises state intervention into the lives of children and families to safeguard and promote child welfare. Under Section 47 of the Children Act 1989 social workers as employees of 'local authorities' have a duty to 'make enquiries' or begin investigations, undertaking assessments and gathering information to inform decision-making regarding actions that may need to be taken to protect a child who is suffering, or at risk of suffering, significant harm. As part of this process where the age of the child is relevant to the recent or current work of health visitors, social workers will communicate with health visitors in the investigation process and may draw from health or other assessments. As a result of such activities led by social workers, courts may subsequently make a care order (whereby the child is committed to the care of the local authority) or supervision order (whereby the child is put under the supervision of a social worker or probation officer) where the threshold criteria is reached. Figure 5.1 specifies the threshold criteria and breaks down the concept of significant harm. What is clear from this is the important contribution that health visitors have to make to child protection processes in respect of sharing their well-documented assessments of children's circumstances and experiences, their physical and mental health and all aspects of their development; physical, emotional, behavioural, intellectual and social.

The concept of significant harm is ambiguous, subjective and open to interpretation by individual practitioners and representatives of various authorities. Its effectiveness in protecting the right children at the right moment in time will thus be inconsistent as individual cases will, by their very nature, vary as will the knowledge, experience, skills and confidence of practitioners working with them. Health visitors should be aware that there are no absolute criteria on which professionals can rely when judging what constitutes significant harm. The interpretation of significant harm as a threshold for

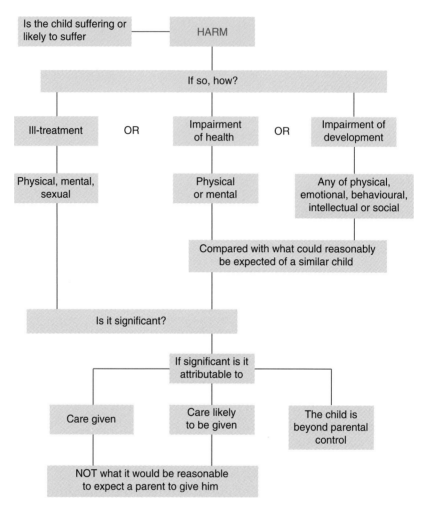

Figure 5.1 Threshold criteria.
Source: White *et al.* (2002). (Reproduced by kind permission from Lexis Nexis.)

intervention is not static and depends on a number of factors that can be explored further in Activity 5.6 (see Appendix 5).

A clear example of the sometimes acutely volatile nature of the threshold for intervention may be seen in response to the case of Peter Connelly (previously known as Baby P) who died in 2007 as a result of extreme physical abuse and neglect. Following Peter's death there was an unprecedented rise in applications for neglected and abused children to be taken into care with March 2010 producing the highest ever number of care applications recorded in an individual month (CAFCASS, 2010). At the time of writing the demand for care applications has remained extremely high. Variations in the threshold for removing the most vulnerable children at risk of, or actually suffering, significant harm from their families presents challenges in practice. When the threshold for intervention is high it may be difficult for professionals to succeed in getting very vulnerable children into care. Such children may be exposed to continuing risk of abuse and neglect and are more dependent on higher levels of support and supervision within the community. Clearly this has an impact on health visiting and other family support services.

The concept of significant harm as a threshold for intervention thus presents challenges, both in theory and practice. Both Nettleton (1998) and Appleton (1994) have identified the stress that occurs for health visitors when working with families in which there are significant concerns about the harms that children may be subjected to, but where a threshold has not been reached to trigger formal intervention by child protection services. The key here is for health visitors to underpin their carefully and clearly written referrals, assessments and reports with reference to research and the evidence base. Such an approach will help to form the basis of collaborative, critical, evidence-based decision-making to determine whether or not a child is being subjected to significant harm. Despite its ambiguities, Harwin and Madge (2010) acknowledge that the concept of significant harm has largely stood the test of time and that the absence of a clear operational definition is both its strength and weakness. They consider that its definition allows for necessary professional discretion acknowledging that its vulnerabilities are associated with external pressures that affect its interpretation and suggest that a more confident workforce and sufficient resources are required.

An advantage of the legal concept of significant harm not being static is of particular interest to health visitors working with families in which there is domestic abuse. Section 120 of the Children and Adoption Act 2002 amended Section 31 of the Children Act 1989 by extending the legal definition of harm to include harm suffered by seeing or hearing the ill treatment of others. This amendment occurred in recognition of society's growing awareness of both the scale of domestic abuse and its negative impact on children and young people. Women suffering domestic abuse may experience multiple forms of abuse; physical, psychological, sexual and financial. It has been estimated that at least 750 000 children witness domestic abuse each year (DH, 2002) and that in homes where domestic abuse occurs children witness approximately three-quarters of incidents (Royal College of Psychiatrists, 2004). Hughes (1992) found that in 90% of cases when domestic abuse is occurring the children are in the same or next room. Thus even when children do not directly see violent or abusive incidents, they are likely to be exposed to hearing both the acts of abuse as well as the reaction of the victim. Furthermore, they will subsequently be exposed to its physical and emotional impact. Being exposed to domestic abuse can cause children harm in a number of ways; for example seeing and hearing a parent (most likely their mother) being abused can cause children emotional distress; children may sustain physical injuries during violent physical assaults when they attempt to intervene to protect a parent; and children may be forced to take part in various forms of abuse or witness it (DH, 2009). Forcing children to take part in or witness abuse reduces them to being used as tools. This behaviour dehumanises children and increases both their own and their mother's suffering. Threats are often made to harm or kill children in an attempt to exert power and control over women. In 30–60% of cases where women are being abused, children are also being physically and/or sexually abused (Edelson, cited in DH, 2009). This is significant when working with families where domestic abuse occurs. Health visitors need to consider that children may be at risk of suffering or actually suffering significant harm through both their exposure to it or additional forms of abuse. Likewise when working with families where there is suspected or known child abuse the possibility that domestic abuse may be occurring should be considered and explored.

Amendments to the Children Act 1989 in respect of domestic abuse demonstrate the importance of updating legislation to reflect society's growing understanding of concepts of abuse. However, it should be acknowledged that society and legislators may take some time to respond to and accept the changing knowledge base about what constitutes child abuse. Take as an example many failed attempts to make child smacking an offence. The repercussions are that the law may not be terribly explicit in safeguarding children from contentious or newly emerging forms of child abuse, leaving some children inadequately provided for. It is vital therefore that health visitors place themselves in a position to influence policies affecting health (CETHV, 1977) by lobbying for changes in national legislation to safeguard children whilst keeping abreast of legislative changes that impact on their everyday practice.

Incidence and prevalence of child abuse

The terms incidence and prevalence hold their own distinct features and can provide useful information on the extent of a given condition in the population. Incidence has been defined as the number of new events occurring within a given population within a specified period of time (Last, 2001). Within the context of child abuse, this refers mainly to those cases of child abuse that are reported and recorded (Creighton, 2007). Prevalence, however, refers to the number of events in a given population at a designated time (Last, 2001). Again, within the context of child abuse this says more about the extent of child abuse in the community and includes both unreported and reported cases. Data on prevalence is mainly reliant on survey based studies to identify the 'hidden' unreported cases. This could be done for example by asking a sample of adults or young people whether they were abused during their childhood regardless of whether it was reported or not. Consequently the nature and outcomes of such studies can only provide estimates of the extent of child abuse in the community or population as a whole.

Prevalence studies have been conducted in the USA, UK and Netherlands over the last 30 years or so and are mostly confined to child sexual abuse (Creighton, 2007). By virtue of the problems associated with these studies and their inherent biases, the prevalence estimates range markedly across studies. For example, in relation to child sexual abuse, the percentage of adults and adolescents affected varies from 6.8-20.4% (women and girls) and 1-16.2% (men and boys) (Creighton, 2007). Some international studies have shown that, depending on the country, between a quarter and a half of all children

Table 5.1 Section 47 enquiries and initial child protection conferences in England which started during the year 1 April, 2008–31 March, 2009.

	Numbers
Children subject to Section 47 enquiries	84 100
Children who were the subject of an initial child protection conference	43 700

Source: DCSF(2009) Statistical First Release 22/2009.
(Reproduced with kind permission).

report severe and frequent physical abuse, which includes being beaten, kicked or tied up by parents (WHO & ISPCAN, 2006).

In relation to socioeconomic status, some studies have suggested a relationship between income and harm to children (DH, 1995; Baldwin & Caruthers, 1998; Corby, 2000). This predominantly relates to physical harm and neglect. However, whilst there may be more known cases of physical abuse or neglect amongst families with lower socioeconomic status, it does not appear to be true of sexual and emotional abuse. Studies have been consistent in failing to find differences in the prevalence of sexual abuse according to socioeconomic status (Parton, 1997). Given that most statistics associated with child abuse are based on known and reported cases, it may only reflect that low income families are more likely to have contact with state agencies and professionals, in a variety of contexts and as such are susceptible to a greater level of state surveillance than families on higher incomes. Caution also needs to be applied when considering data at a population level that are not directly attributable to individuals, i.e. not every parent on a low income abuses their children and vice versa.

A starting point for determining the threshold at which child abuse is reported can be the numbers of Section 47 enquiries that take place. As an example, Table 5.1 shows the number of enquiries that took place in England over a one-year period and the subsequent number of these enquiries that led to initial child protection conferences. The table also shows that whilst section 47 places a duty on social services departments to investigate whether there is a need for further action to safeguard a child's welfare, almost half of these cases did not lead to an initial child protection case conference. This is further evidence of the extent to which health visitors will find themselves working with families with vulnerable children who are exposed to an environment which at the very least lies close to the threshold for recognition as child abuse.

Figure 5.2 demonstrates the rising trend in the recording of child abuse cases from 26 / 10 000 to 34 / 10 000 children under 18 years between 2000 and 2009. The trend of course is not completely linear and suggests that the recording of abuse is linked to other factors besides the actual numbers of abused children. For example, the rises in 2002/3 and 2008/9 may be associated with the response of children's services to the Victoria Climbié and Peter Connolly cases respectively.

Figure 5.3 presents another perspective on the numbers of children recognised as abused and subject to a child protection plan between 2000 and 2009. Health visitors particularly will note the largest group of children is aged under four. School age children in total present an even larger group which in itself presents challenges for school nursing services. Again, the trend is not linear, with a slight 'U' shape, with a decrease up to 2002 but with particular rises in the under-four age group again around 2003 and most steeply from 2008. Again, the reasons are not entirely clear as to why this is. Changes in trend can be as a result of particular events that occur, e.g.

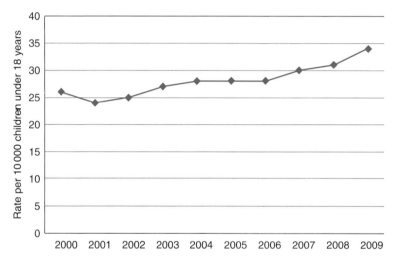

Figure 5.2   Children who became subject to a Child Protection Plan in England during the years 2000–2009.
Source: DCSF (2009), Statistical First Release 22/2009. (Reproduced by kind permission.)

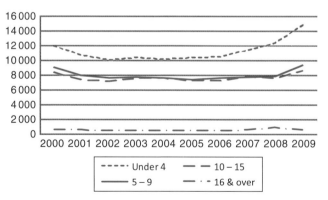

Figure 5.3   Number of children who were the subject of a Child Protection Plan in England, by age group at 31 March 2000–2009.
Source: DCSF (2009), Statistical First Release 22/2009. (Reproduced by kind permission.)

- As above, a possible response by services to high profile cases with a resultant tendency to acknowledge behaviour as abusive, where it may not previously have been perceived so.
- Changes in policy:
  - o The introduction of the Framework for Assessment of Children in Need in 2000 meant that some children who would have been previously placed on the Child Protection Register could now be defined as 'in need'.
  - o The categorisation of abuse, e.g. the acknowledgement of domestic abuse as a form of child abuse may have contributed to an increase in cases in recent years.

Figure 5.4, goes further and breaks down the age groups into the recognised categories of abuse. It is clear across all the age groups that the predominant form is that of neglect, followed by emotional abuse. The incidence of physical abuse appears to decline with age. Health visitors therefore face difficult challenges of working with families with abused young children, where clearly the emphasis is on fostering good parenting skills and positive, warm relationships between parents and their children.

Despite the variation across studies there is a large group of children who are subjected to different forms of abuse that never come to the attention of the authorities. Those that are reported and subsequently recorded as abuse form the 'tip of the iceberg'. The figures above have to be placed within the context of the total population of children where the majority of children are not abused. For health visitors and school nurses this reinforces the importance of the fundamental and universal nature of their provision which should remain pivotal to their work with children and families.

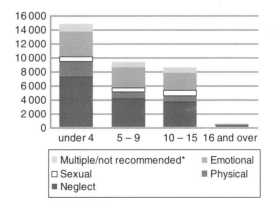

*'Multiple' refers to instances where there is more than one main category of abuse. These children are not counted under the other abuse headings, so a child can appear only once in this table. 'Not recommended' refers to classificatory categories not recommendated by *Working Together* (1999).

Figure 5.4 Number of children who were the subject of a Child Protection Plan in England, by age and category of abuse at 31 March, 2009.
Source: DCSF (2009), Statistical First Release 22/2009. (Reproduced by kind permission.)

Assessment of vulnerable children

Section 17 of the Children Act is concerned with the duty of local authorities including health authorities and health visitors to safeguard and promote the welfare of children in their area deemed to be 'in need'. In Section 17 a child in need is defined as:

(a) He is unlikely to achieve or maintain, or have the opportunity of achieving or maintaining, a reasonable standard of health or development without appropriate provision for him of services by a local authority under this Part;

(b) His health or development is likely to be significantly impaired, without the provision for him or her of services by a local authority under this Part; or

(c) He is disabled.

(Children Act 1989)

In line with the duty of authorities to safeguard and promote the welfare of children in need, local authorities are required to promote the upbringing of children in need by their families by providing a range and level of services appropriate to those children's needs. This provision reflects an underlying principle of the Children Act 1989 that wherever possible children should be brought up by their families. It is important to bear in mind though that this duty is not absolute. The cost implications of meeting identified needs through resources are huge and resources need to be allocated effectively. As a result there is an acknowledgement that resources need to be prioritised according to the assessment of need. Authorities are not required to meet the needs of every single child but are required to take reasonable steps to do so and make provisions as they consider appropriate. Section 17 is clearly significant to the work of health visitors in that it seeks to acknowledge the importance of the safety, health, development and emerging potential of vulnerable children. Health visitors are trained to work with children and families to search for health needs, stimulate awareness of health needs and facilitate health enhancing activities (CETHV, 1977). However, the effectiveness of this provision in the context of health visiting is weakened by both inadequate resourcing of both Section 17 generally and the retention of health visiting services.

The Framework for the Assessment of Children in Need and Their Families

The allocation of resources both to those children in need of support under Section 17 and those in need of possible and actual protection are dependent on effective assessment of children's needs. As highlighted in Chapters 2 and 3, a key element of the health visitor's role relates to the assessment of health needs of children and their families. To support professionals in the process of assessing vulnerable children, the Framework for the Assessment of Children in Need and Their Families was introduced to ensure accurate and effective assessment and a timely response by services (DH & DfEE, 2000).

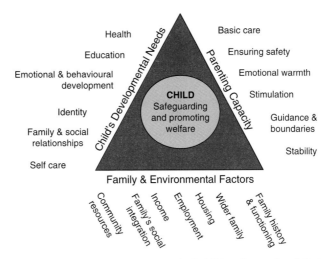

Figure 5.5 Framework for the assessment of children in need and their families.
Source: DH (2000) © Crown copyright. (Reproduced by kind permission.)

The Framework requires consideration of the child's health and development needs, parenting capacity and relevant social and environmental factors (see Figure 5.5). These are described as three domains, each of which contains a number of critical dimensions (DH & DfEE, 2000).

Health visitors need a working understanding of this framework and to maintain relevant, contemporaneous records that detail not only areas of concern but also areas of strength and positivity within a child's life that reflect these critical dimensions. Behaviours or events that cause concern or constitute significant harm may emerge suddenly or surface gradually over time. Sudden major concerns relating to significant harm may occur as a result of a single significant event, for example the violent shaking of a neonate, or the beating or rape of a child. Conversely, a temporal, gradually unfolding picture of concern may emerge through a compilation of seemingly less significant events occurring over a much longer period of time. The corrosive impact of neglect as a form of child abuse on children's health and wellbeing is a good but not exclusive example of how significant harm occurs in this way. A further example from a parenting perspective relates to those parents who exhibit low warmth towards and high criticism of their children (DH, 1995). In such cases the realisation that significant harm may be occurring is based on reflection of the significance of both retrospective and current events and knowledge. The Framework above is useful therefore in assisting health visitors to articulate their knowledge of unmet need and possible child abuse within a chronological context and supports both their referrals to other agencies and any statutory assessments undertaken by social workers.

The Framework for the Assessment of Children in Need and Their Families clearly can provide a useful mechanism to support practice. However, where there are health visitors carrying large and/or complex caseloads, practice shifts from the larger population of children who may have some degree of unrecognised, unmet need and who are possibly at risk to a smaller distinct group of vulnerable children whose needs have already been recognised and prioritised. A silent escalation of risk can occur in the larger population of children that eventually crosses the threshold from children in need of support to children in need of protection resulting in even heavier demands upon services. The utility of the Framework therefore lies within the opportunity for contact with children for early intervention. However, where there is no contact there is no opportunity to assess and meet unmet need and a greater likelihood of practice becoming crisis-led. Furthermore, even when contact between health visitors and families occurs, barriers to the opportunistic recognition of abuse within practice exist and should be considered. For example 'routine' top-to-toe examinations of babies during primary visits may no longer occur and babies may be seen and weighed less frequently than they once were. Good leadership and decision-making becomes an essential part of the health visiting role in these circumstances that call for innovative practice, political awareness and confidence to work in different settings. An example of good leadership might be a health visitor working in partnership with a local faith group to raise awareness of children's needs for safety and protection in a faith setting with the aim of establishing a safeguarding policy. A strength of such an approach would be that the faith leaders may themselves become partners in identifying vulnerable children at risk of suffering or suffering actual harm.

Common Assessment Framework (CAF)

The Every Child Matters Strategy (DfES, 2004) introduced the Common Assessment Framework (CAF) following Lord Laming's (2003) report into the death of Victoria Climbié in 2000. The CAF is a useful shared assessment and planning framework for use across children's services and local areas in England (for an example of a CAF form see http://www.cwdcouncil.org.uk/caf). At face value the introduction of 'another' assessment framework may appear confusing. Some clarity on the relationship between the CAF and the Framework for the Assessment of Children in Need and their Families is therefore of value at this point.

The CAF is recognised as a supplement to the Framework for the Assessment of Children in Need and their Families and as its name suggests provides a common framework to needs assessment that is recognised and used by the whole range of children's services. Its purpose is to provide a more efficient approach to assessing children's needs by avoiding unnecessary duplication and promoting integration of frontline services (CWDC, 2008). It is for practitioners who may be concerned that a child is at risk of not achieving one or more of the five outcomes of every child matters and where the support of one or more agencies is required when the practitioner perceives that the child's additional needs cannot be met by the existing service.

The CWDC (2008) provides a helpful breakdown of the CAF components:

- a pre-assessment checklist to help practitioners identify children who may benefit from a common assessment;
- a three-step process for undertaking the common assessment;
- a standard form for practitioners to record and where appropriate, share information from the assessment with others.

The CAF is *not* for a child when practitioners have concerns that the child may be suffering, or may be at risk of suffering harm. In these cases the practitioner's local safeguarding children's board (LSCB) safeguarding procedures should be followed immediately and if necessary advice sought from the local safeguarding or child protection team. In these cases health visitors and other professionals may find it useful to refer to guidance such as *Working Together* (DCSF, 2010) and *What to Do if You're Worried a Child Is Being Abused* (DfES, 2006). However, where there have been long-standing problems or concerns in families where child protection concerns emerge it is likely that other services have been involved with a child or young person and their family and that a CAF is in place. Clearly assessments undertaken as part of the CAF process should inform work undertaken to protect children who are suffering or likely to suffer significant harm.

The CAF is a voluntary process and given the requirements of the Data Protection Act 1998 children and/or their parents/carers must give their consent at the start of the CAF process for the assessment to take place. The CAF may be opened before, or in support of a referral or subsequent specialist assessment. However, it is not a referral form per se. CAFs can be useful in the referral process to ensure that the referral to a specialist service is relevant and should help to reduce the duplication of repeated assessment. Furthermore a CAF may assist in building up a holistic picture of needs and as such is likely to carry greater weight in a referral process than a series of partial isolated snapshots. Whilst on the one hand the CAF can be a tool that supports health visitors' work with children and families, it also presents challenges for health visitors. In Brandon *et al.*'s (2006) early evaluation of the introduction of the CAF, health and education services are cited as carrying the bulk of common assessments. In addition, Brandon *et al.*'s work identified that some workers highlighted their confidence/skills gap in taking up the role of Lead Professional and chairing meetings. Working with vulnerable children and the CAF process is a good opportunity for health visitors to build their confidence and develop and demonstrate effective leadership skills in a multidisciplinary arena. It is important to recognise that whilst assessment tools such as the CAF and the Framework for the Assessment of Children in Need and their Families are the mainstay of effective assessment in safeguarding practice, a range of other assessment tools exist. Such tools have been and continue to be developed to respond to specific forms and contexts of abuse and may be used in an integrated way to compliment assessments undertaken using the frameworks discussed above. One tool which is being increasingly adopted by Local Safeguarding Children's Boards and practitioners for use in practice is the Graded Care Profile (GCP), an assessment tool designed specifically for use in cases of suspected and actual neglect.

Graded Care Profile

It is important to recognise that neglect may take various forms (Howe, 2005) and that different perspectives of these forms will influence how it is assessed by practitioners. As highlighted earlier in the text, neglect has a significant impact on health visitors' practice and workload. Ayre (2007) acknowledges that despite knowledge of the deleterious impact of neglect on children, practitioners continue to apply alarmingly high thresholds for intervention. This had been highlighted as a particular concern within health (Srivastava et al., 2003) for some time.

The Graded Care Profile is a tool developed by Dr Prakash Srivastava, a community paediatrician, and aims to assist practitioners to quantify in an objective manner, the different levels of care offered by any caregiver (for an example of the GCP see http://www.lutonlscb.org/index.php?option=com_con tent&view–article&id–183&Itemid–52). The tool is based on Maslow's (1943, 1954) Hierarchy of Needs and focuses on four domains of care; Physical Care, Safety, Love and Esteem. Assessment outcomes are scored on a summary sheet and are useful in helping to form a baseline assessment, set targets for improvements in parenting and set an agreed threshold for referral to children's services. Srivastava et al.'s (2003) account of early evaluation highlights a number of strengths in respect of the Graded Care Profile, including:

- cost effectiveness;
- leads to interventions being targeted;
- appropriate and easy to use across professions and agencies;
- popular with professionals and families as caregivers, children and young people; may contribute their own evaluations of care given;
- identifies strengths as well as weaknesses of care giving;
- decreased subjectivity, increased objectivity associated with the assessment of neglect.

Success of the Graded Care Profile to date suggests that it has worked well at a local level; more substantive research into its use is eagerly awaited. Evidence-based assessment tools are essential if assessment in practice is to be acceptable to children, families and the professionals involved in safeguarding children effectively from neglect.

Working together

Evidently, one of the strengths of assessment frameworks is that they provide a mechanism for professionals and agencies to engage with each other to understand the needs of children and assess the degree to which a child might be at risk of harm. Indeed, Section 10 of the Children Act 2004 introduced a requirement of agencies to cooperate for the best outcomes for children.

This is clearly very important, as the outcomes from public inquiries and serious case reviews following the deaths of children have consistently highlighted the fact that professionals and agencies from health, children's services and the police fail to work together effectively. There have been gross errors in communication that may have contributed to a child suffering harm. Take for example the case of Peter Connelly.

> Poor communication and lack of detailed background information about the case also led to delays in making appropriate assessments. For example, at the child protection case conference on 16 March 2007, it was stated in the action points of the case conference that a paediatric assessment was needed. However, the health visitor did not complete a referral for assessment until 10 April 2007. We do not have any information that indicates why the referral took almost a month to be undertaken. It was then delayed further because insufficient information was provided on the referral form. The referral was subsequently rejected by the clinic at St Ann's Hospital until further information was supplied.
>
> (Care Quality Commission, 2009: 16)

Despite constant messages from inquiry reports that stress the importance of inter-agency working this failure suggests that professionals and agencies need to 'learn to learn' from such failures if those children most at risk are to be adequately protected. All too often assumptions are made between professionals without clarification or evidence of understanding. The case study in Box 5.2 relates to the death of Khrya Ishaq and highlights this point.

Box 5.2   Case study: Khyra Ishaq (extracts in *italics* from Serious Case Review (Radford, 2010)

Khyra was the second youngest child in a family of six children, all born to the same parents. She was seven years old when she died in May 2008; her mother and mother's partner were later convicted of manslaughter, causing/allowing the death of a child and five other offences of cruelty in relation to the other children. At post mortem Khrya was described as severely malnourished with severe wasting. The evidence indicated that severe malnutrition was due to inadequate nutrition and that she had suffered starvation over a period of several months.

Para 11.39
26th February 2007 – During Health Visitor 8's contact with mother at the Medical Centre the mother informed the Health Visitor she was very frightened of her ex husband who was very abusive and was inflicting emotional abuse on the children which was having a severe impact on their behaviour. He had asked the children to be uncooperative to their mother and has physically abused them by hitting them if they do not

(Continued)

Box 5.2 *(Continued)*

obey him ... Health Visitor was clear given the information provided she would need to make a referral to Children's Social Care.

Para 11.40
28th February 2007 - Referral made by Health Visitor 8 to Children's Social Care letter read 'I have referred this family because of concerns raised by the children's mother there is a history of domestic violence in this family the parents are no longer married or have any intimate relations according to mother however, persistent abuse still occurs when he visits children ... The letter continues 'mother feels that her ex spouse's behaviour has had a severe impact on her children's behaviour and in my opinion this family needs an urgent assessment and investigation into father's second family.'

[Paragraphs 11.41-11.84 related to incidents or concerns arising from other agencies including the school)

Para 11.85
30th Jan 2008 Referral and Advice Officer, Children's Social Care contacted the Health Visitor who stated she had had no contact with the family since her referral in 2007 despite her own concerns. Health Visitor was requested to check whether a sibling had received the correct immunisations and discussed issues in relation to mother's mental health.

Para 12.3.9
The health visitor did not maintain any contact or support to the family following the referral, although the health visitor made two unsuccessful attempts to contact mother by telephone following the referral. The health visitor had received a letter from Children's Social Care stating that they had completed an assessment and there were no concerns as the mother was able to protect the children and herself. The father was no longer living with the family at that time.

Confidentiality and information sharing

In the context of multi-agency working and safeguarding children of those challenges listed above, the issues of communication, confidentiality and information sharing are those that may seem most contentious and anxiety provoking to professionals in practice. Indeed Lord Laming's progress report (2009) noted that in some situations practitioners remain uncertain about when they can share information. There is, however, a range of legislation and policy that helps to guide professional practice. A broad platform for this includes relevant sections of:

- The Human Rights Act 1998;
- The Data Protection Act 1998;

- The Crime and Disorder Act 1998;
- The Children Act 2004;
- The NHS Act 2006;
- The Common Law Duty of Confidentiality.

Clear guidance on information sharing such as *Information Sharing: Guidance for Practitioners and Managers Guide* (DCSF, 2008) is particularly useful to practitioners. All legislation and policy underpins the professional guidance offered by the Code (NMC, 2008) which states:

- You must respect people's right to confidentiality;
- You must ensure people are informed about how and why information is shared by those who will be providing their care;
- You must disclose information if you believe someone may be at risk of harm in line with the law of the country in which you are practising.

The use of higher level communication skills is an essential part of health visiting practice and the nature of the health visitor client relationship is that sensitive information may be disclosed by the client during contacts. In many cases the health visitor will be able to respect and maintain the client's confidentiality; however, health visitors must not give an absolute guarantee of confidentiality as there are times when confidentiality cannot be kept and information must be shared. Information does need to be shared when practitioners have reasonable cause to believe that a child or adult may be suffering or at risk of suffering significant harm. Information sharing should be carried out preferably with the client's consent. However, where consent cannot be obtained it is possible to share information to protect others. In some cases court orders are made which require practitioners to share confidential information unless their employing organisation is prepared to challenge the court order. In all cases where information needs to be shared, health visitors must ensure that they follow the most up-to-date guidance and seek support where necessary. Of particular interest to health visitors working with a wide age range of children in a safeguarding arena are guidelines around not only obtaining the consent of adults but children and young people too. Where children have the capacity to consent or not to information sharing, the process of seeking their views and opinions on matters concerning their welfare may be deemed as children's rights compliant. Where information sharing is necessary it is important that only relevant information is shared appropriately, with only those other professionals and agencies who need to know.

Supervision

The need for health visitors to work safely and effectively together with vulnerable children and their families in a safeguarding context cannot be overstated. Indeed, safety and effectiveness demands key skills from health visitors which also depend upon good interagency working and partnerships. Over recent years, supervision in the health visitors' safeguarding role has been increasingly recognised as crucial for achieving these aims. It has been described as an elementary requirement of each service (Laming, 2009) and a 'right' of those working with children at all levels of intervention (Brandon *et al.*, 2009). Supervision has been defined as, 'an accountable process which supports assures and develops the knowledge, skills and values of an individual, group or team' (Skills for Care & Children's Workforce Development Council, 2007: 5). Supervision aims to help health visitors develop the necessary skills, confidence and judgement and should be regular and proactive (DCSF, 2010). The extracts below in Box 5.3, taken from high profile Inquiry Reports demonstrate that whilst the nature of supervision from the 1980s to the present date has changed, the deaths of these children were underpinned by services that evoked a sense of apathy and lack of prioritisation towards the supervision of staff for protecting children.

Box 5.3 Supervision

Jasmine Beckford: Extracts in *italics* from the Panel of Inquiry Report by London Borough of Brent (1985: 143)

Jasmine was the oldest of three children who was four years old when she died in July 1984 after being subjected to severe physical abuse over a period of time. Her stepfather, Morris Beckford was found guilty of manslaughter and jailed for 10 years. Her mother, Beverley Lorrington, was jailed for 18 months for neglect.

Miss Tyler, Senior Nurse, told us that the health visitors under her supervision ... were expected to recognise their own areas of weakness and of doubt about their responses to individual cases, and to approach her for guidance and assistance. She considered that there was no obligation on her part to monitor the performance of a health visitor. The crux of supervision to her was self-monitoring by the supervised of his or her own performance; once problems were so identified, to seek help from the supervisor.

This Inquiry recommended the need for *'establishing the practice of planning regular discussions between health visitors and their senior nurses, even if she does not consider there to be a problem with which she is able to deal'*.

Peter Connelly: Extract in *italics* from the Review of the involvement and action taken by health bodies in relation to the case of Baby P (Care Quality Commission, 2009)

Peter Connelly (known previously as Baby P) died in August 2007 aged 17 months after suffering months of severe physical abuse including a fracture / dislocation of the thoraco-lumbar spine. Peter's mother pleaded guilty to causing or allowing his death, her partner and a lodger was also found guilty of the same charge. Following the Serious Case Review into Peter's death the CQC visited four trusts involved in his care and found an absence of child protection supervision.

The Whittington Hospital NHS Trust

Staff reported that there is no formal safeguarding supervision system in place that incorporates reflective practice. However, there are weekly multidisciplinary team meetings for safeguarding and child protection staff. In addition, named professionals have the opportunity to attend monthly peer support meetings but, at present, these meetings have not been given priority due to work commitments.

Paediatric services managed by Great Ormond Street Hospital at North Middlesex University Hospital NHS Trust

While there are weekly multidisciplinary team meetings for safeguarding and child protection staff at the trust, staff reported a lack of safeguarding supervision. In addition, they disclosed a lack of formal one-to-one meetings with their line managers or supervisors. While staff reported having good working relationships, particularly in the A&E department, some staff reported feeling isolated in their role, and that such supervision would provide an element of support to them.

Paediatric services managed by Great Ormond Street Hospital at Haringey Teaching PCT

A number of staff reported that they were not currently receiving any form of safeguarding supervision. Despite this, staff were aware of the appropriate person to approach if they wanted to discuss a case or raise concerns. In general, staff reported that they felt able to access supervision if they needed it. However, due to time constraints, supervision was not being made a priority. Staff reported feeling isolated at St Ann's Hospital and, due to the low staffing levels, reported that there is little sense of team working. In addition, due to the shortage of staff within St Ann's Hospital, peer supervision does not appear to be a viable option at this time.

The Royal College of Nursing (RCN) (2007) recognise that professionals must 'have the skills to acknowledge, examine and work through their own feelings, experiences, values and beliefs regarding children, child abuse and safeguarding children' (p. 9). Clinical supervision is the mechanism which allows this process. Clearly, in relation to the skills outlined above, the ability of practitioners to reflect honestly, critically and analytically is crucial if they wish to develop their safeguarding knowledge, skills and expertise and make critical judgements. Such skills can only develop with time and experience but form the basis for strong and effective leadership for safeguarding practice. However, the quality and thus effectiveness of supervision will be dependent upon a number of factors not least the knowledge, skills and expertise of the supervisor who may be a peer, manager, named or designated professional. Other important factors are the frequency and time allocated to supervisory sessions. Too often, health visitors have been reliant upon informal, peer led supervision that occurs where there is no formal supervision (Nettleton, 1998). Brandon *et al.*'s (2009) study cited one health visitor receiving six monthly safeguarding supervision. Clearly this is inadequate, especially in the context of the current challenges within the health visiting services including low numbers of health visitors, large complex caseloads and health visitors carrying child protection issues that would once have been referred onto children's social care services. These are all issues raised by Lord Laming (2009) in his latest report.

Key findings from interviews held as part of Brandon *et al.*'s (2009) analysis into serious case reviews highlighted:

- the need for regular and sufficiently frequent supervision;
- that key issues are monitored and followed up (including missed appointments);
- that supervision should consider continuity of approach to the family;
- that extra support for less experienced workers should be provided;
- the creation of a structured sharing of uncertainty in order to reach the best possible response to concerns.

Whilst these points are a very necessary aspect of child protection supervision that is led by experts in safeguarding, there is also another aspect of supervision that is essential for the practitioner to have the right level of knowledge and skills for the 'working together' arena. A supervisory relationship that encourages the practitioner to be critically reflective is most likely to be productive where the protection of children is concerned. It is important to consider what is actually meant by 'critical' reflection. It is not just a superficial discussion of practicalities around a case. Critical reflection has been defined as 'A process of reflection which incorporates analysis of individuals' thinking with regard to the influence of socially dominant thinking' (Fook & Askeland, 2006: 41). Therefore health visitors need to be open to new perspectives on how they work with children who are at risk or have been abused and be ready to challenge their pre-existing, dominant assumptions about abuse and the need for a child-focused response. If utilised effectively within supervision, the health visitor becomes more aware of how broader social factors impact upon the family, develops skills to challenge appropriately and equally crucial, understands the boundaries within which they can practise safely and effectively.

Therefore, experience alone is not the only prerequisite for a good child protection supervisor. Child protection supervision requires critical thinking and communication skills that take the supervisory relationship to a new level. In a supportive environment the supervisee is enabled to confront their own values, perceptions and practice to form a robust approach to safeguarding. This raises issues and challenges for organisations that need to develop those individuals who may take on a supervisory role. Indeed, supervision training should not be a one-off event; rather, there should be opportunities for supervisors to develop their knowledge and skills on an ongoing basis. This leads further to the vital consideration *'quis custodiet ipsos custodes'* – who will guard the guardians? Or who supervises the supervisors? Child protection supervision requires a structured framework within an organisation with appropriate resourcing in order to safeguard not only the children it aims to protect but also the wellbeing of staff and the integrity of the organisation.

Summary

This chapter has highlighted some of the challenges that may confront health visitors and other practitioners in their safeguarding practice. In recent decades child abuse and the protection of children under the umbrella term 'safeguarding' has received a higher prominence in society and as a result the health visitor's role is underpinned with a plethora of policy and guidance from an international to local level. The extent and patterning of child abuse across society has enabled an understanding of the burden of child protection work that health visitors face. There is a history of health visiting's association with child welfare and the protection of children from abuse which has become reinforced with the development of the profession and its duties under the auspices of the NMC.

Key concepts have been considered here as a means of highlighting the tensions that exist when working with vulnerable children. An understanding of those tensions assists health visitors in working their way through the ambiguities of everyday practice. Furthermore, with a working knowledge of legislation and policy health visitors are able to undertake the safeguarding role in a safer and more effective way. The importance of agreed definitions of what constitutes child abuse has been highlighted alongside the need for health visitors to keep up to date with emerging forms of child abuse.

Case study material has been utilised to support the discussion and highlight the extent to which poor communication continues to blight the lives of children with gross errors and mis-assumptions between professionals. There is a need for assimilation of messages from serious case reviews and Inquiries into child deaths. The role of the health visitor is acknowledged in recent reports as giving added value to safeguarding services. The profession has a duty to respond to that acknowledgement by seeking to develop through research evidence the effectiveness of its function in safeguarding. Furthermore, the importance of supervision that enables health visitors to develop their knowledge, skills and expertise has been explored with an emphasis on the quality of supervision and the responsibilities of organisations to support this. At the time of writing there is significant change occurring within public sector organisations and it is vital over the coming years that safeguarding children remains a key focus of policy and health visiting practice and that the profession makes the most of every opportunity to advocate for the rights of children in an increasingly challenging world.

References

Appleton, J. (1994) The concept of vulnerability in relation to child protection: health visitors' perceptions. *Journal of Advanced Nursing*, **20**, 1132–1140.

Atkinson, M., Doherty, P. & Kinder, K (2005) Multi-agency working: models, challenges and key factors for success. *Journal of Early Childhood Research*, **3**(1), 7–17.

Ayre, P. (2007) Common ground: Child neglect. *Community Care*, 29 March–4 April, 36–37.

Baldwin, N. & Caruthers, L. (1998) *Developing Neighbourhood Support and Child Protection Strategies: The Henley Safe Children Project*. Ashgate Publishing Ltd, Farnham.

BBC News (2010) Facebook and Bebo child sex abuse postman jailed. 24 September. British Broadcasting Corporation, London. Available from: http://www.bbc.co.uk/news/uk-england-cornwall-11403984 (accessed 30 September, 2010).

Bradford Hill, A. (1965) The environment and disease: Association or causation? *Proceedings of the Royal Society of Medicine*, **58**, 295–300.

Brandon, M., Bailey, S., Belderson, P., *et al.* (2009) *Understanding Serious Case Reviews and their Impact A Biennial Analysis of Serious Case Reviews 2005–07*. DCSF, University of East Anglia.

Brandon, M., Howe, A., Dagley, V., Salter, C. & Warren, C. (2006) What appears to be helping or hindering practitioners in implementing the Common Assessment Framework and lead professional working? *Child Abuse Review*, **15**, 396–413.

Bremner, J.D. (1999) Does stress damage the brain? *Biological Psychiatry*, **45**, 797–805.

Briere, J.N. & Elliot, D.M. (1994) Immediate and long-term impacts of child sexual abuse. *The Future of Children*, **4**, 54–69.

Briere, J.N. & Runtz, M. (1987) Post sexual abuse trauma: Data and implications for clinical practice. *Journal of Interpersonal Violence*, **2**, 367–379.

Butler-Sloss, Dame E. (1988) *Report of the Inquiry into Child Abuse in Cleveland 1987*. Her Majesty's Stationery Office, London.

CAFCASS (2010) *Cafcass Care Demand – Latest Figures for April–August 2010* Children and Family Court Advisory Service. Available from: http://www.cafcass.gov.uk/publications/care_demand_statistics.aspx (accessed 30 September, 2010).

Caraher, M. & McNab, M. (1997) Using lessons from health visiting's past to inform the public health role. *Health Visitor*, **70**, 380–384.

Care Quality Commission (2009) Review of the involvement and action taken by health bodies in relation to the case of Baby P. CQC, London. Available from: http://www.cqc.org.uk/_db/_documents/Baby_Peter_report_FINAL_12_May_09_(2).pdf (Accessed 30 September, 2010).

CETHV (1977) *An Investigation into the Principles of Health Visiting*. Council for the Education & Training of Health Visitors, London.

Children's Workforce Development Council (2008) *Common Assessment Framework* CWDC, London.

Corby, B. (2000) *Child Abuse: Towards a Knowledge Base*. Open University Press, Milton Keynes.

Cowley, S. (1996) Reflecting on the past; preparing for the next century *Health Visitor*, **69**, 313–316.

CPHVA (2007) *Community Practitioners' and Health Visitors' Association Response to 'Facing the Future – A Review of the Role of Health Visitors'*. Available from:

http://www.dodsdata.com/Resources/epolitix/Forum%20Microsites/Amicus-Unite/Appendix%203.pdf (accessed 30 September, 2010).

Creighton, S. (2007) Patterns and outcomes. In: *The Child Protection Handbook* (eds K. Wilson & A. James), 3rd edn, pp. 31–48. Bailliere Tindall, London.

Department for Children, Schools and Families (2008) *Information Sharing: Guidance for Practitioners and Managers*. Department for Children, Schools and Families, London.

Department for Children, Schools and Families (2009) *Referrals, Assessment and Children and Young People Who Are the Subject of a Child Protection Plan, England – Year Ending 31 March 2009*. Available from: http://www.dcsf.gov.uk/rsgateway/DB/SFR/s000873/index.shtml (accessed 30 September, 2010).

Department for Children, Schools and Families (2010) *Working Together to Safeguard Children: A Guide to Inter-agency Working to Safeguard and Promote the Welfare of Children*. Department for Children, Schools and Families, London.

Department for Education and Skills (2004) *Every Child Matters: Change for Children*. Department for Education and Skills, London.

Department for Education and Skills (2006) *What to Do if You're Worried a Child Is Being Abused*. Department for Education and Skills, Nottingham. Available from: http://www.dh.gov.uk/en/Publicationsandstatistics/Publications/PublicationsPolicyAndGuidance/DH_4010283 (accessed 15 January, 2011).

Department of Health (1995) *Child Protection Messages from Research*. HMSO, London.

Department of Health (2002) *Women's Mental Health: Into the Mainstream*. Department of Health, London.

Department of Health (2004a) *Best Practice Guidance for Doctors and Other Health Professionals on the Provision of Advice and Treatment to Young People under 16 on Contraception, Sexual and Reproductive Health*. The Stationery Office, London.

Department of Health (2004b) *The Chief Nursing Officer's Review of the Nursing, Midwifery and Health Visiting Contribution to Vulnerable Children and Young People*. Department of Health, London.

Department of Health (2007) *Facing the future: A review of the role of health visitors* Stationery office, London. Available from: http://www.dh.gov.uk/en/Publicationsandstatistics/Publications/PublicationsPolicyAndGuidance/DH_075642 (accessed 20 September, 2010).

Department of Health (2009) *Improving Safety, Reducing Harm. Children, Young People and Domestic Violence: A Practical Toolkit for Front-line Practitioners*. TSO, London.

Department of Health, Department for Education and Employment, Home Office (2000) *Framework for the Assessment of Children in Need and their Families*. The Stationery Office, Norwich.

Elkan R., Kendrick D., Hewitt M. *et al.* (2000) The effectiveness of domiciliary health visiting: a systematic review of international studies and a selective review of the British literature. *Health Technology Assessment*, **4**(13), 199–230.

Family & Parenting Institute (2007) *Health Visiting an Endangered Species*. Family & Parenting Institute, London.

Felitti, V.J. (1991) Long-term medical consequences of incest, rape, and molestation. *Southern Medical Journal*, **84**, 328–331.

Felitti V.J., Anda, R.F., Nordenberg, D., *et al.* (1998) Relationship of childhood abuse and household dysfunction to many of the leading causes of death in adults: The Adverse Childhood Experiences (ACE) Study. *American Journal of Preventive Medicine*, **14**(4), 245–258.

Felitti, V.J., Anda, R.F., Nordenberg, D. *et al.* (2001) Relationship of childhood abuse and household dysfunction to many of the leading causes of death in adults. In: *Who Pays? We All Do: The Cost of Child Maltreatment* (eds K. Franey, R. Geffner, R. Falconer), pp. 53–69, Family Violence and Sexual Assault Institute, San Diego, CA.

Fergusson, D.M., Horwood, J., Lynskey, M.T. (1996) Childhood sexual abuse and psychiatric disorder in young adulthood; II: Psychiatric outcomes of childhood sexual abuse. *Journal American Academy Child Adolescent Psychiatry*, **34**, 1365-1374.

Fook, J. & Askeland, G.A. (2006) The 'Critical' in critical reflection. In: *Critical Reflection In Health & Social Care* (eds S. White, J. Fook, F. Gardner). Open University Press, Berkshire.

Glaser, D. (2000) Child abuse and neglect and the brain – a review. *Journal of Child Psychology and Psychiatry and Allied Disciplines*, **41**(1), 97-116.

Harwin, J. & Madge, N. (2010) The concept of significant harm in law and practice. *Journal of Children's Services*, **5**(2), 73-83.

Health Select Committee (2009) *Health Inequalities – Third Report*. The Stationery Office, London.

HM Government (2003) Every Child Matters. Presented to Parliament by the Chief Secretary to the Treasury by Command of Her Majesty, September 2003 (Cm 5860). The Stationery Offlce, London. Available from: http://www.education.gov.uk/consultations/downloadableDocs/EveryChildMatters.pdf (accessed 18 March, 2011).

Home Office (1945) *Report by Sir Walter Monckton KCMG KCVO MC KC on the Circumstances which Led to the Boarding Out of Dennis and Terence O'Neill at Bank Farm, Minsterly and the Steps Taken to Supervise Their Welfare.* Cmd 6636 London: Home Office.

Howe, D. (2005) *Child Abuse and Neglect: Attachment, Development and Intervention,* Palgrave Macmillan, Basingstoke.

Hughes, H. (1992) Impact of spouse abuse on children of battered women, *Violence Update*, August, 9-11.

Hulme, P.A. (2000) Symptomatology and health care utilization of women primary care patients who experienced childhood sexual abuse. *Child Abuse Neglect*, **24**, 1471-1484.

Kempe, H. & Helfer, R.E (1972) *Helping the Battered Child and his Family*. Lippincott, Philadelphia.

Kempe, R.S. & Kempe, H. (1978) *Child Abuse, the Developing Child*. Fontana, London.

Kendall-Tackett, K.A. (2000) Physiological correlates of childhood abuse: Chronic hyperarousal in PTSD, depression and irritable bowel syndrome. Invited review. *Child Abuse & Neglect*, **24**, 799-810.

Kendall-Tackett, K.A. (2002) The health effects of childhood abuse: four pathways by which abuse can influence health. *Child Abuse & Neglect*, **6/7**, 715-730.

Kendall-Tackett, K.A. & Marshall, R. (1999) Victimization and diabetes: An exploratory study. *Child Abuse & Neglect*, **23**, 593-596.

Laming, Lord H. (2003) *The Victoria Climbié Inquiry: Report of an Inquiry by Lord Laming*, CM5730. The Stationery Office, London.

Laming, Lord H. (2009) *The Protection of Children in England: A Progress Report*. The Stationery Office, London.

Last, J.M. (2001) *A Dictionary of Epidemiology*. Oxford University Press, Oxford.

London Borough of Brent (1985) *A Child in Trust. The Report of the Panel of Inquiry Investigating the Circumstances Surrounding the Death of Jasmine Beckford.* London Borough of Brent, London.

Marmot, M., Atkinson, T., Bell, J., *et al.* (2010) *Fair Society, Healthy Lives. The Marmot Review,* Marmot Review Team, University College London.

Martell, R. (1999) 'Getting it right'. *Community Practitioner,* **72**(5), 121-122.

Maslow, A.H. (1943) A theory of human motivation. *Psychological Review,* **50**(4), 370-396.

Maslow, A.H. (1954) *Motivation and Personality.* Harper, New York.

Nettleton, R. (1998) Child protection: health visiting and supervision. In: *Clinical Supervision and Mentorship in Nursing* (eds T. Butterworth, J. Fauguer, P. Burnard), 2nd edn, pp. 132-152. Stanley Thornes, Cheltenham.

NSPCC (2009) *Children Subject to Child Protection Plans - England 2005 - 2009* NSPCC, London. Available from: http://www.nspcc.org.uk/Inform/research/statistics/england_wdf49858.pdf (accessed 30 September, 2010).

Nursing and Midwifery Council (2004) *Standards of Proficiency for Specialist Community Public Health Nurses.* NMC, London.

Nursing and Midwifery Council (2008) *The Code: Standards of Conduct, Performance and Ethics for Nurses and Midwives.* Nursing and Midwifery Council, London.

Parton, N. (1997) *Child Protection Risk and the Moral Order.* Macmillan, Basingstoke.

Perry, B. (2002) Childhood experience and the expression of genetic potential: what childhood neglect tells us about nature and nurture. *Brain and Mind,* **3**, 79-100.

Pine, D.S. & Cohen, J.A. (2002) Trauma in children and adolescents: risk and treatment of psychiatric sequelae. *Biological Psychiatry,* **51**(7), 519-531.

Pinheiro, P.S. (2006) *World Report on Violence against Children.* United Nations, New York.

Puffett, N. (2010) Government clarifies ban on *Every Child Matters. Daily Bulletin Children and Young People Now.* 10 August. Available from: http://www.cypnow.co.uk/bulletins/Daily-Bulletin/news/1021116/?DCMP=EMC-DailyBulletin (accessed 30 September, 2010).

Radford, J. (2010) *Serious Case Review under Chapter VIII 'Working Together to Safeguard Children' in Respect of the Death of a Child, Case Number 14.* Birmingham Safeguarding Children Board, Birmingham.

Roberts, R., O'Connor, T., Dunn, J., Golding, J. & ALSPAC Study Team (2004) The effects of child sexual abuse in later family life; mental health, parenting and adjustment of offspring. *Child Abuse and Neglect,* **28**, 525-545.

Robinson, J. (1982) *An Evaluation of Health Visiting.* CETHV, London.

Royal College of Nursing (2007) *Safeguarding Children and Young People: Every Nurses's Responsibility.* RCN, London.

Royal College of Paediatrics & Child Health (2006) *Safeguarding Children and Young People: Roles and Competences for Health Care Staff. Intercollegiate Document.* RCPCH, London. Available from: www.rcpch.ac.uk/doc.aspx?id_Resource=1535 (accessed 3 February, 2010).

Royal College of Psychiatrists (2004) *Domestic Violence: Its Effects on Children, Factsheet for Parents and Teachers.* Royal College of Psychiatrists, London. Available from: http://www.rcpsych.ac.uk/mentalhealthinfo/mentalhealthand growingup/domesticviolence.aspx (accessed 31 August, 2010).

Scheeringa, M.S., Wright, M.J., Hunt, J.P. & Zeanah, C.H. (2006) Factors affecting the diagnosis and prediction of PTSD symptoms in children and adolescents. *American Journal of Psychiatry,* **163**, 644-651.

Skills for Care & Children's Workforce Development Council (2007) *Providing Effective Supervision: A Workforce Development Tool, Including a Unit of*

Competence and Supporting Guidance. Skills for Care and Children's Workforce Development Council, Leeds.

Smith, M.A. (2004) Health visiting: the public health role. *Journal of Advanced Nursing*, **45**(1), 17-25.

Smith, R. (2010) *A Universal Child?* Palgrave Macmillan, Basingstoke.

Srivastava, P., Fountain, R., Ayre, P. & Stewart, J. (2003) The Graded Care Profile: a measure of care. In: *Assessment in Child Care: Using & Developing Frameworks for Practice* (eds M.C. Calder & S. Hackett), Russell House Publishing, Lyme Regis.

Symonds, A. (1991) Angels and interfering busy bodies: the social construction of two occupations. *Sociology of Health & Illness*, **13**, 249-264.

Talley, N.J., Fett, S.L. & Zinsmeister, A.R. (1995) Self-reported abuse and gastrointestinal disease in outpatients: Association with irritable bowel-type symptoms. *American Journal of Gastroenterology*, **90**, 366-371.

Teegen, F. (1999) Childhood sexual abuse and long-term sequelae. In: *Posttraumatic Stress Disorder: A Lifespan Developmental Perspective* (eds A. Maercker, M. Schutzwohl & Z. Solomon), pp. 97-112. Hogrefe & Huber, Seattle.

Unite/CPHVA (2008) *Omnibus Survey*. Unite/Community Practitioners and Health Visitors Association, London.

United Nations International Children's Emergency Fund (UNICEF) (1989) The United Nations Convention on the Rights of the Child. Available from: http://www2.ohchr.org/english/law/crc.htm (accessed 16 January, 2011).

Van der Kolk, B.A. (1984) *Post-Traumatic Stress Disorders: Psychological and Biological Sequelae*. American Psychiatric Press, Washington D.C.

White, R., Carr, P. & Lowe, N. (2002) *The Children Act in Practice*, 3rd edn. Butterworths, London.

Wohl, A.S. (1986) *Endangered Lives: Public Health in Victorian England*. Dent, London.

World Health Organization (2006) *Preventing Child Maltreatment: A Guide to Taking Action and Generating Evidence*. World Health Organization, Geneva.

World Health Organization (WHO) & International Society for Prevention of Child Abuse and Neglect (2006) *Preventing Child Maltreatment: A Guide to Taking Action and Generating Evidence*. World Health Organization and International Society for Prevention of Child Abuse and Neglect, Geneva. Available from: http://whqlibdoc.who.int/publications/2006/9241594365_eng.pdf (accessed 20 March, 2011).

Appendix 5　Activities for Chapter 5

Activity 5.1

Defining 'Child'

Reflect on your own past experiences as a child, young person and professional.

- What additional tensions or ambiguities exist in respect of defining 'child'?
- What implications do these have in respect of the health visitor's role in working with children?

Activity 5.2

Defining 'Safeguarding'

- How would you define safeguarding?
- As you network with colleagues from other professional groups or agencies ask them how they define safeguarding
- Reflect on the value of this activity. How might gaining different views be helpful?

Activity 5.3

Accessing the UNCRC

Take the opportunity to access the UNCRC online (http://www2.ohchr. org/english/law/crc.htm). Consider which of the articles underpin the health visitor's safeguarding role and why.

Activity 5.4

Accessing local safeguarding children's policies

Locate, list and read the local safeguarding children's policies that are relevant to your practice.

Activity 5.5

Defining 'Child Abuse'

Child abuse is broadly categorised as:

- physical abuse
- emotional abuse
- sexual abuse
- neglect

Review *Working Together to Safeguard Children* (DCSF, 2010) and make sure that you are able to define each of the above categories. Identify the abusive behaviours and signs of abuse associated with each category.

Activity 5.6

Analysing the threshold criteria for 'significant harm'

In relation to Figure 5.1, the threshold criteria:

- consider the meaning of the term 'significant' in relation to harm of children;
- what factors make finding a 'similar child' challenging in contemporary society?
- what factors may influence the threshold for intervention?
- what do you consider constitutes 'reasonable care' in respect of the health of pre-school children?

Activity 5.7

Reflecting on a case study

In relation to Box 3, the Case study of Khyra Ishaq:

- What positive actions were undertaken by the health visitor?
- What assumptions have been made and by whom?
- What could have been done better?
- What is the significance of domestic abuse allegedly perpetrated by Khyra's natural father in the context of her death by manslaughter at the hands of her mother and mother's partner?

6
Evaluating Practice

Karen A. Luker and Gretl A. McHugh

The University of Manchester, Manchester, UK

Introduction

Evaluation as a component of care planning is examined in the general context of health visiting and public health. Healthcare can be described as the application of best current knowledge to the condition and values of an individual patient or client, family or population, sometimes referred to as evidence-based practice or policy-making (Muir Gray, 2004). Healthcare and health maintenance can be seen to be the concern of the individual especially in a society where self-care is advocated for the management of a number of long term conditions (DH, 2005b, 2005c, 2010a). In addition a number of professional groups including health visitors have a responsibility to provide health advice and healthcare services to individuals and families.

Over the last decade there has been an enhanced emphasis on skill mix in the community (Buchan & Dal Poz, 2002) and parts of the traditional work of the health visitor are now undertaken by community staff nurses, nursery nurses and healthcare assistants. Given that roles are evolving but titles in the UK are not consistent, we have tended to use the term health visitor. The greater emphasis now placed on the evaluation of healthcare services stems from the escalating public demand for quality services and costs brought about by the increased expectations and complexity of the service plus the decreasing purchasing power of the pound (DH, 2005a, 2010a). The increased complexity of the service has in part been a response to the political pressure to improve the efficiency and quality of the NHS. In addition, medical and technical advances together with new career structures especially in Nursing (DH, 2006, 2008a) and the focus on modernising nurses' careers has resulted in a proliferation of the numbers of allied health staff, some of whom are working as community practitioners. Moreover, the increase in allied health staff has influenced the practice of other professional groups, most notably nurses. The increasing trend towards specialisation initiated by medicine and

Health Visiting: A Rediscovery, Third Edition. Edited by Karen A. Luker, Jean Orr and Gretl A. McHugh.

mirrored in nursing has resulted in greater competition for limited resources. The uncertainty generated by the fact that demand exceeds supply, in terms of finance, has meant that doctors and nurses alike are forced to look for verifiable facts to assist them in establishing a convincing case worthy of continued or additional financial support. Historically, the majority of policy decisions in the healthcare field have simply followed a logical appraisal of the options of the people involved in the decision-making and may not have involved the analysis of available data. In order to justify society's continued support and commitment to healthcare it is necessary to demonstrate effectiveness. Over the past several years, there has been an increase in funding for effectiveness research.

Sources of evidence

The National Institute for Health and Clinical Excellence (NICE) is the expert panel which evaluates new and existing medicines, treatments and procedures in the UK and recommends or otherwise their adoption by the NHS. It also provides evidence-based guidance on treatment and caring for people with specific diseases and conditions (see www.nice.nhs.uk). Clinical guidelines of relevance to health visiting practice around postnatal care of women and their babies was developed by the National Collaborating Centre for Primary Care on behalf of NICE (NCCPC, 2006). There has also been a considerable amount of guidance from NICE around public health with several of its published guidelines of relevance to health visitors, such as *Community Engagement, Maternal and Child Nutrition, Reducing Differences in the Uptake of Immunisations* (NICE, 2008a, b, 2009a, 2010a). Joint publications from NICE and the Social Care Institute for Excellence (see www.scie.org.uk) such as *Looked-after Children and Young People* and *Strategies to Prevent Unintentional Injuries among Children and Young People Aged Under 15* (NICE & SCIE, 2010a, b) will also be relevant guidance to health visitors in their practice. Another guideline which extends into the domain of health visiting is the guidance on helping people to change their behaviour at the population, community and individual level (NICE, 2007). NICE also offers health professionals guidance on the way to implement changes in practice, which is often difficult to do. In addition some of the guidelines have 'audit guidance' on achieving improved standards for example, improving immunisation targets (NICE, 2009b). New topics in the area of public health and social care are emerging on a regular basis. It is clearly important for health and social care practitioners to regularly check the NICE and SCIE websites to keep up to date with evidence-based practice guidance. It might be useful to locate some of the existing guidance of relevance to health visitors and this can be explored by completing Activity 6.1 (see Appendix 6 at the end of the chapter).

Since 2009, NHS Evidence (see www.evidence.nhs.uk) provides individuals working in health and social care access to information, guidelines, and NHS policy so as to improve quality of care for patients. The NHS is driving forward this agenda to improve quality. NHS Evidence – QIPP (Quality, Innovation, Productivity and Prevention) is a collection of evidence to support quality and productivity (see http://www.library.nhs.uk/qipp/). QIPP is a wider NHS initiative enabling the NHS to work in different ways to deliver the highest quality of care.

In addition, another good source of evidence was the *Effective Healthcare Bulletin*, produced by the NHS Centre for Reviews and Dissemination (NHS CRD) which provided information on the development and promotion of evidence-based care, including health promotion interventions in terms of what was and was not effective (see www.york.ac.uk/inst/crd/ehcb.htm). This bulletin ceased publication in 2004. However, the NHS CRD continues to publish high quality systematic reviews, which evaluate the effects of health and social care interventions (see http://www.york.ac.uk/inst/crd/index.htm). Included in the CRD database are: Database of Abstracts of Reviews of Effects (DARE), which includes abstracts of systematic reviews, quality assessment of reviews, and details of Cochrane reviews and protocols; NHS EED (Economic Evaluation Database), and Health Technology Assessment (HTA), which provides completed and ongoing health technology assessments (see http://www.crd.york.ac.uk/crdweb/). These organisations are important sources of evidence for health visitors and can be explored further in Activity 6.2 (see Appendix 6).

There is very little evidence concerning the effectiveness of health visiting interventions (discussed below and in Chapter 3) when compared to interventions provided by other team members. A national scoping exercise of the contribution of nurses, midwives and health visitors to child health and child health services was undertaken and for some activities, e.g. health promotion interventions, there was very little outcome data demonstrating that these health professionals have sustained effects on negative health behaviours or other health outcomes (While *et al.*, 2005). There have been a number of systematic reviews around health visiting practice which have found conflicting evidence concerning the interventions delivered by health visitors, public health nurses and other community health workers (Elkan *et al.*, 2000; Ciliska *et al.*, 2001; Shaw *et al.*, 2006).

Elkan *et al.* (2000) conducted a Health Technology Assessment systematic review of the effectiveness of health visiting. They found a limited amount of evidence supporting some of the interventions which health visitors undertook but found there was positive evidence about home visiting to support parents in improving breastfeeding and immunisations rates. Another systematic review reported that nurses visiting pre- and postnatal clients in their own homes can produce significant benefits especially with interventions of high intensity with clients at 'risk' (Ciliska *et al.*, 2001). A review of nine systematic reviews on home visiting programmes found some evidence to support home visiting in the antenatal and postnatal periods namely in reducing rates of childhood injury and in the identification and management of postnatal depression (Bull *et al.*, 2004). However, home visiting is only one aspect of what health visitors' do and there is variability in what health visitors do and who they visit by employing authority, hence there is a need to examine further the role and functions of health visitors in the UK.

For over 20 years, and highlighted in the 1990 National Health Service and Social Care Act evaluation has been firmly on every professional's agenda, but unfortunately evaluation has been a very neglected area especially in community nursing services and health visiting. According to the Queen's Nursing Institute (QNI) (2008) there are a number of reasons why community nurses and health visitors need to be skilled in evaluating their services or changes to services namely:

> As registered professionals, they have a duty to provide the best possible care, and to do this they need to know the impact of their work on those it's intended to benefit. The increase in competition to provide services means that professionals need to be able to show how and why their service, or new way of working is effective. (p. 1)

The Nursing and Midwifery Council (NMC) has standards of proficiency for specialist public health nurses and several focus on the need for health visitors to be involved in evaluation (NMC, 2004). They are based on ten key public health principles (Skills for Health, 2008) and the four domains of health visiting (CETHV, 1977; Twinn & Cowley, 1992). There are three public health principles, which focus on evaluation within health visiting practice covering two domains in health visiting (see Table 6.1).

The recognition of evaluation as a neglected area of practice alone will not be sufficient to promote the activity. However a better understanding of what

Table 6.1 NMC standards of proficiency for entry onto register.

Principle	Domain: Influence on policies affecting health
Developing health programmes and services and reducing inequalities	Work with others to plan, implement and evaluate programmes and projects to improve health and wellbeing. Identify and evaluate service provision and support networks for individuals, families and groups in the local area or setting.
Research and development to improve health and wellbeing	Develop, implement, evaluate and improve practice on the basis of research, evidence and evaluation.
Principle	**Domain: Facilitation of health-enhancing activities**
Strategic leadership for health and wellbeing	Apply leadership skills and manage projects to improve health and wellbeing. Plan, deliver and evaluate programmes to improve the health and wellbeing of individuals and groups.

Source: NMC (2004).

evaluation may entail is discussed below and may encourage health visitors to focus on this element of their work.

Evaluation – the problem of definition

The word 'evaluation' is widely used and for the most part its meaning is taken for granted. Few attempts have been made to formulate a conceptually rigorous definition of evaluation or to analyse the meanings behind its use. The lack of a clear definition has meant that the word 'evaluation' is used interchangeably with other terms such as 'assessment' and 'appraisal'. We talk of assessment or evaluation in the context of client or community needs and indeed assessment is said to be the first stage in care planning and evaluation the last. We hear nurse managers talk of staff appraisal, performance and development reviews or evaluation and this relates to how well individual practitioners are functioning in their particular role. It is evident then that confusion may arise if we use the word evaluation in a casual way. In addition there may be confusion about the difference between evaluation, research and audit (QNI, 2008).

Taking into account the common usage of the term evaluation there is a distinction to be made between 'evaluation' of everyday practice by a practitioner and evaluation research such as the evaluation of a pilot scheme such as Sure Start or an evaluation trial such as RIPPLE (randomised intervention of pupil peer led sex education) (Oakley *et al.*, 2006).

Evaluation when used in a general way is said to refer to the everyday occurrence of making judgments of worth. Although this interpretation implies some form of logical or rational thought it does not presuppose any systematic procedures for presenting objective evidence to support the judgment. Evaluation when used in this way refers only to the process of assessment or appraisal of worth. Evaluation has been defined by St Leger *et al.* (1992) as:

> The critical assessment, on as objective a basis as possible, of the degree to which entire services or their component parts (e.g. diagnostic tests, treatments, caring procedures) fulfil stated goals. (p. 1)

The authors discuss two key elements of the definition. Firstly, the reference to goals explicitly requiring a comparison with some standard and secondly, the importance of objectivity, ensuring findings of the evaluative process are independent of judgements or prejudices from those undertaking the evaluation and commissioning the evaluation.

Evaluative research on the other hand implies the utilisation of scientific methods and techniques for the purpose of making an evaluation. Inherent in the terms evaluative research is an emphasis on the measurement of change. The distinction made between evaluation and evaluative research may seem irrelevant or daunting to some practitioners who consider that they will never become involved in research as a primary activity, but nevertheless practitioners may be involved in generating research questions or become engaged in data collection for others. Many research questions are developed from an observation in practice. However, in our everyday work as health visitors we are constantly involved in making judgments of worth. For example, if we simply say that we believe that visits to families with a disabled child are a good idea, this is an unsubstantiated judgment. If on the other hand we say that visits to families with a disabled child are good because they reduce the incidence of loneliness and depression in the mother then this is a substantiated judgment. If we have some insight into the criteria used as the basis of the statement this does not make it research but it does imply that we have some evidence to support our position, and may suggest possible outcome measures to be used in research. Other health visitors may not agree with our criteria but this is not essential.

During the past five years a great deal has been written about the importance of being able to measure the outcomes of care. This has largely been driven by the evidence-based practice movement and the financial situation. There is a desire to measure the effectiveness or adequacy of care (DH, 2008c). The Darzi report emphasised the need to improve effectiveness of care throughout the patient journey with personal care, quality and safety high on the agenda (DH, 2008c). In addition, there have been developments in the NHS in the use of Patient Related Outcome Measures (PROMS) to measure the effectiveness of care (DH, 2008b). Recent policy has highlighted the need to focus on improving healthcare outcomes with a more widespread use of PROMS where available, and also learning from patient/client experience surveys and real-time feedback (DH, 2010a). The important insights provided by patient/client experiences of healthcare and information collected about services on what's good and what could be improved ultimately assists in forming judgements about performance and accountability. Before reading on, take some time to consider your own practice and begin to complete Activity 6.3 (see Appendix 6).

Conceptualising evaluation

In conceptualising the various approaches to evaluation the goal attainment model stands out as being particularly appealing to those involved in the evaluation of healthcare. The notion of goal attainment is embodied in the target setting approach adopted by many Trusts; a good example is the immunisation and cervical screening targets which are set as goals for General Practices to attain. Target setting is useful and is also used in identifying service priorities. Targets should be: Specific, Measurable, Achievable, Realistic and Time bound, summarised to the mnemonic SMART targets (Denis *et al.*, 1994).

The starting point for any evaluation is to be clear about the aims of the service that is the benefits expected to be accrued by the recipients of the service. There is general agreement amongst those concerned with evaluation that the most important and yet most difficult phase of the process of evaluation is the clarification of objectives. The emphasis on objectives or goals stems from a conceptualisation of evaluation as measurement of the success or failure of an activity in so far as it reaches its predetermined objectives. One way to avoid this conundrum is to evaluate the service from the perspective of the service user or client. This is a more open-ended approach to evaluation which seeks to capture the experience of the service user in terms of perceived benefits and disbenefits of the service. An example of this approach is Russell and Drennan's (2007) web-based study of 4665 mothers' views of the health visiting service in the UK. Using *Netmums* (http://www.netmums.com/), an online parenting organisation with currently 840 000 members, mostly mums, a survey was conducted following concern that the health visiting service was increasingly difficult to access. The study found that mums valued the health visiting services, in particular their knowledge and expertise around child development and parenting (Russell & Drennan, 2007). However, some of the changes to the service, such as a focus on families most in need, were making the health visitors less accessible to other families. Another example was an evaluation of the health visiting service by questionnaire to examine the parents' perceptions and experiences of the health visiting services. Although the service was valued by those who received it and health visitors provided much needed support and advice, it also highlighted the high expectations from clients asking for more information based on research and evidence so as to deliver higher quality services in the community (McHugh & Luker, 2002). The Department of Health's (2011) service vision for health visiting is to increase the number of health visitors so as to provide increased support to all families and this may ensure that the health visiting service is accessible to all families, in addition to offering evidence-based programmes to vulnerable children and families.

The process of evaluating can be complex and it is always subjective. Different people want to know different things (DH, 2001). Evaluation involves a combination of basic assumptions underlying the activity to be evaluated and the personal values of those engaged in the activities being evaluated. Hence the process of evaluation always starts with recognition of values and these values may be either explicit or implicit. The complexities involved in defining health as either individual or collective are explored. Despite evaluation being problematic in the field of health visiting, the evaluation process as described initially by Suchman (1967) is a useful starting point, which has yet to be superseded; this is represented with slight modification in Figure 6.1.

Example: Weight Management Programme

With reference to the evaluation process (see Figure 6.1), we will explore possible ways of evaluating a health programme. Let us suppose that we are health visitors responsible for health promotion in a school. We have observed that there appear to be a number of overweight children in the classes we teach. Our observations will reflect our values. Firstly, we believe that to be overweight in adolescence is not good; we may also hold different views on why this is undesirable. Some of us may believe that overweight adolescents experience more upper respiratory tract infections and may be more prone to

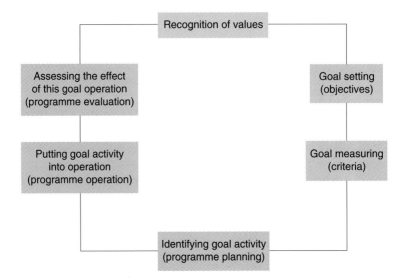

Figure 6.1 Evaluation process.
Source: E.A. Suchman. Figure 1, 'Evaluation process', In: *Evaluative Research: Principles and Practice in Public Service and Social Action Programs.* © 1967 Russell Sage Foundation, 112 East 64th Street, New York, NY 10065. (Reprinted by kind permission.)

develop coronary artery disease in later life. Others may be of the opinion that fat adolescents do not look as attractive as those of average or light build and this may lead to an internalisation of a negative self-image. In part these value judgments reflect the beliefs and values of the society in which we live and work. In response to this perceived need we decide to set up a slimming club. The underlying rationale of this action is that we believe that it would be beneficial to the individuals concerned to lose weight and furthermore we believe it would benefit society if the next generation of parents were fit and healthy.

The objectives of the weight management programme will probably be wider than just getting the children to lose weight, although this will, of course, be the major focus. Firstly we may have to convince the overweight adolescents that to be obese is undesirable and a potential threat to future health and wellbeing. But this approach presupposes that they will place a value on health; we may instead have to appeal to their vanity and suggest that they will feel better in themselves if they were slimmer. As health visitors we see ourselves as health promoters and facilitators and it is likely that we will use the weight management programme to teach the children about the nutritional value of food and the value of a balanced diet. We may even go so far as teaching the children or even family members how to cook nutritious food. There is scope for individual practitioners to think of additional objectives which may be more or less important than those already stated. After identifying our objectives or goals the next stage of the evaluation process is to clarify how we will determine when the goal has been achieved. Looking back at our objectives, we can identify a number of possible criteria on which we will base our judgment concerning the success or failure of the weight management programme. Firstly, the number of children who attend the programme, and the frequency of their attendance. This may give us some indication as to whether the programme was seen as useful by the children. However, we have to be careful how we interpret these data because whether children attend the programme or not depends to some extent on structural factors and we will come back to this topic when thinking about programme planning. Secondly, unlike most areas of health visiting in this context we are fortunate in having one truly objective criteria and that is the amount of weight that each child actually loses. In addition, once a child has attained his or her target weight then we would expect the weight to remain constant and not continue to fall. It goes almost without saying that in order to measure weight accurately we need a reliable pair of scales and the children should be weighed in the same or similar clothes each week. Thirdly, given that our objectives suggest that we want the children to understand something about the nutritional value of food, it may therefore be useful to compare what the children knew before they attended the slimming club with what they know after they have been exposed to learning materials and other teaching sessions on the nutritional value of food. This data or information may best be obtained by giving the children a questionnaire to fill in on the first visit to the programme and then a follow-up questionnaire after the sessions on nutrition. This would give us some indication of their knowledge level and some feedback as to whether or not our teaching sessions have been successful.

In order to achieve our goals, the evaluation process suggests that we devise a strategy for setting up our weight management programme. It is important to work with children and parents in the planning and implementation of this initiative. First it would be helpful to know how many children would be interested in coming to the programme. We could find out this information by putting a poster in each of the classrooms inviting children who consider themselves to be overweight to attend a meeting either at lunchtime or immediately after school. Given that there is some interest at the subsequent meeting, discussion could take place about the time and location for the proposed meetings (obviously if the meetings are held at inconvenient times and places then attendance will be poor). Involving potential users of the programme, the next step is to decide how the programme will be run. Will there, for example, be a health promotion input every week? Will other health professionals be asked to take part such as the dietician or physiotherapist? Will there be an exercise session? It is also important to look at the evidence around the effectiveness of weight management interventions and those studies which take into account the child's perspective around obesity and weight management, such as the systematic reviews by: Whitlock *et al.*, 2008, 2010; *Rees et al.*, 2009. Once this is done we then have to meet the challenge of putting the programme into action.

We may find that in the early stages we need to make modifications. For example, we may find that it is better to put the formal talk or demonstration before rather than after the exercise session; perhaps it will be necessary to enlist the support of some colleagues and do more group work. There are always teething problems when launching any new programme and time is well spent in the early stages making adjustments and modifications. Once the programme is well established we begin to think more carefully about the final stage of the evaluation process, i.e. judging the effects of the programme. It is important to remember that it is usual to evaluate a programme in terms of its goals and the goal measuring criteria are the key to the evaluation. In addition we may wish to collect supplementary information which might help us with future planning. We could, for example, ask those attending the sessions to suggest ways in which we could improve the weight management programme. Our evaluation, that is our judgment about whether or not the programme was a success or failure, feeds back into our value system and the whole process is repeated. Activity 6.4 (see Appendix 6) provides you with an opportunity to start thinking about designing a new programme to be implemented within health visiting practice.

The care planning process

It would appear that the goal attainment approach towards evaluation is applicable to health visiting at an individual and family level since goal setting and evaluation are operationalised through the care planning process. Fundamentally care planning is a problem-solving or needs-led approach to care and this has a tendency to make it appear alien to traditional health visitors since they perceive it as diminishing their preventive function. This approach is enshrined in the DH (2001) health visitor practice development resources pack (see Figure 6.2). Activity 6.5 (see Appendix 6) provides you with an opportunity to start using a record of action plans.

Other approaches to care planning involve: identifying the needs of both child and family; agree actions; expected outcome; timescale and actual outcome (see Figure 6.3). Care planning is a continual process. The SMART

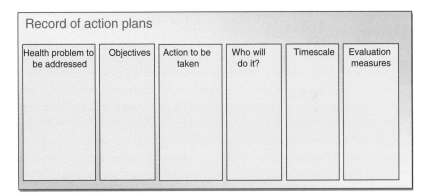

Figure 6.2 Record of action plans.
Source: DH (2001), © Crown copyright. (Reproduced by kind permission.)

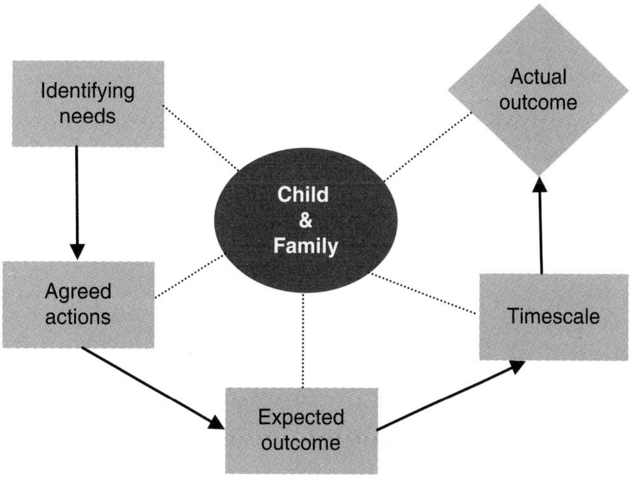

Figure 6.3 Care planning.

approach, described previously can be used to ensure activities are directed towards achieving the required outcome.

Using these or a similar approach enables a systematic approach to the care planning process and what needs to done in order to tackle the issues/problems identified. It's important to ensure there are regular reviews of the progress. The evaluation process will determine whether objectives are being met, if amendments are required but also in terms of the success of the plan of action. Gaining experience in using the SMART approach is explored in Activity 6.6 (see Appendix 6).

Actual and potential problems

In the past, health visitors were reluctant to consider themselves as involved in dealing with clients' health problems. Instead they have reiterated their uniqueness in so far as they claim to visit families many of whom have no apparent health problems. However, the role of the health visitor has evolved into one where the average family may only receive a birth visit so that the families visited are more likely to fall into the category of needy. The focus on 'proportionate universalism' (previously referred to as 'progressive universalism') ensures that health visitors provide a service according to need at a neighbourhood and individual level achieving greater equity of outcomes for all children (DH, 2007, 2010b; Marmot *et al.*, 2010). Those families with greater risks and needs will receive more health visiting input. The word 'problem' is often associated by many health visitors with that nebulous term 'problem family'. However, in this context, a health problem or health need, following a healthcare needs analysis, is defined as a matter which concerns the health visitor or client about the client's health at the time of the visit or assessment. Actual problems are those which are present at the time of the assessment or follow-up visits. Potential problems are not present;

instead there are indicators or cues which suggest that an actual problem may develop if no action is taken.

An example of an actual problem at an assessment visit may be that of a baby with a sore eye, a baby who refuses to suck at the breast, or a child who has regressed to soiling himself. Health visitors are more concerned with potential problems, i.e. preventing actual problems occurring. An example of a potential problem for a couple expecting a baby who already have a two-year-old child might be jealousy on the part of the toddler after the baby is born. The health visitor would be keen to assist the parents in preventing this problem occurring. She would, therefore, discuss ways in which the family might begin to prepare the two year old for the birth of the new baby. Discussion may also follow concerning the management of the toddler during his first separation from his mother which is, of course, inevitable if the birth is to take place in hospital. By intervening before there is an actual problem the health visitor tries to promote the wellbeing of the whole family. This is getting back to the core health visiting function of early intervention and prevention.

Health visitors used to visit families from conception to the grave; however, this is no longer the case. The main focus of the health visitors' work is on the pre-school child and the family, although in many parts of the UK it may be that it is largely around child protection issues and focusing less on preventative and public health issues. If we view life as a developmental time span then theoretically it can be argued that the younger one is, the more potential health problems one has and the fewer actual problems. Conversely, the older one is, the more actual problems one experiences and the relative risk of potential problems developing is reduced. However, a potential problem is usually only considered by the health visitor if it has a higher than average probability of becoming an actual problem. For example, all babies are at risk of developing obesity; the infant whose siblings or parents are obese, however, would be considered by the health visitor to have a potential problem in this area. Similarly, all elderly people could be said to be at risk from falling. However, this may only be recorded as a potential problem if there were factors present which suggested that there was an above average risk of the client falling. For example, if the elderly person had failing vision due to senile cataracts or dizzy spells as a result of Ménière's disease or had been reported to have had previous falls then the client may be deemed to have a potential problem in this area.

Problem-solving

The care planning process is made up of a number of components:

- data collection;
- goal setting;
- care planning;
- intervention;
- evaluation.

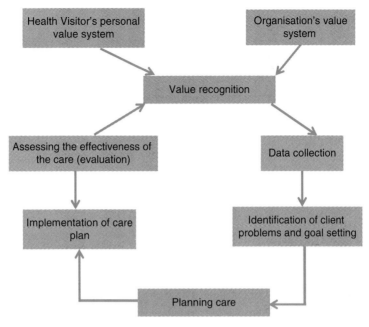

Figure 6.4 Evaluating practice.

It is noteworthy that problem-solving is subjective and value laden in so far as health visitors collect data and identify problems which they or the recipients of their care consider to be important. Hence the care planning process, like the evaluative process, begins with recognition of values (see Figure 6.4).

Evaluation and evaluative research

Although the evaluation component of the care planning process is able to substantiate its claims, there are two reasons why it cannot be said to constitute evaluative research. Firstly, in evaluative research the main thrust of the activity is directed towards measuring how far intervention has achieved or not achieved its goals whereas in the care planning process the measurement of the effectiveness of care is subsidiary to the primary goal of giving care. Owing to the secondary purpose of evaluation in the care planning process goal statements may not be recorded; however, health visitors and other practitioners are involved in making judgments of worth about the care which they give whether they record it or not. Many of these value judgments will be made on the basis of systematically collected data and experience, and the evaluation criteria may vary between individuals. Secondly, in evaluative research, data are collected on a predetermined target population and therefore findings may be related to more than one individual, whereas in the evaluative component of the care planning process the health visitor evaluates the care she gives to each individual and is not in a position to determine her clients in the same way as a researcher determines the sample.

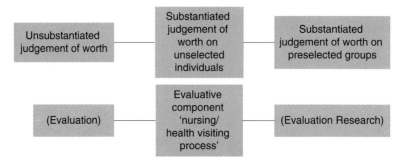

Figure 6.5 Continuum of evaluation.

All in all, evaluation may best be viewed as a continuum. The evaluation component of the care planning process can be placed almost anywhere along this continuum depending upon the way the data are collected (systematically or otherwise) and recorded (see Figure 6.5). Data which have been systematically collected and recorded during the execution of care planning may be used retrospectively by health practitioners for research purposes. The retrospective use of the material may be referred to as 'evaluative research' because evaluation and not care giving has become the main thrust of the activity and the researcher is able to determine the population to be studied.

Evaluation of healthcare

Concern for the measurement of the quality of healthcare provided to patients/clients and attempts at evaluating care are not new. It may be possible to get agreement on the importance of evaluation. There is less agreement, however, about what will be evaluated and how the evaluation should be done. The US Agency for Healthcare Research and Quality (AHRQ) provides guidance on improving quality through guidance to those involved in designing or evaluating new interventions to improve care coordination. They discuss five key elements: (1) assessment of needs for coordination; (2) identification of options for improving coordination; (3) selection and implementation of one of the alternatives; (4) evaluation to determine effects on care coordination and outcomes of care; and (5) amendments if required (McDonald *et al.*, 2007).

The North American literature on evaluation dates back to Derryberry (1939) who, in a report concerning the accomplishments of nursing, stated:

> In the past, evaluation of nursing services have been based upon volume and intensity of service ... Evidence of the more elusive quality of service as expressed by the changing state of the patient has been sought in the present analysis. (p. 2035)

It is interesting that more than seventy years have passed since Derryberry made this plea to move away from evaluations based on volume and intensity of service in favour of focusing on patient/client outcome. However, within the context of health visiting we have unfortunately failed to move very far forward. It is only with policy recommendations on improving and measuring the effectiveness of care and the drive towards quality in healthcare that there has been a push to using defined outcomes measures or patient-related outcome measures (PROMS). This has been taken up by the NHS Health and Social Care Information Centre in measuring quality from the patients' perspective, largely focusing on clinical procedures, using PROMS to measure health gain after surgical treatment, this will be expanded to more areas of healthcare in the future (www.ic.nhs.uk/proms).

Data which is of relevance to health visiting work is often limited. The data most commonly used to provide insight into the work of health visitors at both a national and local level are the statistical data which relate to frequency of health visitor visits to particular client groups (see Table 6.2). It is possible for these statistics to be used to demonstrate how health visitors spend some of their time and this information may be useful to managers and policy-makers. There is often little feedback to health visitors on the activity data they record for client contact. At a national level, however, the format in which the data were collected changed and comparisons beyond 2003–04 are no longer possible. Suffice it to say here that the data collected in 2003–04 indicated a reduction in face-to-face contacts (from 3 826 000 in 1988–89 to 3 010 000 in 2003–04) (DH, 2004). Local statistics produced by strategic health authorities appear to be available until 2004 (DH, 2004). From this data it appears, not surprisingly, that the majority of first contacts by health visitors are made to the under-fours with little contacts made to older people. Recent data was not available to see any change in pattern to first contact, but due to a reduction in numbers of health visitors from 12 800 in 1999 to 10 959 in 2009 (NHS Information Centre, 2010), this places more pressure on health visitors in their workload priorities especially if we assume that some time is needed to supervise ancillary staff and community staff nurses.

Other sources of data that would assist health visitors and others with their work are some of the routinely collected statistics from the Office for National Statistics and the Public Health Observatories, which provide statistical data pertaining to the health of the population and an overview of the health problems within specific communities. Local councils also provide information on health and housing. Practice-based information such, as immunisation rates, or quality outcomes framework data, which are practice specific, and can be compared with other areas in the UK. With all sources of routinely collected data, there are limitations and biases often associated with it. Table 6.3 provides some sources of routinely collected information which is available. To gain experience in locating routine sources of information, complete Activity 6.7 (see Appendix 6).

Structure, process and outcome evaluation

In the context of healthcare evaluation the classic reference of Donabedian (1969), a pioneer in this field, has not been superseded. He described three approaches to evaluation: structure evaluation, process evaluation and

Table 6.2 First contacts with health visitors by age.

Year	Under 1	1	2-4	5-15	16-24	25-34	35-44	45-54	55-64	65-74	75-84	85 and over
	Percentage											
1999-2000	25	12	24	4	7	17	6	1	0	1	2	1
2000-01	25	11	24	5	7	16	6	1	0	1	2	1
2001-02	26	12	24	4	7	17	6	1	0	1	2	1
2002-03	27	12	22	4	7	17	7	1	0	1	2	1

Source: DH (2004): (KC55 DH statistics Division, 2003). (© Crown Copyright. Reproduced by kind permission.)

Table 6.3 Routine sources of data and information.

Data and information	Source
Neighbourhood Statistics: Statistics about local area of interest.	Office for National Statistics: URL: http://neighbourhood.statistics.gov.uk
National statistics online provides information in areas such as: Census data, Population; Health & Care – Health Inequality; Health Expectancy; Life Expectancy etc.	Office for National Statistics: URL: http://www.statistics.gov.uk/default.asp
Department of Health provides: Indicators of Nation's Health: Health profile of England; Local indicators on breastfeeding, smoking, obesity etc.; mortality target monitoring; health inequality data etc.	Department of Health- Public Health statistics URL: http://www.dh.gov.uk/en/ Publicationsandstatistics/Statistics/StatisticalWorkAreas/ Statisticalpublichealth/index.htm
Hospital Episode Statistics, providing data of all admissions and outpatient appointments in the NHS.	Hospital Episode Statistics: URL: http://www.hesonline.nhs.uk
Patient-related outcome measures (PROMS) – data on health gains after e.g. surgical treatment with pre and post operative measures.	NHS information centre: URL: http://www.ic.nhs.uk/proms
GP data; Quality & Outcomes Framework (QOF) of the GP contract – provides disease prevalence across the UK or by local GP practice.	QOF database: URL: http://www.gpcontract.co.uk
The NHS Information Centre provides useful data on: Health & Lifestyles; Primary care: Prescriptions etc.	URL: http://www.ic.nhs.uk
National guidelines, relating to public health and management of specific diseases	National Institute for Health & Clinical Excellence: URL: http://www.nice.nhs.uk Scottish Intercollegiate Guidelines Network: URL: http://www.sign.ac.uk Social Care Institute for Excellence: URL: http://www.scie.org.uk/
Health profiles: highlights of local health issues	Association of Public Health Observatories URL: http://www.apho.org.uk/
Child and Maternal Health Observatory (ChiMat): Knowledge hub around topics of safeguarding children; child health profiles; infant mortality profiles; healthy schools profiles; needs assessment tools – breastfeeding data ; obese children data etc. (can compare with localities).	ChiMat URL: http://www.chimat.org.uk

outcome evaluation. Donabedian's approach to evaluation is as valid today as it was in the 1970s. The framework is also used as a basis for assessing quality of care (Donabedian, 1988). Others have built on his work (see QNI, 2008) and used slightly different language, but in reality the approach to evaluation and assessing quality is the same.

Structure evaluation

Structure evaluation involves the study of factors in the organisation system, the availability of facilities and equipment, staffing levels, styles of management and the characteristics of the care givers. The assumption underlying this approach to evaluation is that if the facilities, staff and equipment reach specified standards then the care which follows will be 'good' and clients will benefit. In keeping with this approach it would be assumed that Trusts that have achieved their health visitor client ratio target of 250–400 children per health visitor should be providing a better service than areas which are not achieving this target. Research by the Family and Parenting Institute (2009) found that the ratio of children under five to health visitors ranged from 165.00 to 894.25 children under per health visitor for each Primary Care Trust (PCT) surveyed. Community Practitioners' Health Visitors' Association (CPHVA) and Unite recommend that the average and more normal caseload size for health visitors should be no more than 250, with health visitors working in areas of high vulnerability being much less, and 400 should be the absolute maximum caseload size (Unite/CPHVA, 2009). With the health visitor implementation plan of 2011–15, the vision to expand and strengthen the health visiting service should reduce caseload size (DH, 2011).

Skill mix is clearly embedded in health visiting. We have grown accustomed to the notion of nurses trained to work in a particular speciality, e.g. traditionally health visiting and district nursing. The demographic changes, that is growing numbers of elderly people and fewer school leavers, coupled with the economic imperative, have forced us to rethink how best to use resources. We therefore expect to see more healthcare assistants, nursery nurses and staff nurses working in the community and a refocusing of the priorities of health visitors as specialist public health practitioners.

Process evaluation

Process evaluation focuses on the staff, who give the care to clients in terms of whether or not the care was appropriate and carried out in the correct manner. The emphasis is firmly on what the health visitor does and may also include decision-making. This may be considered as the traditional or taken-for-granted approach to evaluation. In health promotion interventions, process evaluation enables questions such as: was the intervention applied in the manner intended? did other factors come into play that might have affected the result? what did the participants think about the process? (Speller et al., 1997).

If we ask health visitors about the effects of their work they usually begin by telling us what they do. Hence the success of the visit is measured in terms of whether the health visitor has achieved what she set out to do. For example, did she successfully complete the health needs assessment or carry out a developmental assessment on a two year old – or identify and support a mother with postnatal depression? The emphasis is on what the health visitor has done and this can be partially accounted for by reflecting on the type of information that health visitors are required to keep, although this now varies by Trust. The Department of Health used to publish national statistics on health visiting activity but it is up to local services to collect information on activity within health visiting. There are still problems with recording activity as the complexities of health visiting mean that it is difficult to categorise visits under a single heading.

Each Trust tends to have its own system for recording information. There are usually several records which the health visitor will complete as part of the child health recording system. Universally the Personal Child Health Record, known as the 'Red Book' is the primary record for information pertaining to a child's health and development. Other forms of record-keeping involve health-care needs analysis, family assessment, care planning and evaluation, ensuring the needs of the families are identified to achieve the best outcomes of care. These may be recorded on a family record or active intervention card. Computerised systems also vary in Trusts but client contacts either face to face or by telephone are recorded; also information on health checks and immunisation are often entered into the child health computer record systems. Yet despite these systems for recording health visiting activity and intervention, little outcome data is available.

In the future, there will be more of a focus on enabling individuals to have control of their own health records; initially this will be through access to their GP record, but will extend to records held by other healthcare providers. Clients/patients will be able to give permission to other agencies to view their GP records to assist with their care (DH, 2010a).

Statistics concerning community healthcare are needed for many reasons and these have been summarised from the Korner report (DHSS, 1983) and are still relevant to this day:

- planning and monitoring;
- evaluation and research;
- operational control;
- treatment of individual patients/clients;
- legal requirements;
- accountability.

A further example of process evaluation is an audit of records, which is also sometimes confused with evaluation research; here, the focus is on not just what the health visitor does but may also include some notion of how well she performs in her role as evidenced in record-keeping or by observation at work. In the context of health visiting an audit for evaluating the performance of students or health visitors could be developed from the skills outlined in a validated curriculum (NMC, 2004). To use an example, if we look at the skills involved in interviewing we see that the 'attitudinal set' for this skill can be is itemised as follows:

- Be nonjudgmental both orally and nonverbally.
- Be willing to listen and empathise.
- Value objectivity as appropriate.
- Value subjectivity as appropriate (show human warmth).
- Value clients' rights to privacy and confidentiality.
- Value goal of clients having independence.
- Value own listening role.
- Affirm the principles of the practice of health visiting.

As a manager, community practice teacher or mentor involved in the appraisal of health visitors or students we could use the above as a checklist against which we could evaluate interviewing skills in either staff or students. The assumption underlying process evaluation is that what the health visitor does is of primary importance and evaluations are made concerning health visitor rather than client-orientated, objectives. Furthermore this example reiterates the subjective nature of evaluation.

Outcome evaluation

Outcome evaluation on the other hand refers to the end-result of intervention or care in terms of its affect upon the client. In brief, a judgment is made about the achievement of client-orientated objectives with no regard as to the reason why the observed outcome occurred. The assumption underlying outcome evaluation is that the care a person receives is of secondary importance to its effects – hence the emphasis is placed upon the client and not the health visitor or other health practitioner.

Outcome evaluation is implicit in care planning where client-orientated goals or objectives are set and act as the criteria against which the success or failure of intervention is evaluated. This was also made clear in the Health Visitors Practice Development Resources Pack (DH, 2001). In the context of health visiting, it is usually assumed that the goals of care are commonly understood, although this is seldom the case. Where possible the expected outcome of intervention should be written down in the client or family record. The expected outcome of an intervention can take many forms. It may relate to the acquisition of new knowledge as a result of a one-to-one teaching, or a behavioural change as in potty training or visiting the family planning clinic. Whatever the expected outcome or criteria for judging the success of the intervention, it should be clearly stated so that what constitutes success or failure can be readily understood by any practitioner.

Let us now consider an example: all newborn babies are at risk from developing gastroenteritis. This risk is increased if the infant is bottle-fed, if the bottle is made up for two feeds and then reheated, and if the parents have little understanding of the need for sterilisation. In such circumstances the health visitor may list gastroenteritis as a potential problem.

Goal statement A:

the mother/father will demonstrate that they understand the preparation of bottle feeds and the way to sterilise bottles.

This statement has limitations because it does not indicate how the parents will demonstrate their understanding and we have no indication of the time perspective. Will it be at the next visit, next feed or for the next baby? Goal statement B gives us this additional information.

Goal statement B:

the mother/father will discuss the way in which they make up the bottle feeds and their method of sterilisation and will give a practical demonstration at the next visit which has been arranged for, say, 10.00 hours on 4 April 2011.

The process of goal setting can be further explored in Activity 6.8 (see Appendix 6).

In the context of outcome evaluation it can be argued that in some respects health visiting is rather more complex to evaluate than hospital nursing. In the community we are dealing with families not individuals; however, this is not intended to imply that the hospital nurses do not consider the family as important. When health visitors visit clients in their own homes the focus of their work is on the family. The initial reason for the visit may have been precipitated by a referral from a general practitioner reporting the failing mental state of an elderly person. Despite the fact that the elderly person is in one sense the client, it may well be that the health visitor directs most of her intervention towards the daughter who feels that she cannot go on indefinitely caring for her mother. In the context of hospital nursing, a care plan is usually only made for the patient – that is, the person who occupies the bed in the ward. Hence the outcome of care is only evaluated in this context.

In health visiting it is not always so clear cut as to who the client is and it may well be necessary to make more than one care plan. Similarly, goals may be in conflict with each other and many compromises will need to be made. If, for example, a woman feels she can no longer care for her mentally confused mother-in-law because she is getting little or no support from her husband then there are three individuals to consider. Any attempts to evaluate the outcome of intervention would have to take into account the conflicting needs of these three individuals. In order to begin to deal with this problem, i.e. the family's perceived inability to care for a mentally confused elderly person, the health visitor might initially try to uncover the reason for the apparently sudden feelings of not being able to cope on the part of the daughter-in-law. The health visitor has certain beliefs and values about the function of the family and male and female roles within it. She has acquired this knowledge from her roles as a woman, as a nurse and perhaps as a carer herself.

Let us say that on taking a family history from the female carer we learn that she used to work as a cleaner and gave up work six months ago to be at home with her mother-in-law. She is in many respects happily married but considers that her husband has put pressure on her to give up work to take care of his mother. She feels that her husband is rather old-fashioned about women working and prefers her to be at home. The husband has never helped in the house but he does do all the gardening and decorating. The situation in this household was tolerable until the husband's mother began getting up in the night and wandering around the house and out into the street. Because the husband has to be at work by 8 am each morning the wife felt it was her duty to get up to keep an eye on her mother-in-law. This practice has resulted in her feeling very tired and unable to cope with the housework, shopping and cooking. The problem has been further compounded by the recent onset of urinary incontinence in the elderly person and it was when this happened that she went to her general practitioner. When speaking to the mother-in-law the health visitor finds that she is disorientated in time and place and that she repeatedly asks to be taken home to her mother. She seems not to know the name of her daughter-in-law but does remember the name of her son. Towards the end of the interview the husband returns from work and makes it quite plain that he has no intention of letting his mother go into a home or a hospital. He also considers that his wife exaggerates the problem. Clearly there is no right or obvious answer to this family's problems. Indeed, it would be interesting to identify the actual and potential problems of each family member and try to write goal statements for each. Let us say that the health visitor in question considers that it is the female carer that has the most dominant or pressing needs, then what can she do to ameliorate the situation?

Decisions concerning intervention are not made in a social vacuum; they are made in the context of service cutbacks and an awareness of the constraints of time. Let us say that it is decided that a possible solution to the problem would be day care five days a week for the elderly person (something the husband is in agreement with). The problem then becomes one of getting the placement and the transport. In the first instance there may be no vacancy at all. As an interim measure the health visitor somehow has to offer support to the female carer to enable her to carry on a little longer. This support may be given by providing an opportunity for her to talk about how she feels both about her marriage and caring for her mother-in-law. In addition, time may be spent with the husband to try to give him some insight into his wife's situation in the hope that he will be willing to help more in the house. The health visitor may also give some practical advice and assistance with the management of the incontinence such as arranging for the laundry service and the provision of incontinence aids such as Kanga pads and pants or arrange for the specialist continence nurse to visit. There may also be financial benefits that the family are entitled to such as attendance or carer's allowance.

Obviously there are a number of other interventions that we might try but our intention here is not to provide an exhaustive list but instead to provide some insight into the complexities of dealing with families. An example of this nature introduces another problem in the context of evaluation in so far as it is not possible to evaluate what you are unable to provide, in this case, day care. Nevertheless all health practitioners are in a position to collect data concerned with existing services that fall short in meeting the needs of the community. We contend that all practitioners have a moral responsibility to collate this information if they are to be serious about meeting community needs.

To return to evaluation, it is incumbent upon the evaluator to decide whether to use structure, process or outcome criteria, or a combination of two or more of these. In choosing a particular approach to evaluation, certain assumptions have to be made. If it is possible in terms of time and financial resources it may be advantageous to attempt an evaluation incorporating structure, process and outcome goals and it might be expected that there would be a positive correlation between the three approaches.

Against the background of resource constraints in the NHS and the embedding of the evidence-based practice movement it is expected that a greater emphasis will be placed on outcome evaluation as evidenced by health gain. The DH (2009a) emphasises the need for measurement and evaluation in achieving continuous improvement. As previously stated, NHS Trusts are charged with the responsibility of assessing the health needs of their resident population. Priorities will be set and services targeted accordingly. Performance will be measured by comparing health outcomes within and between health providers. By focusing on client or patient outcomes, the contribution of individual practitioners in the primary healthcare team becomes less important since it is the collective effort that will be the measurable input in most cases. However, if health visiting and community services are to survive and develop, it is essential that individual practitioners are in a position to identify, quantify and evaluate their own input in terms of client outcomes. The section that follows addresses the particular issues involved in evaluating health visiting.

Additional issues in evaluating the practice of health visiting

When seeking to evaluate health visiting practice there is a basic problem in that the goals of health visiting are broadly stated and as such cannot easily act as criteria against which the effectiveness of practice can be measured. A review of the role of health visitors (DH 2007) described a renewed role that:

- delivers measurable health outcomes for individuals and communities and provides a rewarding and enjoyable job for nurses;
- has the support of families and communities;
- commissioners will commission;
- delivers government policies for children and families, improving health and reducing inequalities and social exclusion;
- fits the new system of providing choice and contestability through new providers, that promotes self-care, service integration, improved productivity and local decision-making;
- can adapt and respond to changing needs and aspirations;
- attracts a new generation to the profession.

The significance of the above focus is the priority given to evaluation in terms of measurable outcomes. The core elements of health visiting were identified in the same report and provide an extended role as discussed in earlier chapters. The overall goal of health visiting remains as 'the promotion of health and prevention of ill-health' in its broadest sense and embraces the principles of public health. However, this is too broad and unrealistic a goal to be considered as a single outcome criterion for health visiting practice.

Health visiting places an emphasis on prevention and therefore it shares the problems inherent in the evaluation of all preventive techniques or programmes; namely, if something does not occur because it has been prevented, how can it be measured? 'Prevention' embraces a wide variety of programmes and activities. Some community health programmes, such as sewage disposal or screening for phenylketonuria, can be said to be highly effective or at least cost effective. Some programmes, on the other hand, such as screening for breast cancer are controversial with respect to the target population and efficacy. Programmes which depend for their success on the adherence or compliance of the client may in some circumstances not be effective. The importance of lifestyle is pre-eminent in the promotion of health (Bandura, 2004). Health visitors are involved in health promotion both at a group and an individual level. Health visitors engage in one to one health education when they visit people in their own homes or see individual clients at the clinic. Similarly if they visit schools or participate in antenatal classes they teach groups rather than individuals and this requires a different set of skills. Very little evidence exists concerning the effectiveness of teaching undertaken by health visitors. Hobbs, as long ago as 1973, commented on the lack of evidence regarding the effectiveness of one-to-one teaching undertaken by the health visitor; almost forty years later we are no further forward. It can be argued that the successful outcome of the health visitor's work depends to a large extent upon the cooperation and partnership with the client. The extent to which patients follow doctors' orders has been investigated, but little or no work has been carried out concerning the clients' concordance with health visiting advice.

In the context of medicine the adherence studies carried out have usually focused on the extent to which patients have followed their drug prescription. Since non-adherence has been a problem to general practitioners in so far as it has hindered the efficacy of their drug treatments, the quest has been to search out the potential non-adherer so that he or she can be dealt with. The emphasis in these studies has been to see the problem – that is, non-adherence – from the doctor's point of view rather than the patient or client's point of view. Over the years there has been a shift in emphasis from the practitioner's viewpoint to that of the patient or service user. It is now accepted that patients/service users make decisions about whether or not to follow the advice in the light of the discussions they have with people who share their own social and cultural background and we still need to know more about how to influence lifestyle choice of at risk groups. While to the best of our knowledge no work of this nature has been carried out concerning whether or not clients follow the advice given to them by health visitors, intuitively we feel that there is a high incidence of noncompliance with health visitors' advice. It would be interesting to investigate the clients' perception of health visitor advice since this may assist in improving the service to the clients.

In the days of the sanitary missionary through primary prevention, it was possible to lower the infectious disease mortality and morbidity rates. Today, in the era of the generic family visitor, we are in the position of choosing among interventions which have much lower levels of effectiveness. The reason for this is that today we are dealing with more problems where the resolution can only be achieved by a fundamental change in client lifestyle or behaviour. The example of obesity makes this point. In order to lose weight it is necessary to alter one's eating patterns and consequently one's shopping and exercise habits. Food and the sharing of food also have social meaning and, therefore, reducing weight may require an adjustment to be made in many aspects of everyday life. Few people would be willing to alter their behaviour to this extent. The apparent lack of dramatic opportunities to measure the effects of prevention is one estimate of how far we have come in community health. Although there are underserved groups within society who still exhibit dispro-portionate levels of ill health. A review of deaths between 1921 and 2007 shows inequality increasing with the poorest people more likely to die prematurely than the more affluent (Thomas *et al.*, 2010). There is a major policy drive to tackle health inequalities in health (DH, 2009b; Marmot *et al.*, 2010). In discuss-ing a possible model for assessing the work of the health visitor, Luker over 35 years ago stated:

> Some health visitors believe that the effects of health visiting are too subtle, intangible or elusive to be realistically assessed. If this were so there would be little reason for health visitors to offer a service, since no one, including the client, would be aware of its effects. Intangible and elusive changes can hardly be worthwhile goals or a reason for continuing profes-sional practice. Moreover in the context of the present economic climate it would seem urgent to assess the care given by health visitors in order to demonstrate its effectiveness and to justify the provision of the service. (Luker, 1978)

Health visitors have been content to avoid studying the process of health visitor intervention in terms of its benefit to the client by dismissing it as methodologically impractical. Researchers have focused instead on describing health visiting in terms of what health visitors say they do, the result has been that the numbers of health visitors have fallen over the last thirty years and the shortfall has hardly been commented upon. This lack of focus on outcome evaluation has resulted in the government via the Department of Health seizing the initiative to reconstruct health visiting and to reconfigure its boundaries. *Facing the Future* (DH, 2007) and *Getting It Right for Children and*

Families: Maximising the Contribution of the Health Visiting Team (DH, 2009b) clearly set out the direction of travel, much of which has been discussed in earlier chapters. The health visitor's contribution falls into three main areas: (1) needs assessment; (2) programme delivery (delivery the Healthy Child Programme (HCP)); and (3) a wider public health function, including supplying information on vulnerable groups to enable commissioners to create services (DH, 2009a). All this is underpinned by the best evidence and demonstrating and measuring achievement.

The preventive aspects of health visiting are still important but are difficult to measure because of the long-term nature of the work and the lack of data other than for specific programmes such as immunisation and developmental screening. However, health visitors do deal with clients and families who have tangible problems which are amenable to short-term intervention. In attempting to solve short-term problems health visitors may affect the future health of the client or family in an unknown way since problems which are prevented from developing because of health visitor intervention cannot readily be assessed. Nevertheless, it is thought that evaluation of health visitor intervention in terms of its effect upon the client might begin in the area of tangible problems. There have been some attempts to evaluate the effectiveness of health visitor intervention; however, the studies that have been done are likely to be viewed as no longer relevant given the changing focus of health visiting (Luker, 1978; Elkan *et al.*, 2000; Watson *et al.*, 2004). Getting health visitors involved in 'new' activities such as identifying postnatal depression using validated tools and then delivering a psychologically informed intervention to postnatal mothers has been found to be effective (Morrell *et al.*, 2009) but not all health visitors employ this approach.

In fact little research effort in nursing generally has been directed at evaluation, possibly because of the difficulties involved in demonstrating a cause and effect relationship. Ethical issues are often raised when considering the design of a study to demonstrate a cause and effect relationship. The usual scientific approach has been to use an experimental method which may necessitate denying a control group access to the service. Health visitors have seemed reluctant to deny their service in the interest of scientific enquiry and this reluctance to evaluate practice in addition to the methodological and ethical problems raises the question 'can health visitor intervention be evaluated?'

Attempts have been made in North America to evaluate the effects of 'public health nurse' interventions (Brooten *et al.*, 1986; Casiro *et al.*, 1993; Olds *et al.*, 1986, 1997; Macmillan *et al.*, 2005). These studies have been randomised controlled trials (RCTs) of new interventions such as parenting programmes; intensive home visiting to reduce child physical; rehospitalisation of low birth weight babies. Work by McLennan and Lavis (2006) on evaluating 12 parenting interventions in Canada found that only three had been evaluated by at least one RCT. There was a distinct lack of evidence supporting these parenting interventions but no doubt parenting interventions continue to be a regular feature of health visiting work.

The problems of evaluating social casework are similar to the problems involved in evaluating health visiting. Social workers initially were somewhat more adventurous than health visitors in using the experimental methods. The first such study was conducted by Goldberg *et al.* (1970) who attempted the first controlled field experiment in Britain in the complex and diffuse area known as social casework. The target population of her study was elderly people and the study involved a comparison of the outcome of one group of clients who received the services of a trained social worker with another group who received the services of an untrained social worker. Goldberg *et al.* addressed some of the key problems in evaluation which are shared by health visitors and other community nurses, namely:

- What constitutes success?
- How might success be measured?
- What is an improvement or deterioration and for whom is it for, the client or their family?
- Over what time-scale should the effects of intervention be assessed?
- Whose judgment should be final, the client's or the professional's?

The questions posed by Goldberg are central to any attempt at evaluation. These questions have no straightforward answers but could usefully form the basis of seminar or group work for both students and experienced health visitors. To date there is little evidence to suggest where health visitors might most usefully be deployed. It is suggested here that the opinions of experienced health visitors, concerned with where they consider they have been the most and the least successful in realising their objectives, may shed some light on the goals of health visiting practice at an individual level.

Record-keeping

It may at first glance appear out of place in a chapter on evaluation to include a section on record-keeping. However, it is our contention that a problem-orientated recording system may be used as an adjunct to evaluation. This section is intended to assist students in presenting information in a system-atic and logical way. We do not advocate that health visiting records should necessarily always follow this format. Indeed, given the growing popularity of client-held records it would not be feasible for all records to follow the problem-orientated format. However, in terms of acquainting students with some of the issues involved in evaluation, we advocate this approach. Students often comment that they have received little or no instruction on how to keep client or family records. This is often due to the fact that the tutors in universities assume that community practice teachers (CPTs) give instruction on record-keeping and yet all too often the CPTs assume that record-keeping has been part of the university curriculum.

Information management is one of the core components of health visiting and community practice. Records are important and are therefore transferred to other Trusts and providers when clients move. Records form the basis for confidential reports to other agencies and indeed act as evidence in court. In addition, they are important to managers and may be subject to audit which, as we have already mentioned, is a form of process evaluation. Unlike hospital nursing work, health visitors work in isolation; hence their work is virtually invisible to quality assurance. Health visitors, for example, are seldom observed on home visitors and this provides much scope for individual variations in practice. The only area of a health visitor's work which can readily be monitored is her record-keeping. Thus, it is essential and a legal requirement that a health visitor keeps adequate records which can verify that she has operated in an organisationally and professionally correct manner. This is even more important with the introduction of corporate working in health visiting and school nursing where the records may be written up by any of the team members. The introduction of the Common Assessment Framework (CAF) form (discussed in Chapter 5) has assisted health practitioners to record using a structured form which can be shared as appropriate with other agencies (DES, 2003). The NMC, CPHVA, and each local Trust provide guidance on record-keeping and procedures for auditing records (NMC, 2009; Unite/CPHVA, 2007).

Problem-orientated recording

Health visitors will often record their records in a narrative format or using problem-orientated recording. If health visitors collect information from their clients in accordance with their personal philosophy of healthcare it does not necessarily follow that recordings other than the initial assessment will be organised in a logical way. Doctors have been using formal problem-solving for much longer than nurses; however, if we look at medical records, we invariably find that systematic recording is usually only apparent in the initial assessment, and not in the subsequent progress notes.

The concept of problem-orientated medical records was pioneered by Dr Lawrence Weed. The original intention was to use problem-orientated medical records as a means of logically organising information around the patient's medical problem. Weed (1969) uses the patient's medical records as a tool which facilitates the accomplishment of goals for and with the patients. In Weed's (1969) problem-orientated recording system the mnemonic SOAP stands for Subjective and Objective information about an individual's problem, Assessment and Planning. To make this recording format more applicable to health visiting we suggest that subjective information should relate to what the client says about the problem. Here it is important to stress that the recording should use the client's own words rather than the health visitors' interpretation of what the client meant. The term objective should be replaced by the word observation and here the health visitor records what she observes about the problem; thus observation may be objective or subjective, which of course will depend to some extent on the nature of the problem.

Since within the context of health visiting there is no obvious format for the systematic recording of progress notes, we believe that a modified problem-orientated recording system, using the SOAP system, can be used to assist the health visitor to become more objective about her work and this approach may also assist her in evaluating the outcome of intervention. The other alternative is to use the SMART approach to realistic objective setting (discussed earlier in Care Planning).

The word assessment may be confused with the initial information giving or assessment visit which is sometimes regarded as the first stage in the care process. Hence it is suggested that the word analysis be used instead. This implies that the practitioner places an interpretation on her observations; in doing this she takes account of what the client has said and also what she has observed. At the initial assessment visit it is likely that the analysis section of the records will contain only a statement of the problem. It is reasonable to assume that at a first visit the health visitor will identify an actual and potential problem on the basis of what she observes and by what the client says about a particular issue or area of concern. For the second and subsequent visits the analysis section of the records should contain a statement indicating, on the basis of the evidence, whether or not the problem is the same, better, or worse than before. A plan is then developed of how to deal with the client's problem, or, alternatively, how to help the client deal with his or her own problem.

When writing about problem-orientated recording we are mindful of health visitors' general reluctance to consider that they are dealing with clients with problems. This approach does not ignore the preventive aspect of the work, but enhances the preventive function by requiring the health visitor to make explicit her intentions in the planning section of the records. This approach also encourages health visitors to evaluate their work, since they are obliged to write a substantiated judgment of 'worth' into the analysis section of the records.

It is worth pointing out that new record cards are not necessary when the SOAP format for recording progress notes is used. It is not essential to write out the problem and goal each time an entry is made. If the problems and goals are numbered then the number will be all that is required. It may be helpful at this point to include an example of problem-orientated records using the modified SOAP format.

Example 6.1

This example concerns a mother with a four-year-old child who was referred to the health visitor by the general practitioner. Her problem was identified as having 'difficulty in coping' with the child's behaviour. This was having an affect on relationship with her new partner.

Activity 6.10 (see Appendix 6) will provide the opportunity to practise using SOAP for recording activity.

Front of record card

Problem: Behaviour management
Goal: To cope better with child's behaviour

First visit – 1.2.11

S: 'I am at my wits' end. I don't know how to cope with Ben (child). I am now with a new partner and it is affecting our relationship. I don't like taking him (Ben) places in case he has a tantrum. I thought this happened more at the age of two not when he's four.'

O: Mother appears stressed, near to tears.

A: Really does want to learn how to cope better with child's behaviour; Mother doesn't feel there is anything medically wrong with child.

P: (1) Get the mother to keep a diary to see if anything triggers the outbursts of behaviour;

    (2) Provide information to mother on behaviour management;

    (3) Get the mother to reward the child for positive behaviour (e.g. star chart).

Progress Note 3.4.11

S: 'I have been keeping a diary of Ben's outbursts and it seems to be related to when I am giving attention to my partner'.

O: Has found a 'trigger' to Ben's outbursts.

A: Has been using the 'star chart'; also has been trying to spend time doing things with Ben.

P: (1) Discussed involving partner with doing things as a family; and the partner doing something on his own with Ben.

    (2) Continue with rewarding Ben for positive behaviour.

Progress Note 4.5.11

S: 'I have managed to encourage my partner to take more of an interest in Ben and this seems to have helped. They went fishing together the other day.'

O: Less temper outbursts from Ben; Mother is happier.

A: Positive rewards to Ben for his good behaviour. Has started to go swimming on her own with Ben each week.

P: (1) No further home visits necessary. Mother to contact health visitor again if needs further guidance and information.

    (2) Discussed the support groups and parenting programmes available in area.

This example gives a good insight into how the health visitor was attempting to work with the mother in dealing with her child's behaviour and the record also clearly states the progress the mother has made. Some health visitors feel that this type of record-keeping is too time consuming to be used on day-to-day practice. Those of us who have used this method have found it time consuming at first but once we have become used to the approach we are surprised at how adept we become. It is suggested that health visitors might be encouraged in the first instance to use this style of recording for selected problems such as infant feeding problems, bedwetting, or behaviour management. This would mean that they would develop some competence in recording in this way and may then think it worthwhile to extend it to other aspects of their work. It is thought that as a learning exercise students should be encouraged to use problem-orientated recording in their family or care studies. This approach to record-keeping can also provide useful data about how health visitors approach particular client problems. If the analysis section of the record is filled in adequately we may also gain an insight into the outcome of the intervention. This type of information can be used retrospectively and may in some cases constitute evaluative research.

Summary

This chapter has provided insight into some of the ways that health visitors might approach evaluation. It has highlighted some key sources of evidence available to health visitors in evaluating their practice, including suggested ways to approach evaluation, such as the 'care planning process', target setting using the 'SMART' approach and goal attainment using the 'SOAP' format.

In the context of the 'purchaser provider ideology', value for money as evidenced by health gain is the currency in the marketplace. Health visitors have thus been required to reflect on their contribution to healthcare. It is evident that in the past health visitors have been reluctant to evaluate their work. Instead they have been content to claim that a meaningful evaluation was impossible, due to the individual nature of client problems and the centrality of the relationship with the client. Owing to competing demands on services and restricted financial resources at a national and local level there is an inherent danger in health visitors being replaced by other workers since there is little evidence to support the contention that health visiting makes a difference to the health of the population that could not be achieved using less well-qualified workers.

We have seen a reduction in the numbers of health visitors (NHS Information Centre, 2010) at a time when the health needs of the population are rising and the health differential between social classes increasing. This will change with the Department of Health's implementation plan to increase the health visitor workforce by 37.5% by 2013/14 (DH, 2011). Historically health visitors have been spread thinly across a range of client groups hence minimising their own visibility and potential impact. Latterly health visitors have been redeployed to work with high-risk families which in some respects minimises the preventive health function and makes the work difficult to differentiate from other groups such as social workers. Whilst health visitors might believe that they do 'good work' this is no longer sufficient evidence to be convincing to others who may be sceptical about the benefit of the service. In order to secure continued or additional resources, all health visitors should be prepared to generate information about what they do and the outcome of their work.

References

Bandura, A. (2004) Health promotion by social cognitive means. *Health Education & Behaviour*, **31**(2), 143-164.

Bloch, D. (1975) Evaluation of nursing care in terms of process and outcome. Issues in research and quality assurance. *Nursing Research*, **24**(4), 256-263.

Brooten, D., Kumar, S., Brown, L.P., *et al.* (1986) A randomised clinic trial of early discharge and home follow-up of very-low-birth-weight infants. *New England Journal of Medicine*, **315**, 934-939.

Buchan, J. & DalPoz, M.R. (2002) Skill mix in the health care workforce: reviewing the evidence. *Bulletin of the World Health Organization*, **80**(7), 575-580.

Bull, J., McCormick, G., Swann, C. & Mulvihill, C. (2004) *Ante- and Post-natal Home-visiting Programmes: a Review of Reviews: Evidence Briefing.*, NHS Health Development Agency, London.

Casiro, O.G., McKenzie, M.E., McFadyen, L., *et al.* (1993) Earlier discharge with community-based intervention for low birth weight infants: a randomized trial. *Paediatrics*, **92**, 128-134.

Ciliska, D., Mastrilli, P., Ploeg, J., Hayward, S., Brunton, G. & Underwood, J. (2001) The effectiveness of home visiting as a delivery strategy for public health nursing interventions to clients in the prenatal and postnatal period: A systematic review. *Primary Health Care Research & Development*, **2**(1), 41-54.

Council for the Education and Training of Health Visitors (1977) *An Investigation into the Principles of Health Visiting*. CETHV, London.

Denis, J.L., Langley, A. & Lozeau, A. (1994) Setting priorities in public hospitals: the paradoxes of strategic planning. In: *Setting Priorities in Health Care* (ed. M. Malek). John Wiley & Sons, Ltd, Chichester.

Department for Education and Skills (2003) *Every Child Matters*. Stationery Office, London.

Department of Health (2001) *Health Visitor Practice Development Resource Pack*. DH, London.

Department of Health (2004) *NHS Health Visiting: Professional Advice and Support in the Community: Summary Information for 2003-04 England*. DH, London.

Department of Health (2005a) *Choosing Health: Making Healthy Choices Easier*. DH, London.

Department of Health (2005b) *Self-Care: A Real Choice*. DH, London.

Department of Health (2005c) *Supporting People with Long-Term Conditions. An NHS and Social Care Model to Support Local Innovation and Integration*. DH, London.

Department of Health (2006) *Modernising Nursing Careers - Setting the Direction*. DH, London.

Department of Health (2007) *Facing the Future: A Review of the Role of Health Visitors*. DH, London.

Department of Health (2008a) *Framing the Nursing and Midwifery Contribution: Driving up the Quality of Care*. DH, London.

Department of Health (2008b) *Guidance on the Routine Collection of Patient Reported Outcome Measures (PROMs)*. DH, London.

Department of Health (2008c) *High Quality Care for All: NHS Next Stage Review Final Report*. DH, London.

Department of Health (2009a) *Getting it Right for Children and Families: Maximising the Contribution of the Health Visiting Team: 'Ambition, Action, Achievement'*. DH, London.

Department of Health (2009b) *Tackling Health Inequalities: 10 Years On*. DH, London.

Department of Health (2010a) *Equity and Excellence: Liberating the NHS*. DH, London.

Department of Health (2010b) *White Paper – Health Lives, Healthy People: Our Strategy for Public Health in England*. DH, London.

Department of Health (2011) *Health Visitor Implementation Plan 2011-15: A Call to Action February 2011*. DH, London.

Department of Health and Social Security. Steering Group on Health Services Information (1983). *A Report from a Working Group on Community Health Services*. DHSS, London.

Derryberry, M. (1939) Nursing accomplishments as revealed by case records. *Public Health Report*, **54**(46), 2035-2043.

Donabedian, A. (1969) Some issues in evaluating the quality of nursing care. *American Journal of Public Health*, **59**(10), 1833-1836.

Donabedian, A. (1988) The quality of care: How can it be assessed? *Journal of the American Medical Association*, **260**, 1743-1748.

Elkan, R., Kendrick, D., Hewitt, M., *et al.* (2000) The effectiveness of domiciliary health visiting: a systematic review of international studies and a selective review of the British literature. *Health Technology Assessment*, **4**(13), 1-339.

Family & Parenting Institute (2009) *Health Visitors: A Progress Report*. National Family and Parenting Institute, London.

Goldberg, E.M., Mortimer, A. & Williams, B. (1970) *Helping the Age: a Field Experiment in Social Work*. Allen & Unwin, London.

Hobbs, P. (1973) *Aptitude or Environment*. Royal College of Nursing, London.

Luker, K.A. (1978) Goal attainment: a possible model for assessing the work of the health visitor. *Nursing Times*, **75**(35), 1488-1490.

McDonald, K.M., Sundaram, V., Bravata, D. M., *et al.* (2007) *Care Coordination*. Vol. 7 of: *Closing the Quality Gap: A Critical Analysis of Quality Improvement Strategies. Technical Review 9* (eds K.G. Shojania, K.M. McDonald, R.M. Wachter & D.K. Owens). (Prepared by the Stanford University-UCSF Evidence-based Practice Center under contract 290-02-0017), AHRQ Publication No. 04(07)-0051-7, Agency for Healthcare Research and Quality, Rockville, MD.

McHugh, G. & Luker, K. (2002) Users' perceptions of the health visiting service. *Community Practitioner*, **75**(2), 57-61.

McLennan, J.D. & Lavis, J.N. (2006) What is the evidence for parenting interventions offered in a Canadian community? *Canadian Journal of Public Health*, **97**(6), 454-458.

Macmillan, H.L., Thoms, B.H., Jamieson, E., *et al.* (2005). Effectiveness of home visitation by public-health nurses in prevention of the recurrence of child physical abuse and neglect: a randomized controlled trial. *The Lancet*, **365**, 1786–1793.

Marmot, M., Atkinson, T., Bell, J., *et al.* (2010) *Fair Society, Healthy Lives. The Marmot Review*, Marmot Review Team, University College London.

Morrell, C.J., Slade, P., Warner, R., *et al.* (2009) Clinical effectiveness of health visitor training in psychologically informed approaches for depression in postnatal women: pragmatic cluster randomised trial in primary care. *British Medical Journal*, **338**, a3045; doi 10.1136/bmja3045.

Muir Gray, J.A. (2004) Evidence based policy making: Editorial. *British Medical Journal*, **329**, 988–989.

National Collaborating Centre for Primary Care (2006) *Routine Postnatal Care of Women and Their Babies. NICE Clinical Guideline 37*. NICE, London.

National Institute for Health & Clinical Excellence (2007). *Behaviour Change at Population, Community and Individual Levels: Public Health Guidance 6*. NICE, London.

National Institute for Health & Clinical Excellence (2008a) *Community Engagement*. NICE, London.

National Institute for Health & Clinical Excellence (2008b) *Maternal and Child Nutrition*. NICE, London.

National Institute for Health & Clinical Excellence (2009a) *Reducing the Differences in the Uptake of Immunisations*. NICE, London.

National Institute for Health & Clinical Excellence (2009b) *Reducing the Differences in the Uptake of Immunisations: Audit Support*. NICE, London.

National Institute for Health & Clinical Excellence & Social Care Institute for Excellence (2010a) *Looked After Children and Young People*. NICE, London.

National Institute for Health & Clinical Excellence & Social Care Institute for Excellence (2010b) *Strategies to Prevent Unintentional Injuries among Children and Young People Aged Under 15*. NICE, London.

NHS The Information Centre Workforce and Facilities Team (2010) *NHS Hospital and Community Health Services: Non-medical staff England 1999–2009*. The Health and Social Care Information Centre, London.

Nursing and Midwifery Council (2004) *Standards of Proficiency for Specialist Community Public Health Nurses*. NMC, London.

Nursing and Midwifery Council (2009) *Record Keeping: Guidance for Nurses and Midwives*. NMC, London.

Oakley, A., Strange, V., Bonell, C., Allen, E., Stephenson, J., RIPPLE Study Team. (2006) Process evaluation in randomised controlled trials of complex interventions. *British Medical Journal*, **332**, 413–416, doi:10.1136/bmj.332.7538.413.

Olds, D.L., Eckenrode, J., Henderson, C.R., Jr, *et al.* (1997) Long-term effects of home visitation on maternal life course and child abuse and neglect. Fifteen year follow-up of a randomized trial. *Journal of the American Association*, **278**(8), 637–643.

Olds, D.L., Henderson, C.R., Chamberlin, R. & Tatelbaum, R. (1986) Preventing child abuse and neglect: a randomized trial of nurse home visitation. *Pediatrics*, **78**, 65–78.

Queen's Nursing Institute (2008) *Briefing: Evaluating Outcomes*. QNI, London.

Rees, R., Oliver, K., Woodman, J. & Thomas, J. (2009) *Children's Views about Obesity, Body Size, Shape and Weight: A Systematic Review*. EPPI-Centre, London.

Russell, S. & Drennan, V. (2007) Mothers' views of the health visiting service in the UK: a web-based survey. *Community Practitioner*, **80**(8), 22–26.

St Leger, A.S., Schnieden, H. & Walsworth-Bell, J.P. (1992) *Evaluating Health Services' Effectiveness*. Open University Press, Buckingham.

Shaw, E., Levitt, C., Wong, S., Kaczorowski, J., & The McMaster University Postpartum Research Group (2006) Systematic review of the literature on postpartum care: Effectiveness of postpartum support to improve maternal parenting, mental health, quality of life, and physical health. *Birth*, **33**(3), 210-220.

Skills for Health (2008) *Public Health Skills and Career Framework*, Skills for Health, Bristol.

Speller, V., Learmonth, A. & Harrison, D. (1997) The search for evidence of effective health promotion. *British Medical Journal*, **315**, 361-363.

Suchman, E.A. (1967) *Evaluation Research*. Russell Sage Foundation, New York.

Thomas, B., Dorling, D. & Davy Smith, G. (2010) Inequalities in premature mortality in Britain: Observational study from 1921 to 2007. *British Medical Journal*, **341**, C3639.

Twinn, S. & Cowley, S. (1992) *Principles of Health Visiting: A Re-examination*. CPHVA, London.

Unite/CPHVA (2007) *Record Keeping and the Law*. Unite/CPHVA, London.

Unite/CPHVA (2009) *What Size Caseload Should a Health Visitor Have?* Unite/CPHVA, London.

Watson, M., Kendrick, D., Coupland, C., Woods, A., Futers, D. & Robinson, J. (2004) Providing child safety equipment to prevent injuries: randomised controlled trial. *British Medical Journal*, doi:10.1136/bmj.38309.664444.8F.

Weed, L.L. (1969) *Medical Records, Medical Education and Patient Care*. Press of Case Western Reserve University, Ohio.

While, A., Forbes, A., Ullman, R. & Murgatroyd, B. (2005) *The Contribution of Nurses, Midwives and Health Visitors to Child Health and Child Health Services: a Scoping Review*. NCCSDO, London.

Whitlock, E.P., O'Connor, E.A., Williams, S.B., Beil, T.L. and Lutz, K.W. (2008) *Effectiveness of Weight Management Programs in Children and Adolescents*. Agency for Healthcare Research and Quality, Rockville, MD USA.

Whitlock, E.P., O'Connor, E.A., Williams, S.B., Beil, T.L. and Lutz, K.W. (2010) Effectiveness of weight management interventions: a targeted systematic review for the USPSTF. *Paediatrics*, **125**(2):e396-418. Epub 2010, 18 Jan.

Appendix 6   Activities for Chapter 6

Activity 6.1

Using guidelines

- Go onto the following websites: National Institute for Health and Clinical Evidence (NICE) (www.nice.nhs.uk) and Social Care Institute for Excellence (www.scie.org.uk).
- Select a guideline, which is of relevance to your practice.
- Compare this national guidance to your local guidelines (if they exist) in your workplace or compare them to your own current practice so as to identify any similarities and differences.
- What recommendations would you make for changing your current practice after reading the national guideline?

Activity 6.2

Locating sources of evidence

Take the opportunity to explore the relevant websites:

- NHS Evidence: www.evidence.nhs.uk
- NHS Evidence QIPP: http://www.library.nhs.uk/qipp/
- Effective healthcare bulletin: www. york.ac.uk/inst/crd/ehcb.htm
- Centre for Reviews and Dissemination Publications: http://www.york. ac.uk/inst/crd/index_publications.htm
- Centre for Reviews and Dissemination Databases: http://www.crd. york.ac.uk/crdweb/.
  - o Database of Abstracts of Reviews of Effects (DARE);
  - o NHS EED (Economic Evaluation Database);
  - o Health Technology Assessment (HTA) (see also: http://www.hta.ac.uk)

Activity 6.3

Thinking about your practice

- Think about a specific area of your practice, what are the aims of this area of practice?
- How do you know the aims are being met?
- After integrating new guidance or research evidence (if available), is there anything you would change about this area of practice?
- How would you go about assessing whether the change has had any impact on improving your practice or service delivery?

Activity 6.4

Developing new programmes

- Design a programme which could be delivered in your practice (e.g. weight management; weaning programme; behaviour management).
- Start to identify the evaluation criteria (e.g. what are the aims of the programme; what do you want to achieve; how do you know it is of benefit?)

Activity 6.5

Action planning

- Think of a health problem(s) to be addressed with one of your families
- Complete the record of action plan table:

Health problem to be addressed	Objective	Action to be taken	Who will do it?	Evaluation measures
1)				
2)				
3)				
4)				

Activity 6.6

Using the SMART approach

Think of a common issue you encounter in practice and complete the SMART approach to goal setting. An example is provided below of a mother who wishes to lose weight using the SMART approach to goal setting.

SMART	Client problem
Specific goal	Mother will lose half stone
Measurable goal	Mother will lose 3 lbs in a month and a further 4 lbs 2 months later
Achievable goal	Mother will weigh herself fortnightly Mother will follow diet plan provided
Realistic goal	By the end of the year the mother wishes to be able to fit into pre-pregnancy clothes.
Time-bound	Mother will have lost $1/2$ stone by December 2012.

Please complete your own example:

SMART	Client problem
Specific goal	
Measurable goal	
Achievable goal	
Realistic goal	
Time-bound	

Activity 6.7

Locating sources of information

The Association of Public Health Observatories provide useful data for assessing health need and planning resources for a range of public health issues. Visit the Child and Maternal Health Observatory (ChiMat) (http://www.chimat.org.uk) and see if you can locate the child health profiles for your specific area (click on *Tools and Data*; then *Interactive Child Health Profiles* then on your *geographical region* then on *area*). This can also be done to find out the *breastfeeding profiles* on your area (see: http://atlas.chimat.org.uk/IAS/dataviews/breastfeedingprofile).

Activity 6.8

Developing goals

Consider your visit to a new mother who has the problem of sore breasts. Goal A is the more general goal and goal B will helps you specify the activities to achieve the goal (e.g. watch how baby latches on to nipple). This activity helps you to understand how specific goals should be so as to be achievable and then evaluated more easily.

Goal statement A

Goal statement B

Activity 6.9

Using SOAP for an approach to record-keeping

In Chapter 6 you were provided with an example of a mother's contact with the health visitor concerning her child's behaviour. Select an example of a problem a family may be having and complete your records using the SOAP format (Subjective and Objective information about a client's problem, Assessment and Planning).

Front of record card

Problem:

Goal:

First visit – Date:

S:

O:

A:

P:(1)

  (2)

  (3)

Bibliography

Alaszewski, A. (2006) Managing risk in community practice: nursing, risk and decision-making. In: *Risk and Nursing Practice* (ed. P. Godin), pp. 24–41. Palgrave, London.

Allen, G. & Duncan Smith, I. (2010) *Early Intervention: Good Parents, Great Kids, Better Citizens*. The Centre for Social Justice and The Smith Institute, London. Available from: http://www.centreforsocialjustice.org.uk/default.asp?pageRef=269 (accessed 8 March, 2011).

Andrew, N., Tolson, D. & Ferguson D. (2008) Building on Wenger: communities of practice in nursing. *Nurse Education Today.* **28**, 246–252.

Angus, J., Kontos, P., Dyck, I., McKeever, P. & Poland B. (2005) The personal significance of home: habitus and the experience of receiving long-term home care. *Sociology of Health and Illness*, **27**(5), 161–187.

Antonovsky, A. (1996) The salutogenic model as a theory to guide health promotion. *Health Promotion International*, **11**(1), 11–18.

Appleby, J., Walshe, K. & Ham C. (1995) *Acting on the Evidence*. National Association of Health Authorities & Trusts, Birmingham.

Appleton, J. (1994) The concept of vulnerability in relation to child protection: health visitors' perceptions. *Journal of Advanced Nursing*, **20**, 1132–1140.

Arnstein, S. (1969) A ladder of citizen participation. *American Institute of Planners Journal*, **35**(4), 216–224.

Ashton, J. & Seymour, H. (1988) *The New Public Health*. Open University Press, Milton Keynes.

Association of Public Health Observatories (2010) Health Profiles. Available from: www.apho.org.uk (accessed 3 February, 2011).

Atkinson, M., Doherty, P. & Kinder, K (2005) Multi-agency working: models, challenges and key factors for success. *Journal of Early Childhood Research*, **3**(1), 7–17.

Audit Commission (2010) *Giving Children a Healthy Start: Health Report*. Available at: www.audit-commission.gov.uk (accessed 9 March, 2011).

Ayre, P. (2007) Common ground: Child neglect. *Community Care*, 29 March–4 April, 36–37.

Baggott, R. (2000) *Public Health: Policy & Politics*. Palgrave Macmillan, Basingstoke.

Baldwin, N. & Caruthers, L. (1998) *Developing Neighbourhood Support and Child Protection Strategies: The Henley Safe Children Project*. Ashgate Publishing Ltd, Farnham.

Bandura, A. (1977) Self-efficacy: towards a unifying theory of behavioural change. *Psychological Review*, **84**, 191–215.

Health Visiting: A Rediscovery, Third Edition. Edited by Karen A. Luker, Jean Orr and Gretl A. McHugh.
© 2012 Blackwell Publishing Ltd. Published 2012 by Blackwell Publishing Ltd.

Bandura, A. (2004) Health promotion by social cognitive means. *Health Education & Behaviour*, **31**(2), 143-164.

Barker, D.J.P. (ed.) (1992) *Fetal and infant origins of adult disease*. BMJ Publishing, London.

Barker, W. (1984) *Child Development Programme*, Early Childhood Development Unit, Senate House, University of Bristol, Bristol.

Barker, W. & Anderson, R. (1988) *Child Development Programme: An Evaluation of Process and Outcomes*. Early Child Development Unit, University of Bristol.

Barlow, J., Coren, E. & Stewart-Brown, S. (2002) Meta-analysis of the effectiveness of parenting programmes in improving maternal psychosocial health. *British Journal of General Practice*, **52**(476), 223-233.

Barlow, J., Coren, E. & Stewart-Brown, S. (2003) Parent-training programmes for improving maternal psychosocial health (Review). *Cochrane Database of Systematic Reviews*, **76**, 223-233.

Barlow, J., Kirkpatrick, S., Wood, D., Ball, M., & Stewart-Brown, S. (2007) *Sure Start National Evaluation Summary: Family and Parenting Support in Sure Start Local Programmes*. Available from: http://www.education.gov.uk/research/data/uploadfiles/NESS2007SF023.pdf (accessed 9 March, 2011).

Barrett, G., Naidoo, J. & Orme, J. (2007) Capacity and capability in public health. In: *Public Health for the 21st Century* (eds J. Orme, J. Powell, P. Taylor & M. Grey), 2nd ed, Ch. 5, pp. 83-97. Open University Press McGraw-Hill Education, Maidenhead.

Bauld, L. (2011) *The Impact of Smokefree Legislation in England: Evidence Review, March 2011*. Department of Health, London.

BBC News (2008) 'MMR: Mothers divided'. Available from: http://news.bbc.co.uk/1/hi/health/1804665.stm (accessed 3 March, 2011).

BBC News (2010) Facebook and Bebo child sex abuse postman jailed. 24 September. British Broadcasting Corporation, London. Available from: http://www.bbc.co.uk/news/uk-england-cornwall-11403984 (accessed 30 September, 2010).

BBC News (2011) Cuts 'destroying big society' concept, says CSV head BBC News, London. Available from: http://www.bbc.co.uk/news/uk-politics-12378974 (accessed 8 March, 2011).

Beaglehole, R. & Bonita, R. (1997) *Public Health at the Crossroads*. Cambridge University Press, Cambridge.

Beattie, A. (2003 (1991)) Knowledge and control in health promotion: a test case for social policy and social theory. In: *The Sociology of the Health Service* (eds J. Gabe, M. Calnan & M. Bury), Ch. 7, pp. 162-202. Routledge, London.

Beauchamp, T. & Childress, J. (2001) *Principles of Biomedical Ethics*, 5th edn. Oxford University Press, Oxford.

Bell, C. & Newby, H. (1971) *Community Studies*. Allen & Unwin, London.

Belsky, J., Melhuish, E., Barnes, J., Leyland, A.H. & Romaniuk, H. (2006) The National Evaluation of Sure Start Research Team Effects of Sure Start local programmes on children and families: early findings from a quasi-experimental, cross sectional study. *British Medical Journal*, **332**, 1476. doi:10.1136/bmj.38853.451748.2F (published 16 June, 2006).

Benson, J. (1976) The concept of community. In: *Talking about Welfare* (eds N. Timms & D. Watson). Routledge & Kegan Paul, London.

Birmingham Primary Care Trusts (2007) *Health Visitor and School Health Record Keeping Guidelines*. Available from: www.bpcssa.nhs.uk/policies/_south%5Cpolicies%5C764.pdf (accessed 9 March, 2011).

Bloch, D. (1975) Evaluation of nursing care in terms of process and outcome. Issues in research and quality assurance. *Nursing Research*, **24**(4), 256-263.

Bonnell, C., McKee, M., Fletcher, A., Wilkinson, P. & Haines, A. (2011) One nudge forward, two steps back, *British Medical Journal*, **342**, d401.

Bowlby, J. (1969) *Attachment and Loss. Volume 1. Attachment*. Basic Books, New York.

Bradford Hill, A. (1965) The environment and disease: Association or causation? *Proceedings of the Royal Society of Medicine*, **58**, 295-300.

Bradshaw, J. (1972) The concept of social need. *New Society*, **30**, 640-643.

Bradshaw, J. (1994) The conceptualisation and measurement of need – a social policy perspective. In: *Researching the People's Health* (eds J. Popay & G. Williams), Ch. 3, pp. 45-57. Routledge, London.

Brandon, M., Bailey, S., Belderson, P., *et al.* (2009) *Understanding Serious Case Reviews and their Impact A Biennial Analysis of Serious Case Reviews 2005-07*. DCSF, University of East Anglia.

Brandon, M., Howe, A., Dagley, V., Salter, C. & Warren, C. (2006) What appears to be helping or hindering practitioners in implementing the Common Assessment Framework and lead professional working? *Child Abuse Review*, **15**, 396-413.

Bremner, J.D. (1999) Does stress damage the brain? *Biological Psychiatry*, **45**, 797-805.

Briere, J.N. & Elliot, D.M. (1994) Immediate and long-term impacts of child sexual abuse. *The Future of Children*, **4**, 54-69.

Briere, J.N. & Runtz, M. (1987) Post sexual abuse trauma: Data and implications for clinical practice. *Journal of Interpersonal Violence*, **2**, 367-379.

Bronfenbrenner, U. (1979) *The Ecology of Human Development: Experiments by Nature and Design*. Harvard University Press, London.

Brooten, D., Kumar, S., Brown, L.P., *et al.* (1986) A randomised clinic trial of early discharge and home follow-up of very-low-birth-weight infants. *New England Journal of Medicine*, **315**, 934-939.

Bryans, A., Cornich, E. & McIntosh, J. (2009) The potential of the ecological theory for building an integrated framework to develop the public health contribution of health visiting. *Health and Social Care in the Community*, **17**(6), 564-572.

Bryar, R. & Fisk, L. (1994) Setting up a community health house. *Community Practitioner*, **67**(6), 203-205.

Bryar, R., Kendall, S. & Mogotlane, S.M. (2011) *Reforming Primary Health: A Nursing Perspective: Contributing to Health Care Reform, Issues and Challenges*. ICHRN, ICN, Geneva (In press).

Buchan, J. & DalPoz, M.R. (2002) Skill mix in the health care workforce: reviewing the evidence. *Bulletin of the World Health Organisation*, **80**(7), 575-580.

Bull, J., McCormick, G., Swann, C. & Mulvihill, C. (2004) *Ante- and Post-natal Home-visiting Programmes: a Review of Reviews: Evidence Briefing.*, NHS Health Development Agency, London.

Butler-Sloss, Dame E. (1988) *Report of the Inquiry into Child Abuse in Cleveland 1987*. Her Majesty's Stationery Office, London.

Cabinet Office (2006) *Reaching Out: An Action Plan on Social Exclusion Publication*. Stationery Office, London.

Cabinet Office (2007) *Families at Risk: Background on Families with Multiple Disadvantages*. Stationery Office, London.

Cabinet Office (2009) *Social Exclusion Task Force, Family Nurse Partnership*. Available from: http://webarchive.nationalarchives.gov.uk/+/http:/www.cabinetoffice.gov.uk/social_exclusion_task_force/family_nurse_partnership.aspx (accessed 9 March, 2011).

CAFCASS (2010) *Cafcass Care Demand – Latest Figures for April-August 2010* Children and Family Court Advisory Service. Available from: http://www.cafcass.gov.uk/publications/care_demand_statistics.aspx (accessed 30 September, 2010).

Cameron, S. & Christie, G. (2007) Exploring health visitors' perceptions of the public health nursing role. *Primary Health Care Research and Development*, **8**(1), 80–90.

Campbell, A., Converse, P. & Rodgers, W. (1976) *The Quality of American Life: Perceptions, Evaluations and Satisfaction*. Russell Sage Foundation, New York.

Capewell, S. & Graham, H. (2010) Will cardiovascular disease prevention widen health inequalities? *PLoS Medicine*, **7**(8), e1000320. Available from: http://www.plosmedicine. org/article/info%3Adoi%2F10.1371%2Fjournal.pmed.1000320#pmed.1000320-McLaren1 (accessed 11 March, 2011).

Caraher, M. & McNab, M. (1997) Using lessons from health visiting's past to inform the public health role. *Health Visitor*, **70**, 380–384.

Care Quality Commission (2009) Review of the involvement and action taken by health bodies in relation to the case of Baby P. CQC, London. Available from: http://www.cqc. org.uk/_db/_documents/Baby_Peter_report_FINAL_12_May_09_(2).pdf (Accessed 30 September, 2010).

Carers UK (2008) 2008 Carers UK: National Carers' Strategy. Available from: http:// www.carersuk.org/Aboutus/MoreaboutCarersUK/StrategyAnnualReportAccounts (accessed 18 March, 2011).

Carper, B.A. (1978) Fundamental patterns of knowing in nursing. *Advances in Nursing Science*, **1**(1), 13–23.

Casiro, O.G., McKenzie, M.E., McFadyen, L., *et al.* (1993) Earlier discharge with community-based intervention for low birth weight infants: a randomized trial. *Paediatrics*, **92**, 128–134.

CESCR (2000) *Substantive Issues Arising in the Implementation of the International Covenant on Economic, Social & Cultural Rights: General Comment No. 14*. Committee on Economic, Social & Cultural Rights, New York. Available from: http://www.unhchr. ch/tbs/doc.nsf/(Symbol)/40d009901358b0e2c1256915005090be?Opendocument (accessed 7 March, 2011).

CETHV (1977) *An Investigation into the Principles of Health Visiting*. Council for the Education and Training of Health Visitors, London.

Chalmers, I. (2003) Trying to do more good than harm in policy and practice: the role of rigorous, transparent, up-to-date evaluations. *Annals of the American Academy of Political and Social Science*, **589**, 22–40.

Chalmers, I. (2005) If evidence-informed policy works in practice, does it matter if it doesn't work in theory? *Evidence and Policy*, **1**(2), 227–242.

Chalmers, K.I. (1992a) Giving and receiving: an empirically derived theory of health visiting practice. *Journal of Advanced Nursing*, **17**(11), 1317–1325.

Chalmers, K.I. (1992b) Working with men: an analysis of health visiting practice in families with young children. *International Journal of Nursing Studies*, **29**(1), 3–16.

Chalmers, K.I. (1994) Difficult work: health visitors' work with clients in the community. *International Journal of Nursing Studies*, **31**(2), 168–182.

Chalmers, K.I. & Bramadat, I. (1996) Community development: analysis of the role for community health nurses. *Journal of Advanced Nursing*, **24**, 719–726.

Chalmers, K.I & Luker, K. (1991) The development of the health visitor-client relationship. *Scandinavian Journal of Caring Sciences*, **5**(1), 33–41.

Change4Life (undated) Home Page. Available from: www.nhs.uk/Change4Life/Pages/ change-for-life.aspx (accessed 12 March, 2011).

Children's Workforce Development Council (2008) *Common Assessment Framework* CWDC, London.

Ciliska, D., Mastrilli, P., Ploeg, J., Hayward, S., Brunton, G. & Underwood, J. (2001) The effectiveness of home visiting as a delivery strategy for public health nursing interventions to clients in the prenatal and postnatal period: A systematic review. *Primary Health Care Research & Development*, **2**(1), 41–54.

Clarke, K. (2006) Childhood, parenting and early intervention: a critical examination of the SureStart national programme, *Critical Social Policy*, **26**(4), 699–721.

Corby, B. (2000) *Child Abuse: Towards a Knowledge Base*. Open University Press, Milton Keynes.

Council for the Education and Training of Health Visitors (1965) *Syllabus Examination for Health Visitors in the United Kingdom*. Council for the Education and Training of Health Visitors, London; cited in J. Robinson & R. Elkan (1996) *Health Needs Assessment. Theory and Practice*. Churchill Livingstone, Edinburgh.

Council for the Education and Training of Health Visitors (1967) *The Function of the Health Visitor*. Council for the Education and Training of Health Visitors, London, cited in J. Robinson & R. Elkan (1996) *Health Needs Assessment. Theory and Practice*. Churchill Livingstone, Edinburgh.

Council for the Education and Training of Health Visitors (1977) *An Investigation into the Principles of Health Visiting*. CETHV, London.

Council of Europe (1950) *Convention for the Protection of Human Rights and Fundamental Freedoms (amended, 2010)* Council of Europe, Available from: http://conventions.coe.int/treaty/en/Treaties/Html/005.htm (accessed 6 March, 2011).

Cowley, S. (1996) Reflecting on the past; preparing for the next century *Health Visitor*, **69**, 313–316.

Cowley, S. & Frost, M. (2006) *The Principles of Health Visiting: Opening the Door to Public Health Practice in the 21st Century*. Community Practitioners' and Health Visitors' Association, London.

CPHVA (2007) *Community Practitioners' and Health Visitors' Association Response to 'Facing the Future – A Review of the Role of Health Visitors'*. Available from: http://www.dodsdata.com/Resources/epolitix/Forum%20Microsites/Amicus-Unite/Appendix%203.pdf (accessed 30 September, 2010).

Craig, P.M. (1995) *A Different Role: Health Visiting in a Community Project*. Glasgow City Health Project, Glasgow.

Craig, P.M. (2000) The nursing contribution to public health: In: *Nursing for Public Health. Population-based care* (eds P.M. Craig & Lindsay G.M.). Churchill Livingstone, London.

Craig, P.M. & Lindsay, G.M. (eds) (2000) *Nursing for Public Health. Population-based Care*. Churchill Livingstone, London.

Creighton, S. (2007) Patterns and outcomes. In: *The Child Protection Handbook* (eds K. Wilson & A. James), 3rd edn, pp. 31–48. Bailliere Tindall, London.

Crow, G. (2002) Community Studies: Fifty Years of Theorization. *Sociological Research Online*, **7**(3), 1–13, Available from: www.socresonline.org.uk/7/3/crow.html (accessed 23 March, 2011).

Dahlgren, G. & Whitehead, M. (1991) *Policies and Strategies to Promote Social Equity in Health*. Institute for Futures Studies, Stockholm.

Davey Smith, G., Hart, C., Blane, D., Gillis, C. & Hawthorne, V. (1997) Lifetime socioeconomic position and mortality: prospective observational study. *British Medical Journal*, **314**, 547.

Davey Smith, G., Hart, C., Blane, D. & Hole, D. (1998) Adverse socioeconomic conditions in childhood and cause specific adult mortality: prospective observational study, *British Medical Journal*, **316**, 1631.

Dawley, K., Loch, J. & Bindrich, I. (2007) The Nurse Family Partnership. *American Journal of Nursing*, **107**(11), 60–67.

Delamont, S. (1976) *Interaction in the Classroom*. Methuen, London.

Denis, J.L., Langley, A. & Lozeau, A. (1994) Setting priorities in public hospitals: the paradoxes of strategic planning. In: *Setting Priorities in Health Care* (ed. M. Malek). John Wiley & Sons, Ltd, Chichester.

Dench, G., Gavron, K. & Young, M. (2006) *The New East End: Kinship, Race and Conflict*. The Young Foundation, London.

Department for Children, Schools and Families (2008) *Information Sharing: Guidance for Practitioners and Managers*. Department for Children, Schools and Families, London.

Department for Children, Schools and Families (2009) *Referrals, Assessment and Children and Young People Who Are the Subject of a Child Protection Plan, England – Year Ending 31 March 2009*. Available from: http://www.dcsf.gov.uk/rsgateway/DB/SFR/s000873/index.shtml (accessed 30 September, 2010).

Department for Children, Schools and Families (2010a) *Home Page: Sure Start Children's Centres*. Available from: http://www.dcsf.gov.uk/everychildmatters/earlyyears/surestart/whatsurestartdoes/ (accessed 9 March, 2011).

Department for Children, Schools and Families (2010b) *Working Together to Safeguard Children: A Guide to Inter-agency Working to Safeguard and Promote the Welfare of Children*. Department for Children, Schools and Families, London.

Department for Children, Schools and Families & Department of Health (2008) *Nurse-Family Partnership Programme: First Year Pilot Sites, Implementation in England. Pregnancy and the Post Partum Period*. Research Report DCSF-RW051 (authors: L. Barnes, M. Ball, P. Meadows, J. McLeish, J. Belsky and the FNP Implementation Research Team, Institute for the Study of Children, Families and Social Issues, University of London Birkbeck). Department for Children, Schools and Families, London.

Department for Children, Schools and Families & Department of Health (2009) *Nurse-Family Partnership Programme: Second Year Pilot Sites, Implementation in England. The Infancy Period*. Research Report DCSF-RR166 (authors L. Barnes, M. Ball, P. Meadows, J. McLeish, J. Belsky and the FNP implementation team, Institute for the Study of Children, Families and Social Issues, Birkbeck, University of London). Department for Children, Schools and Families, London.

Department for Education and Skills (2004) *Common Assessment Framework*. Available from: http://www.education.gov.uk/consultations/downloadableDocs/ACFA006.pdf (accessed 15 February, 2011).

Department for Education and Skills (2004) *Every Child Matters: Change for Children*. Department for Education and Skills, London.

Department for Education and Skills (2006) *What to Do if You're Worried a Child Is Being Abused*. Department for Education and Skills, Nottingham. Available from: http://www.dh.gov.uk/en/Publicationsandstatistics/Publications/PublicationsPolicyAndGuidance/DH_4010283 (accessed 15 January, 2011).

Department of Health (1995) *Child Protection Messages from Research*. HMSO, London.

Department of Health (1988) *Public Health in England: the Report of the Committee of Inquiry into the Future Development of the Public Health Function*. Department of Health, London.

Department of Health (1999) *Saving Lives: Our Healthier Nation*. The Stationery Office, London.

Department of Health (2001a) *The Health Visitor and School Nurse Development Programme: Health Visitor Practice Development Resource Pack*. Department of Health, London.

Department of Health (2001b) *Health Visitor Practice Development Resource Pack*. Department of Health, London.

Department of Health (2002) *Women's Mental Health: Into the Mainstream*. Department of Health, London.

Department of Health (2003) *Liberating the Public Health Talents of Community Practitioners and Health Visitors*. Department of Health, London.

Department of Health (2004a) *Best Practice Guidance for Doctors and Other Health Professionals on the Provision of Advice and Treatment to Young People under 16 on Contraception, Sexual and Reproductive Health*. The Stationery Office, London.

Department of Health (2004b) *The Chief Nursing Officer's Review of the Nursing, Midwifery and Health Visiting Contribution to Vulnerable Children and Young People*. Department of Health, London.

Department of Health (2004c) *National Service Framework for Children, Young People and Maternity Services*. Department of Health, London.

Department of Health (2004d) *NHS Health Visiting: Professional Advice and Support in the Community: Summary Information for 2003–04 England*. DH, London.

Department of Health (2005a) *Choosing Health: Making Healthy Choices Easier*. DH, London.

Department of Health (2005b) *Self-Care: A Real Choice*. DH, London.

Department of Health (2005c) *Supporting People with Long-Term Conditions. An NHS and Social Care Model to Support Local Innovation and Integration*. DH, London.

Department of Health (2006a) *Modernising Nursing Careers – Setting the Direction*. DH, London.

Department of Health (2006b) *Our Health, Our Care, Our Say: A New Direction for Community Services*. The Stationery Office, London.

Department of Health (2007a) *Facing the Future: A Review of the Role of Health Visitors*. Department of Health, London. Available from: http://www.phru.net/phn/healthvisitingreview/Literature%20Review%20and%20Evidence/health%20visitor%20review.pdf (accessed 9 March, 2011).

Department of Health (2007b) *The Government Response to Facing the Future: a Review of the Role of Health Visitors*. Department of Health, London. Available from: http://www.dh.gov.uk/en/Publicationsandstatistics/Publications/PublicationsPolicyAndGuidance/DH_075642 (accessed 26 February, 2011).

Department of Health (2007c) *Guidance on Joint Strategic Needs Assessment*. Department of Health, London.

Department of Health (2008a) *Framing the Nursing and Midwifery Contribution: Driving up the Quality of Care*. DH, London.

Department of Health (2008b) *Guidance on the Routine Collection of Patient Reported Outcome Measures (PROMs)*. DH, London.

Department of Health (2008c) *Healthy Child Programme*. Department of Health, London.

Department of Health (2008d) *High Quality Care for All: NHS Next Stage Review Final Report*. DH, London.

Department of Health (2008e) *NHS Next Stage Review: Our Vision for Primary Care and Community Care (Darzi Report)*. Department of Health, London.

Department of Health (2009a) *Getting it Right for Children and Families: Maximising the Contribution of the Health Visiting Team: 'Ambition, Action, Achievement'*. DH, London.

Department of Health (2009b) *Healthy Child Programme: Pregnancy and the First Five Years of Life*. Department of Health, London. Available from: http://www.dh.gov.uk/en/Publicationsandstatistics/Publications/PublicationsPolicyAndGuidance/DH_107563 (accessed 23 February, 2011).

Department of Health (2009c) *Improving Safety, Reducing Harm. Children, Young People and Domestic Violence: A Practical Toolkit for Front-line Practitioners*. TSO, London.

Department of Health (2009d) *Tackling Health Inequalities: 10 Years On*. DH, London.

Department of Health (2009e) *Transforming Community Services: Enabling New Patterns of Provision*. Department of Health, London.

Department of Health (2010a) *Equity and Excellence: Liberating the NHS*. DH, London.

Department of Health (2010b) *Healthy Lives, Healthy People: Our Strategy for Public Health in England*. Stationery Office, London Available from: http://www.dh.gov.uk/en/Publicationsandstatistics/Publications/PublicationsPolicyAndGuidance/DH_121941 (accessed 23 February, 2011).

Department of Health (2010c) *Equity and Excellence: Liberating the NHS*, The Stationery Office, London, Available from: http://www.dh.gov.uk/en/Publicationsandstatistics/Publications/PublicationsPolicyAndGuidance/DH_117353 (accessed 3 March, 2011).

Department of Health (2010d) *Service Vision for Health Visiting in England. CPHVA Conference 20-22 October 2010*. Department of Health, London.

Department of Health (2011a) The Family-Nurse Partnership Programme in England: Wave 1 Implementation in Toddlerhood & a Comparison between Waves 1 and 2a of Implementation in Pregnancy and Infancy. Institute for Study of Children, Families and Social Issues, Birkbeck, University of London.

Department of Health (2011b) *Health Visitor Implementation Plan 2011-15: Call to Action*. Department of Health, London. Available from: http://www.dh.gov.uk/en/Publicationsandstatistics/Publications/PublicationsPolicyAndGuidance/DH_124202 (accessed 23 February, 2011).

Department of Health and Department for Children, Schools & Families (2009) *Healthy Lives, Brighter Futures – The Strategy for Children and Young People's Health,* Department of Health and Department for Children, Schools & Families, Stationery Office, London. Available from: http://www.dh.gov.uk/en/Publications andstatistics/Publications/PublicationsPolicyAndGuidance/DH_094400 (accessed 28 February, 2011).

Department of Health, Department for Education and Employment, Home Office (2000) *Framework for the Assessment of Children in Need and their Families*. The Stationery Office, Norwich.

Department of Health and Social Security. Steering Group on Health Services Information (1983). *A Report from a Working Group on Community Health Services*. DHSS, London.

Department of Health, Social Services and Public Safety (2006) *UNOCINI and the Comprehensive Assessment of Children in Need*. DHSSPS, Northern Ireland.

Department of Health, Social Services and Public Safety (2009) *Review of Health Visiting and School Nursing in Northern Ireland 2009-2011/12*. DHSSPS, Belfast.

Department of Health, Social Services and Public Safety (2010) Redesign of community nursing – *Healthy Futures: The Contribution of Health Visitors and School Nurses in Northern Ireland*. DHSSPS, Belfast. Available from: http://www.dhsspsni.gov.uk/microsoft_word_-_hvsn_review_-_main_report_-_june_2009.pdf (accessed 23 August, 2010).

Department of Health/Unite/CPHVA (2009) *Getting it Right for Children and Families. Maximising the Contribution of the Health Visiting Team. 'Ambition, Action, Achievement'*. Department of Health, London.

Derryberry, M. (1939) Nursing accomplishments as revealed by case records. *Public Health Report*, **54**(46), 2035-2043.

Donabedian, A. (1969) Some issues in evaluating the quality of nursing care. *American Journal of Public Health*, **59**(10), 1833-1836.

Donabedian, A. (1988) The quality of care: How can it be assessed? *Journal of the American Medical Association*, **260**, 1743-1748.

Draper, A.K., Hewitt, G. & Rifkin, S. (2010) Chasing the dragon: Developing indicators for assessment of community participation in health programmes. *Social Science & Medicine*, **71**(6), 1102-1109.

Drennan, V. (ed.) (1988) *Health Visitors and Groups. Politics and Practice*. Heinemann Professional Publishing Ltd, Oxford.

Drew, P. & Heritage, J. (eds) (1992) *Talk at Work*. Cambridge University Press, Cambridge.

Driscoll, J. & Teh, B. (2001) The potential of reflective practice to develop individual orthopaedic nurse practitioners and their practice. *Journal of Orthopaedic Nursing*, **5**, 95-103.

Earle, S. (2007) Exploring health. In: *Theory and Research in Promoting Public Health* (eds S. Earle, C.E. Lloyd, M. Sidell & S. Spurr). Sage, London.

Earle, S. & O'Donnell, T. (2007) The factors that influence health. In: *Theory and Research in Promoting Public Health* (eds S. Earle, C.E. Lloyd, M. Sidell & S. Spurr). Sage, London.

Elkan, R., Kendrick, D., Hewitt, M. *et al.* (2000) The effectiveness of domiciliary health visiting: a systematic review of international studies and a selective review of the British literature. *Health Technology Assessment*, **4**(13), i-v, 1-339.

Emond, A., Pollock, J., Deave, T., Bonnell, S., Peters, T.J. & Harvey, I. (2002) An evaluation of the First Parent Health Visiting Scheme. *Archives of Disease in Childhood*, **86**, 150-157. doi:10.1136/adc.86.3.150.

Estabrooks, C. (1998) Will evidence based nursing practice make practice perfect? *Canadian Journal of Nursing Research*, **30**, 15-36.

Estabrooks, C., Rutakumwa, W., O'Leary, K. *et al.* (2005) Sources of practice knowledge among nurses. *Qualitative Health Research*, **15**(4), 460-476.

Family & Parenting Institute (2007) *Health Visiting an Endangered Species*. Family & Parenting Institute, London.

Family & Parenting Institute (2009) *Health Visitors: A Progress Report*. National Family & Parenting Institute, London. Available from: http://www.familyandparenting.org/Filestore//Documents/Our_work/Campaigns/HealthVisitors_a_progress_report.pdf (accessed 10 March, 2011).

Featherstone, B. & Trinder, L. (2001) New Labour, families and fathers. *Critical Social Policy*, **21**(4), 534-536.

Felitti, V.J. (1991) Long-term medical consequences of incest, rape, and molestation. *Southern Medical Journal*, **84**, 328-331.

Felitti V.J., Anda, R.F., Nordenberg, D., *et al.* (1998) Relationship of childhood abuse and household dysfunction to many of the leading causes of death in adults: The Adverse Childhood Experiences (ACE) Study. *American Journal of Preventive Medicine*, **14**(4), 245-258.

Felitti, V.J., Anda, R.F., Nordenberg, D. *et al.* (2001) Relationship of childhood abuse and household dysfunction to many of the leading causes of death in adults. In: *Who Pays? We All Do: The Cost of Child Maltreatment* (eds K. Franey, R. Geffner, R. Falconer), pp. 53-69, Family Violence and Sexual Assault Institute, San Diego, CA.

Ferguson, H. (2010) Walks, home visits and atmospheres: risk and the everyday practices and mobilities of social work and child protection. *British Journal of Social Work*, **40**, 1100-1117.

Fergusson, D.M., Horwood, J., Lynskey, M.T. (1996) Childhood sexual abuse and psychiatric disorder in young adulthood; II: Psychiatric outcomes of childhood sexual abuse. *Journal American Academy Child Adolescent Psychiatry*, **34**, 1365-1374.

Field, F. (2010) *The Foundation Years: Preventing Poor Children from Becoming Poor Adults*. Cabinet Office, London. Available from: http://www.frankfield.co.uk/review-on-poverty-and-life-chances/ (accessed 8 March, 2011).

Fitzpatrick, P., Molloy, B. & Johnson, Z. (1997) Community mothers' programme: extension to the travelling community in Ireland. *Journal of Epidemiology and Community Health*, **51**(3), 299–303.

Fook, J. & Askeland, G.A. (2006) The 'Critical' in critical reflection. In: *Critical Reflection In Health & Social Care* (eds S. White, J. Fook, F. Gardner). Open University Press, Berkshire.

Fromer, M.J. (1981) *Ethical Issues in Healthcare*. CV Mosby, St Louis.

Frost, M. & Horner, S. (2009) Health visiting. In: *Community Health Care Nursing* (eds D. Sines, M. Saunders & J. Forbes-Burford), 4th edn. Wiley-Blackwell, Chichester.

Gabbay, J. & le May, A. (2004) Evidence-based guidelines or collectively constructed 'mindlines?' Ethnographic study of knowledge management in primary care. *British Medical Journal*, **329**, 1013 (30 October).

Gerrish, K. (2003) Evidence-based practice: unravelling the rhetoric and making it real. *Practice Development in Health Care*, **2**(2), 99–113.

Giddens, A. (2006) *Sociology*, 5th edn. Polity Press, Cambridge.

Gilchrist, A. (2007) *Community Development and Networking for Health*. In: *Public Health for the 21st Century* (eds J. Orme, J. Powell, P. Taylor & M. Grey), 2nd edn, Ch. 8, pp. 135–152. Open University Press McGraw-Hill Education, Maidenhead.

Glaser, D. (2000) Child abuse and neglect and the brain – a review. *Journal of Child Psychology and Psychiatry and Allied Disciplines*, **41**(1), 97–116.

Glass, N. (1999) 'Sure Start: The development of an early intervention programme for young children in the United Kingdom', *Children and Society*, **13**, 257–264.

Glaszious, P., Vandenbroucke, J. & Chalmers, I. (2004) Assessing the quality of research. *British Medical Journal*, **328** (3 January), 39–41.

Goldberg, E.M., Mortimer, A. & Williams, B. (1970) *Helping the Age: a Field Experiment in Social Work*. Allen & Unwin, London.

Gomby, D.S. (1999) Understanding evaluations of home visiting programmes. *Future Child*, **9**, 27–43.

de Graaf, I., Speetjens, P., Smit, F., de Wolff, M. & Tavacchio, L. (2008) Effectiveness of the Triple P- Positive ParentingProgram on behavioural problems in children: meta-analysis. *Behaviour Modification*, **32**(5), 714-35. doi: *10.1177/0145445508317134* Available from: www.triplep.net/cicms/assets/pdfs/pg1as100gr5so142.pdf (accessed 9 March, 2011).

Graham, H. (2007) *Unequal Lives*. Open University Press, Maidenhead.

Gray, J.A.M. (1997) *Evidence-based Healthcare*. Churchill Livingstone, Edinburgh.

Greenwood, J. (1998) On nursing's 'reflective madness'. *Contemporary Nurse*, **7**(1), 3–4.

Greer, S. & Minar, D. (1969) *The Concept of Community*. Aldine Press, Chicago.

Grimshaw, J.M. & Thomson, M.A. (1998) What have new efforts to change professional practice achieved? *Journal of the Royal Society of Medicine*, **S35**(91), 20–25.

Grol, R. & Wensing, M. (2004) What drives change? Barriers to and incentives for achieving evidence-based practice. *The Medical Journal of Australia*. **180**, 15 March, S57–S60.

Gruskin, S. & Tarantola, D. (2004) Health and human rights. In: *Oxford Textbook of Public Health* (eds R. Detels, J. McEwen, R. Beaglehole & H. Tanaka), 4th edn. Oxford University Press, Oxford.

Hall, D.M.B. & Elliman, D. (2006) *Health for All Children*, 4th edn, revised. Oxford University Press, Oxford.

Hall, D.M.B. & Hall, S. (2007) *The 'Family-Nurse Partnership': Developing an Instrument for Identification, Assessment and Recruitment of Clients*. Department for Children, Schools and Families. Ref: DCSF-RW022. Available from: http://www.education.gov.uk/research/data/uploadfiles/DCSF-RW022.pdf (accessed 9 March, 2011).

Hamer, J., Jacobson, B., Flowers, J. & Johnstone, F. (2003) *Health Equity Audit Made Simple: A briefing for Primary Care Trusts and Local Strategic Partnerships. Working Document January 2003*. NICE, London.

Hammersley, M. (2005) Is the evidence-based practice movement doing more good than harm? Reflections on Iain Chalmers' case for research-based policy making and practice. *Evidence and Policy*, **1**(1), 85-100.

Haringey NHS Teaching Primary Care Trust (2004) *Guidelines for Use of New Health Visiting and School Nursing across Haringey TPCT* (authors: J Grant & D Cole). Available from: www.haringey.nhs.uk/.../1789_clinical_records_system_health_visitors_and_school_nurses_1_.pdf (accessed 9 March, 2011).

Hart, J.T. (1971) The Inverse Care Law. *The Lancet*, **I**, 405-412.

Harwin, J. & Madge, N. (2010) The concept of significant harm in law and practice. *Journal of Children's Services*, **5**(2), 73-83.

Health Development Agency (2004a) *Health Needs Assessment*. HDA, NICE, London.

Health Development Agency (2004b) *Clarifying Health Impact Assessment, Integrated Impact Assessment and Health Needs Assessment*. HDA, NICE, London.

Health Select Committee (2009) *Health Inequalities – Third Report*. The Stationery Office, London.

Heaman, M.I., Chalmers, K.I., Woodgate, L. & Brown, J. (2006) Early childhood home visiting programme: factors contributing to success. *Journal of Advanced Nursing*, **55**(3), 291-300.

Heaman, M.I., Chalmers, K.I., Woodgate, R. & Brown, J. (2007) Relationship work in an early childhood home visiting program. *Journal of Paediatric Nursing*, **22**(4), 319-330.

Heath, C. (1986) *Body Movement and Speech in Medical Interaction*. Cambridge University Press, Cambridge.

Heritage, J. & Sefi, S. (1992) Dilemmas of advice: aspects of the delivery and reception of advice in interactions between health visitors and first-time mothers. In: *Talk at Work* (eds P. Drew & J. Heritage), pp. 359-417. Cambridge University Press, Cambridge.

Hillery, G.A. (1955) Definition of community – areas of agreement. *Rural Sociology*, **20** (June), 111-123.

Hillery, G.A. (1982) *Developing and Testing a Community Theory. A Research Odyssey*. Transaction Inc., New Brunswick.

Hilton, S., Petticrew, M. & Hunt, K. (2007) Parents' champions vs. vested interests: who do parents believe about MMR? A Qualitative Study. *BMC Public Health*, 7, 42, published online 28 March, doi 10.1186/1471-2458-7-42.

HM Government (2003) *Every Child Matters*. Presented to Parliament by the Chief Secretary to the Treasury by Command of Her Majesty, September 2003 (Cm 5860). The Stationery Office, London. Available from: http://www.education.gov.uk/consultations/downloadableDocs/EveryChildMatters.pdf (accessed 18 March, 2011).

HM Government (2006) *Reaching Out: An Action Plan on Social Exclusion*. Cabinet Office, Social Exclusion Task Force, London. Available from: http://webarchive.nationalarchives.gov.uk/20061019062131/http://cabinetoffice.gov.uk/social_exclusion_task_force/publications/reaching_out/reaching_out.asp (accessed 4 March, 2011).

Hobbs, P. (1973) *Aptitude or Environment*. Royal College of Nursing, London.

Home Office (1945) *Report by Sir Walter Monckton KCMG KCVO MC KC on the Circumstances which Led to the Boarding Out of Dennis and Terence O'Neill at Bank Farm, Minsterly and the Steps Taken to Supervise Their Welfare*. Cmd 6636 London: Home Office.

Home Office (1998) *Supporting Families: A Consultation Document*. Stationery Office, London.

Hooper, J. & Longworth, P. (2002) *Health Needs Assessment Workbook*. HDA, NICE, London.

Hoskins, R.A.J (2009) Health visiting – the end of a UK service? *Health Policy*, **93**, 93-101.

House of Commons (1990) *The National Health Service and Community Care Act*. HMSO, London.

Howe, D. (2005) *Child Abuse and Neglect: Attachment, Development and Intervention*, Palgrave Macmillan, Basingstoke.

HSC (2009) *Health Inequalities: Third Report of Session 2008-09* Health Select Committee, House of Commons, London. Available from: http://www.publications.parliament.uk/pa/cm200809/cmselect/cmhealth/286/286.pdf (accessed 12 February, 2011).

Hughes, H. (1992) Impact of spouse abuse on children of battered women, *Violence Update*, August, 9-11.

Hulme, P.A. (2000) Symptomatology and health care utilization of women primary care patients who experienced childhood sexual abuse. *Child Abuse Neglect*, **24**, 1471-1484.

Hunt, R. (2009) *Introduction to Community-Based Nursing*, 4th edn. Walters Kluwer, Lippincott Williams & Wilkins, Philadelphia.

Hutching, J., Bywater, T., Daley, D., Gardner, F., Whitaker, C., Jones, K., Eames, C. & Edwards, R.T. (2007) Parenting intervention in Sure Start services for children at risk of developing conduct disorder: pragmatic randomised controlled trial. *British Medical Journal*, **7**(334), 678 doi:10.1136/bmj.39126.620799.55 (published 9 March, 2007).

Hutchinson, S. & Shakespeare, P. (2010) Standard setting, external regulation and professional autonomy: exploring the implications for university education. In: *Education for Future Practice* (eds J. Higgs, D. Fish, I. Goulter, S. Loftus, J. Reid & F. Trede), pp. 75-84. Sense, Amsterdam.

Impicciatore, P., Pandolfini, C., Casella, N. & Bonati, M. (1997) Reliability of health information for the public on the world wide web: systematic survey of advice on managing fever in children at home. *British Medical Journal*, **314**, 1875 (28 June).

Irwin, L., Siddiqi, A., Hertzman, C. (2007) Early child development: a powerful equalizer. *Final Report for the World Health Organization Commission on the Social Determinants of Health*. Available from: http://www.who.int/social_determinants/resources/ecd_kn_report_07_2007.pdf (accessed 10 March, 2011).

ISRCTN Trial registration (2009) *An Evaluation of the Triple P Parent Programme in Birmingham: Support for Parents of 5-11 Year Old Children Displaying Problem Behaviour*. Available from: www.controlled-trials.com/ISRCTN10429692 (accessed 10 March, 2011).

Jack, S.M., DiCenso, A., Lohfeld, L. (2002) A theory of maternal engagement with public health nurses and family visitors. *Journal of Advanced Nursing*, **49**(2), 182-190.

Jefferis, B.J.M.H., Power, C. & Hertzman, C. (2002) Birth weight, childhood socioeconomic environment, and cognitive development in the 1958 British birth cohort study. *British Medical Journal*, **325**, 305.

Johnson, Z., Howell, F., Molloy, B. (1993) Community mothers' programme: randomised controlled trial of non-professional intervention in parenting. *British Medical Journal*, **29**(306), 1449-1452.

Johnson, Z., Molloy, B., Scallan, E., *et al.* (2000) Community Mothers Programme – seven year follow-up of a randomized controlled trial of non-professional intervention in parenting. *Journal of Public Health Medicine*, **22**(3), 337-342.

Joly, L.M.A. (2009) *A mixed method study to explore interagency working to support the health of people who are homeless*. PhD thesis. University College London, London.

Kata, A. (2010) A postmodern Pandora's box: anti-vaccination misinformation on the internet. *Vaccine*, **28**, 1709-1716.

Kelly, M., Morgan, A., Ellis, S., Younger, T., Huntley, J. & Swann, C. (2010) Evidence based public health: a review of the experience of the National Institute of Health and Clinical Excellence (NICE) of developing public health guidance in England. *Social Science & Medicine*, **71**, 1056-1062.

Kempe, H. & Helfer, R.E (1972) *Helping the Battered Child and his Family*. Lippincott, Philadelphia.

Kempe, R.S. & Kempe, H. (1978) *Child Abuse, the Developing Child*. Fontana, London.

Kendall, S. (1993) Do health visitors promote client participation? An analysis of the health visitor-client interaction. *Journal of Clinical Nursing*, **2**(2), 103-109.

Kendall-Tackett, K.A. (2000) Physiological correlates of childhood abuse: Chronic hyperarousal in PTSD, depression and irritable bowel syndrome. Invited review. *Child Abuse & Neglect*, **24**, 799-810.

Kendall-Tackett, K.A. (2002) The health effects of childhood abuse: four pathways by which abuse can influence health. *Child Abuse & Neglect*, **6/7**, 715-730.

Kendall-Tackett, K.A. & Marshall, R. (1999) Victimization and diabetes: An exploratory study. *Child Abuse & Neglect*, **23**, 593-596.

Kerridge, I., Lowe, M. & Henry, D. (1998) Ethics and evidence based medicine. *British Medical Journal*, **316**, 11 April, 1151-1153.

Kitzman, H., Olds, D.L., Henderson, C.R Jr. *et al.* (1997) Effect of prenatal and infancy home visitation by nurses on pregnancy outcomes, childhood injuries, and repeated childbearing. A randomized controlled trial. *Journal of the American Association*, **278**(8), 644-652.

Knai, C. (2009) What is public health? In: G. Thornbory (ed.), *Public Health Nursing: A Textbook for Health Visitors, School Nurses and Occupational Health Nurses*. Wiley-Blackwell, Chichester.

Knight, B. & Hayes, R. (1981) *Self Help in the Inner City*. Voluntary Services Council, London.

Konig, R. (1968) *The Community*. Allen & Unwin, London.

Kretzmann, J.P. & McKnight, J.L. (1993) *Building Communities from the Inside Out: A Path towards Finding and Mobilising a Community's Assets*. Acta Publications, Chicago.

Kristjanson, L. & Chalmers, K.I. (1990) Nurse-client interactions in community based practice: Creating common meaning. *Public Health Nursing*, **7**(4), 215-223.

Krupat, E. & Guild, W. (1980) Defining the city: The use of objective and subjective measures for community description. *Journal of Social Issues*, **36**(3), 9-28.

Laming, Lord H. (2003) *The Victoria Climbié Inquiry: Report of an Inquiry by Lord Laming*, CM5730. The Stationery Office, London.

Laming, Lord H. (2009) *The Protection of Children in England: A Progress Report*. The Stationery Office, London.

Lansley, A. (2010) *Health Committee - Minutes of Evidence Responsibilities of the Secretary of State for Health* Question 38. Available from: http://www.publications.parliament.uk/pa/cm201011/cmselect/cmhealth/380/10072004.htm (accessed 1 March, 2011).

Lantz, P.M., House, J.S., Lepkowski, J.M., Williams, D.R., Mero, R.P. & Chen, J. (1998) Socio-economic factors, health behaviours and mortality *Journal of the American Medical Association*, **279**(21), 1703-1708.

Last, J.M. (2001) *A Dictionary of Epidemiology*. Oxford University Press, Oxford.

Lave, J. & Wenger, E. (2001) *Situated Learning, Legitimate Peripheral Participation*. Cambridge University Press, Cambridge.

Layard, R. & Dunne, J. (2009) *A Good Childhood inquiry: Searching for Values in a Competitive Age*. Penguin Group, London, cited in Y. Roberts, M. Brophy & N. Bacon (2009) *Parenting and Wellbeing: Knitting Families Together*. The Young Foundation, London.

Lock, K. (2000) Health impact assessment. *BMJ*, **320**, 1395-1398, cited in: J. Naidoo & J. Wills (2009) *Foundations for Health Promotion*. 3rd edn. Bailliere Tindall Elsevier, Edinburgh.

Lomax, H. & Robinson, K.S.M. (1998) Evidence base practice: a dilemma for health visiting? In: *The Sociology of the Caring Professions* (eds. P. Abbott & L. Meerabeau), 2nd edn. Routledge, London.

London Borough of Brent (1985) *A Child in Trust. The Report of the Panel of Inquiry Investigating the Circumstances Surrounding the Death of Jasmine Beckford*. London Borough of Brent, London.

Long, A., McCarney, S., Smyth, G., Magorrian, N., Dillon, A. (2001) The effectiveness of parenting programmes facilitated by health visitors. *Journal of Advanced Nursing*, **34**(5), 611-620.

Luker, K.A. (1978) Goal attainment: a possible model for assessing the work of the health visitor. *Nursing Times*, **75**(35), 1488-1490.

Luker, K.A. & Chalmers, K.I. (1990) Gaining access to clients: the case of health visiting. *Journal of Advanced Nursing*, **15**, 74-82.

Luker, K.A. & Orr, J. (eds) (1992) *Health Visiting: Towards Community Health Nursing*. Blackwell Science, Oxford.

Lynch, J.W., Law, C., Brinkman, S., Chittleborough, C. & Sawyer, M (2010) Inequalities in child health development: Some challenges for effective implementation. *Social Science & Medicine*, **71**(4), 1244-1248.

McDonald, K.M., Sundaram, V., Bravata, D. M., *et al.* (2007) *Care Coordination*. Vol. 7 of: *Closing the Quality Gap: A Critical Analysis of Quality Improvement Strategies. Technical Review 9* (eds K.G. Shojania, K.M. McDonald, R.M. Wachter & D.K. Owens). (Prepared by the Stanford University-UCSF Evidence-based Practice Center under contract 290-02-0017), AHRQ Publication No. 04(07)-0051-7, Agency for Healthcare Research and Quality, Rockville, MD.

McDonald, R. & Harrison S. (2004) The micropolitics of clinical guidelines: an empirical study. *Policy and Politics,* **32**(2), 223-239.

McGoldrick, M, Gerson, R, Petry S.S. (2008) Genograms: Assessment and intervention (3rd ed.), W.W. Norton & Co., New York.

McHugh, G. & Luker, K. (2002) Users' perceptions of the health visiting service. *Community Practitioner,* **75**(2), 57-61.

McIntosh, J. (2006) The process of health visiting and its contribution to parental support in the Starting Well demonstration project. *Health and Social Care in the Community*, **15**(1), 77-85.

MacIntyre, S., Chalmers, I., Horton, R. & Smith, R. (2001) Using evidence to inform health policy: a case study. *British Medical Journal*, **322**, January 27, 7280.

MacIver, R.M. & Page, C.H. (1962) *Society. An Introductory Analysis*. Macmillan, London.

McKenna, H., Cutliffe, J. & McKenna, P. (1999) Evidence-based practice: demolishing some myths. *Nursing Standard*, **14**(16), 39-42.

Mackenzie, M. (2008) 'Doing' public health and 'making' public health practitioners: putting policy into practice in 'Starting Well'. *Social Science & Medicine*, **67**(6), 1028-1037. doi:10.1016/j.socscimed.2008.05.021.

McKenzie, M., Shute, J., Berzns, K. & Judge, K. (2004) *The Independent Evaluation of 'Starting Well': Final Report*. Health Promotion Policy Unit, University of Glasgow, Glasgow.

Mackintosh, C. (1998) Reflection: a flawed strategy for the nursing profession. *Nurse Education Today*, **18**(7), 553-557.

McLennan, J.D. & Lavis, J.N. (2006) What is the evidence for parenting interventions offered in a Canadian community? *Canadian Journal of Public Health*, **97**(6), 454-458.

Macmillan, H.L., Thoms, B.H., Jamieson, E., *et al.* (2005). Effectiveness of home visitation by public-health nurses in prevention of the recurrence of child physical abuse and neglect: a randomized controlled trial. *The Lancet*, **365**, 1786-1793.

McNaught, A. (2009) *Leadership in Community Development*, Chapter 12, pp. 165-176. In: *Professional Practice in Public Health* (eds J. Stewart & Y. Cornish). Reflect Press Ltd, Exeter.

Malin, N. & Morrow, G. (2009) Evaluating the role of the Sure Start Plus Advisor in providing integrated support for pregnant teenagers and young parents. *Journal of Health and Social Care in the Community*, **17**(5), 495-503.

Marmot, M. (2006) Status syndrome: a challenge to medicine. *Journal of the American Association*, **295**(11), 1304-1307.

Marmot, M., Atkinson, T., Bell, J., *et al.* (2010) *Fair Society, Healthy Lives. The Marmot Review*. Marmot Review Team, University College London.

Marteau, T.M., Ogilvie, D., Roland, M., Suhrcke, M. & Kelly, M.P. (2011) Judging nudging: can nudging improve population health? *British Medical Journal*, **342**, d228.

Martell, R. (1999) 'Getting it right'. *Community Practitioner*, **72**(5), 121-122.

Maslow, A.H. (1943) A theory of human motivation. *Psychological Review*, **50**(4), 370-396.

Maslow, A.H. (1954) *Motivation and Personality*. Harper, New York.

May, C. (2006) Mobilising modern facts: health technology assessment and the politics of evidence. *Sociology of Health and Illness*, **28**(5), 513-532.

Melhuish, T. & Belsky, J., The National Evaluation of Sure Start Research Team (2008) *The Impact of Sure Start Local Programmes on Three Year Olds and Their Families*. Institute for the Study of Children, Families and Social Issues. University of London, Birkbeck.

Mguni, N. & Bacon, N. (2010) *Taking the Temperature of Local Communities. The Wellbeing and Resilience Measure (WARM)*. The Young Foundation, London.

Midwinter, E. (1973) *Patterns of Community Education*. Ward Lock Publications, London.

Milio, N. (1986) *Promoting Health through Public Policy*. Canadian Public Health Association, Ottawa.

Moore, S., Haines, V., Hawe, P. & Shiell, A. (2006) Lost in translation: a genealogy of the 'social capital' concept in public health. *Journal of Epidemiology and Community Health*, **60**, 729-734.

Moos, R.H. (1976) *The Human Context; Environmental Determinants of Behaviour*. John Wiley & Sons, Inc., New York.

Moos, R.H. (2002) The mystery of human context and coping: an unravelling of clues. *American Journal of Community Psychology*, **30**(1), 67-88.

Morrell, C.J., Slade, P., Warner, R., *et al.* (2009) Clinical effectiveness of health visitor training in psychologically informed approaches for depression in postnatal women: pragmatic cluster randomised trial in primary care. *British Medical Journal*, **338,** a3045; doi 10.1136/bmja3045.

Muir Gray, J.A. (2004) Evidence based policy making: Editorial. *British Medical Journal*, **329**, 988-989.

Mulcahy, H. & McCarthy, G. (2008) Participatory nurse/client relationships: perceptions of public health nurses and mothers of vulnerable families. *Applied Nursing Research*, **21**(3), 169-172.

Mulgan, G. (2010) *Investing in Social Growth. Can the Big Society be More than a Slogan?* The Young Foundation, London.

Mykhalovskiy, E. & Weir, L. (2004) The problem of evidence-based medicine: directions for social science. *Social Science and Medicine*, **59**, 1059-1069.

Naidoo, J. & Wills, J. (2009) *Foundations for Health Promotion*, 3rd edn. Bailliere Tindall Elsevier, Edinburgh.

National Collaborating Centre for Primary Care (2006) *Routine Postnatal Care of Women and Their Babies. NICE Clinical Guideline 37*. NICE, London.

National Evaluation of Sure Start (NESS) (2009) *BBK NESS Site Home Page*. Available from: www.ness.bbk.ac.uk (accessed 9 March, 2011).

National Institute for Health & Clinical Excellence (2007). *Behaviour Change at Population, Community and Individual Levels: Public Health Guidance 6*. NICE, London.

National Institute for Health & Clinical Excellence (2008a) *Community Engagement*. NICE, London.

National Institute for Health & Clinical Excellence (2008b) *Maternal and Child Nutrition*. NICE, London.

National Institute for Health & Clinical Excellence (2009a) *Reducing the Differences in the Uptake of Immunisations*. NICE, London.

National Institute for Health & Clinical Excellence (2009b) *Reducing the Differences in the Uptake of Immunisations: Audit Support*. NICE, London.

National Institute for Health & Clinical Excellence & Social Care Institute for Excellence (2010a) *Looked After Children and Young People*. NICE, London.

National Institute for Health & Clinical Excellence & Social Care Institute for Excellence (2010b) *Strategies to Prevent Unintentional Injuries among Children and Young People Aged Under 15*. NICE, London.

Nettleton, R. (1998) Child protection: health visiting and supervision. In: *Clinical Supervision and Mentorship in Nursing* (eds T. Butterworth, J. Fauguer, P. Burnard), 2nd edn, pp. 132-152. Stanley Thornes, Cheltenham.

NHS Health Development Agency (2004) *Ante-natal and Post-natal Home Visiting Programmes: A Review of Reviews. EVIDENCE BRIEFING* (authors: J. Bull, G. McCormick, C. Swann & C. Mulvihill); available from: http://www.hda.nhs.uk/evidence or https://www.nice.org.uk/niceMedia/documents/home_visiting.pdf (accessed 9 March, 2011).

NHS The Information Centre Workforce and Facilities Team (2010) *NHS Hospital and Community Health Services: Non-medical staff England 1999-2009*. The Health and Social Care Information Centre, London.

NSPCC (2009) *Children Subject to Child Protection Plans - England 2005 - 2009* NSPCC, London. Available from: http://www.nspcc.org.uk/Inform/research/statistics/england_wdf49858.pdf (accessed 30 September, 2010).

Nursing and Midwifery Council (2004) *Standards of Proficiency for Specialist Community Public Health Nurses*. NMC, London.

Nursing and Midwifery Council (2008) *The Code: Standards of Conduct, Performance and Ethics for Nurses and Midwives*. Nursing and Midwifery Council, London.

Nursing and Midwifery Council (2009) *Record Keeping: Guidance for Nurses and Midwives*. NMC, London.

Oakley, A., Strange, V., Bonell, C., Allen, E., Stephenson, J., RIPPLE Study Team. (2006) Process evaluation in randomised controlled trials of complex interventions. *British Medical Journal*, **332**, 413-416, doi:10.1136/bmj.332.7538.413.

O'Dwyer, L.A., Baum, F., Kavanagh, A. & Macdougall, C. (2007) Do area-based interventions to reduce health inequalities work? A systematic review of the evidence. *Critical Public Health*, **17**(4), 317-335, cited in A.K. Draper, G. Hewitt & S. Rifkin (2010)

Chasing the dragon: Developing indicators for assessment of community participation in health programmes. *Social Science & Medicine*, **71**(6), 1102-1109.

Office of Public Sector Information, OPSI (2004) *Carers (Equal Opportunities) Act.* Available from: www.opsi.gov.uk/acts/acts2004/ukpga_20040015_en_1 (accessed 10 March, 2011).

Olds, D.L., Eckenrode, J., Henderson C.R.,Jr. *et al.* (1997) Long-term effects of home visitation on maternal life course and child abuse and neglect. Fifteen year follow-up of a randomized trial. *Journal of the American Association*, 278(8), 637-643.

Olds, D.L., Henderson, C.R., Chamberlin, R. & Tatelbaum, R. (1986) Preventing child abuse and neglect: a randomized trial of nurse home visitation. *Pediatrics*, **78**, 65-78.

Olds, D.L., Henderson, C.R., Jr, Cole, R. *et al.* (1998) Long-term effects of nurse home visitation on children's criminal and antisocial behavior: 15-year follow-up of a randomized controlled trial. *Journal of the American Association*, **280**(14), 1238-1244.

Olds, D.L., Henderson C.R., Jr, Tatelbaum, R. and Chamberlin, R. (1986) Improving the delivery of prenatal care and outcomes of pregnancy: a randomized trial of nurse home visitation. *Pediatrics*, 77(1):16-28.

Olds, D.L, Kitzman, H., Hanks, C. *et al.* (2007) Effects of nurse home visiting on maternal and child functioning: age-9 follow-up of a randomized trial. *Pediatrics*, **120**(4), e832-845.

Olds, D.L., Robinson, J., O'Brien, R. *et al.* (2002) Home visiting by paraprofessionals and by nurses: a randomized controlled trial. *Pediatrics*, **110**(3), 486-496.

Olds, D.L., Robinson, J., Pettitt, L. *et al.* (2004) Effects of home visits by paraprofessionals and by nurses: age 4 follow-up results of a randomized trial. *Pediatrics*, **114**(6), 1560-1568.

Orme, J., Powell, J., Taylor, P. & Grey, M. (2007) Mapping public health. In: *Public Health for the 21st Century: New Perspectives on Policy, Participation and Practice* (eds J. Orme, J. Powell, P. Taylor & M. Grey), 2nd edn. Open University Press, Maidenhead.

Orr, J. (1992a) Assessing individual and family health needs. In: *Health Visiting: Towards Community Health Nursing* (eds K. Luker & J. Orr), pp. 107-158. Blackwell Science, Oxford.

Orr, J. (1992b) The community dimension. In: *Health Visiting: Towards Community Health Nursing* (eds K. Luker & J. Orr), Ch. 2, pp. 43-72. Blackwell Science, Oxford.

Parker, J.M. (2002) Evidence-based nursing: a defence. *Nursing Inquiry, 9*(3), 139-140.

Parton, N. (1997) *Child Protection Risk and the Moral Order*. Macmillan, Basingstoke.

Pearson, L. (2003) Capturing client voices for community development using participatory appraisal. In: *Practice Development in Community Nursing. Principles and Processes* (eds R.M. Bryar & J.M. Griffiths), Ch. 9 pp. 175-193. Arnold, London.

Perry, B. (2002) Childhood experience and the expression of genetic potential: what childhood neglect tells us about nature and nurture. *Brain and Mind*, **3**, 79-100.

Pine, D.S. & Cohen, J.A. (2002) Trauma in children and adolescents: risk and treatment of psychiatric sequelae. *Biological Psychiatry*, **51**(7), 519-531.

Pinheiro, P.S. (2006) *World Report on Violence against Children*. United Nations, New York.

Plastow, L. (2009) Strategic directions for public health nursing. In: *Community Health Care Nursing* (eds D. Sines, M. Saunders & J. Forbes-Burford), 4th edn. Wiley-Blackwell, Chichester.

Poland, B., Lehoux, P., Holmes, D. & Andrews, G. (2005) How place matters: unpacking technology and power in health and social care. *Health and Social Care in the Community*, **13**(2), 170-180.

Prevention Action (2008) *Ireland's Community Mothers Take the Pressure off Family Life*. Available from: http://www.preventionaction.org/what-works/irelands-community-mothers-take-pressure-family-life (accessed 18 August, 2010).

Prinz, R.J., Sanders, M.R, Shapiro, C.J., Whitaker, D.J. & Lutzker, J.R. (2009) Population-based prevention of child maltreatment: the U.S. Triple P system population trial. *Prevention Science,* **10**, 1-12.

Public Health Resource Unit & Skills for Health (2008) *Public Health Skills and Career Framework. Multidisciplinary/Multi-agency/Multi-professional April 2008*. Available from Solutions for Public Health Website*: http://www.sph.nhs.uk/what-we-do/public-health-workforce/outcomes/public-health-skills-and-career-framework/* (accessed 16 March, 2011).

Puffett, N. (2010) Government clarifies ban on *Every Child Matters. Daily Bulletin Children and Young People Now*. 10 August. Available from: http://www.cypnow.co.uk/bulletins/Daily-Bulletin/news/1021116/?DCMP=EMC-DailyBulletin (accessed 30 September, 2010).

Queen's Nursing Institute (2008) *Briefing: Evaluating Outcomes*. QNI, London.

Radford, A. (2009) *Reflections on AI and Their Implications for Sustaining AI as a Way of Life*. www.aradford.co.uk (accessed 23 March, 2011).

Radford, J. (2010) *Serious Case Review under Chapter VIII 'Working Together to Safeguard Children' in Respect of the Death of a Child, Case Number 14*. Birmingham Safeguarding Children Board, Birmingham.

Radley, A. & Billig, M. (1996) Accounts of health and illness: dilemmas and representations. *Sociology and Health and Illness,* **18**(2), 220-240.

Reed, J. (2007) *Appreciative Inquiry – Research for Change*. Sage, London.

Rees, R., Oliver, K., Woodman, J. & Thomas, J. (2009) *Children's Views about Obesity, Body Size, Shape and Weight: A Systematic Review*. EPPI-Centre, London.

Rifkin, S.B. (1985) *Health Planning and Community Participation: Case Studies in Southeast Asia*. Croom Helm Ltd, Beckenham.

Roberts, R., O'Connor, T., Dunn, J., Golding, J. & ALSPAC Study Team (2004) The effects of child sexual abuse in later family life; mental health, parenting and adjustment of offspring. *Child Abuse and Neglect,* **28**, 525-545.

Roberts, Y., Brophy, M., Bacon, N. (2009) *Parenting and Wellbeing: Knitting Families Together*. The Young Foundation, London.

Robinson, J. (1982) *An Evaluation of Health Visiting*. CETHV, London.

Robinson, J. & Elkan, R. (1996) *Health Needs Assessment. Theory and Practice*. Churchill Livingstone, Edinburgh.

Robinson, K.S.M. (1986) *The social construction of health visiting*. PhD thesis, CNAA, Polytechnic of the South Bank.

Royal College of Nursing (2007) *Safeguarding Children and Young People: Every Nurses's Responsibility*. RCN, London.

Royal College of Paediatrics & Child Health (2006) *Safeguarding Children and Young People: Roles and Competences for Health Care Staff. Intercollegiate Document*. RCPCH, London. Available from: www.rcpch.ac.uk/doc.aspx?id_Resource=1535 (accessed 3 February, 2010).

Royal College of Psychiatrists (2004) *Domestic Violence: Its Effects on Children, Factsheet for Parents and Teachers*. Royal College of Psychiatrists, London. Available from: http://www.rcpsych.ac.uk/mentalhealthinfo/mentalhealthandgrowingup/domesticviolence.aspx (accessed 31 August, 2010).

Russell, S. and Drennan, V. (2007) Mothers' views of the health visiting service in the UK: a web-based survey. *Community Practitioner,* **80**(8), 22-26.

Rycroft-Malone, J., Seers, K., Titchen, A., Harvey, G., Kitson, A. & McCormack, B. (2004) What counts as evidence in evidence-based practice? *Journal of Advanced Nursing,* **47**(1), 81–90.

Rycroft-Malone, J., Fontenla, M., Seers, K. & Bick, D. (2009) Protocol-based care: the standardisation of decision -making? *Journal of Clinical Nursing,* **18**, 1490–1500.

Ryan, W. (1976) *Blaming the Victim.* Vintage, New York.

Sackett, D.L., Richardson, W.S., Rosenberg, W. & Haynes, R.B. (1997) *Evidence Based Medicine. How to Practice and Teach EBM.* Churchill Livingstone, Edinburgh.

St Leger, A.S., Schnieden, H. & Walsworth-Bell, J.P. (1992) *Evaluating Health Services' Effectiveness.* Open University Press, Buckingham.

Sanders, M.R. (1999) Triple P-Positive Parenting Program: towards an empirically validated multilevel parenting and family support strategy for the prevention of behavior and emotional problems in children. *Clinical Child Family Psychology Review,* **2**(2), 71–90.

Sanders, M.R. (2008) Triple P-Positive Parenting Programme as a public health approach to strengthening parenting. *Journal of Family Psychology,* **22**(3), 506–517.

Scheeringa, M.S., Wright, M.J., Hunt, J.P. & Zeanah, C.H. (2006) Factors affecting the diagnosis and prediction of PTSD symptoms in children and adolescents. *American Journal of Psychiatry,* **163**, 644–651.

Schön, D. (1983) *The Reflective Practitioner: How Professionals Think in Action.* Temple Smith, London.

Scottish Government (2004) *Independent Evaluation of 'Starting Well' Final Report* (authors: M. Mackenzie, J. Shute, K. Berzins, K. Judge). Available from: www.scotland. gov.uk/Publications/2005/04/20890/55054 (accessed 26 August, 2010).

Scottish Government (2005) *Detailed Plan for Phase Two of the National Health Demonstration Project Starting Well.* Available from: www.scotland.gov.uk (accessed 26 August, 2010).

Scriven, A. (2010) *Promoting Health. A Practical Guide.* Balliere Tindall Elsevier, Edinburgh.

Shaw, E., Levitt, C., Wong, S., Kaczorowski, J., & The McMaster University Postpartum Research Group (2006) Systematic review of the literature on postpartum care: Effectiveness of postpartum support to improve maternal parenting, mental health, quality of life, and physical health. *Birth,* **33**(3), 210–220.

Shorter Oxford English Dictionary (1973) Clarendon Press, Oxford.

Shute, J.L. & Judge, K. (2005) Evaluating 'Starting Well', the Scottish national demonstration project for child health: outcomes at six months. *Journal of Primary Prevention,* **26**(3), 221–240.

Sirkin, S., Iacopeno, V., Grodin, M.A. & Danieli, Y. (2005) The role of health professionals in protecting and promoting human rights. In: *Perspectives on Health and Human Rights* (eds S. Gruskin, M.A. Grodin, S.P. Marks & G.J. Annas), Routledge, Abingdon.

Skills for Care & Children's Workforce Development Council (2007) *Providing Effective Supervision: A Workforce Development Tool, Including a Unit of Competence and Supporting Guidance.* Skills for Care and Children's Workforce Development Council, Leeds.

Skills for Health (2004) *National Occupational Standards for the Practice of Public Health Guide.* Skills for Health, Bristol.

Skills for Health (2008) *Public Health Skills and Career Framework,* Skills for Health, Bristol.

Smith, M.A. (2004) Health visiting: the public health role. *Journal of Advanced Nursing,* **45**(1), 17–25.

Smith, M.K. (2003, 2009) Communities of practice, *the encyclopaedia of informal education*. Available from: www.infed.org/biblio/communities_of_practice.htm (accessed 19 November, 2010).

Smith, R. (2010) *A Universal Child?* Palgrave Macmillan, Basingstoke.

SmithBattle, L., Diekemper, M. & Leander, S. (2004) Moving upstream: Becoming a public health nurse, Part 2. *Public Health Nursing*, **21**(2), 95–102.

Somerville, D. & Keeling, J. (2004) A practical approach to promote reflective practice within nursing. Available from: www.nursingtimes.net/204502.article (accessed 3 March, 2011).

South East Wales Trials Units (SEWTU) (undated website) *Evaluating the Family Nurse Partnership in England: A Randomised Controlled Trial (Building Blocks Study)*. Dr Mike Robling Chief Investigator, Cardiff_University. Available from: http://medic.cardiff.ac.uk/archive_subsites/_/_/medic/subsites/buildingblocks/index.html (accessed 26 July, 2010).

Speller, V., Learmonth, A. & Harrison, D. (1997) The search for evidence of effective health promotion. *British Medical Journal*, **315**, 361–363.

Spijkers, W., Jansen, D., de Meer, G. & Reijneveld, S.A. (2010) Effectiveness of a parenting programme in a public health setting: a randomised controlled trial of the positive parenting programme (Triple P) level 3 versus care as usual provided by the preventive child healthcare (PCH). *BMC Public Health*, **10**, 131 (published online 15 March, 2010), doi: 10.1186/1471-2458-10-131.

Srivastava, P., Fountain, R., Ayre, P. & Stewart, J. (2003) The Graded Care Profile: a measure of care. In: *Assessment in Child Care: Using & Developing Frameworks for Practice* (eds M.C. Calder & S. Hackett), Russell House Publishing, Lyme Regis.

Starfield, B. (1996) Public health and primary care: A framework for proposed linkages. *American Journal of Public Health*, **86**(10), 1365–1369.

Starting Well Demonstration Project (undated) Available from: www.gorbalslive.org.uk/data/community/.../startingwell.htm (accessed 26 August, 2010).

Stewart, J., Cornish, Y., Patel, S. (2009) Health needs assessment. In: *Professional Practice in Public Health* (eds J. Stewart & Y. Cornish), Ch. 10, pp. 133–147. Reflect Press Ltd, Exeter.

Suchman, E.A. (1967) *Evaluation Research*. Russell Sage Foundation, New York.

Swann, B. & Brocklehurst, N. (2004) Three in one: the Stockport model of health visiting. *Community Practitioner*, **77**(7), 251–256.

Sweet, M. (2004) Development of strategies to encourage adoption of best evidence into practice in Australia: workshop overview. *Medical Journal of Australia*, **180**(6) Supplement, S45–S47.

Sweet, M.A. & Applebaum, M.I. (2004) Is home visiting an effective strategy? A meta-analytic review of home visiting programs for families with young children. *Child Development*, **75**(5), 1435–1456. doi: 10.1111/j.1467-8624.2004.00750.

Symonds, A. (1991) Angels and interfering busy bodies: the social construction of two occupations. *Sociology of Health & Illness*, **13**, 249–264.

Talley, N.J., Fett, S.L. & Zinsmeister, A.R. (1995) Self-reported abuse and gastrointestinal disease in outpatients: Association with irritable bowel-type symptoms. *American Journal of Gastroenterology*, **90**, 366–371.

Taylor, C. & White, S. (2000) *Practising Reflexivity in Health and Welfare*. Open University Press, Buckingham.

Teegen, F. (1999) Childhood sexual abuse and long-term sequelae. In: *Posttraumatic Stress Disorder: A Lifespan Developmental Perspective* (eds A. Maercker, M. Schutzwohl & Z. Solomon), pp. 97–112. Hogrefe & Huber, Seattle.

Thaler, R.H. & Sunstein, C.R. (2008) *Nudge: Improving Decisions about Health, Wealth, and Happiness*. Yale University Press, London.

Thomas, B., Dorling, D. & Davy Smith, G. (2010) Inequalities in premature mortality in Britain: Observational study from 1921 to 2007. *British Medical Journal*, **341**, C3639.

Tönnies, F. (1955; first published 1887) *Community and Association*. Routledge & Kegan Paul, London.

Traynor, M. (2002) The oil crisis, risk and evidence-based practice. *Nursing Inquiry*, **9**(3), 162-169.

Traynor M., Boland, M. & Buus, N. (2010) Autonomy, evidence and intuition: nurses and decision-making. *Journal of Advanced Nursing*, **66**(7), 1584-1591.

Tucker, W.H. (1979) The nature of a community. In: *Community Health Care and the Nursing Process* (ed. M.J. Fromer). C.V. Mosby, St Louis.

Twinn, S. & Cowley, S. (1992) *Principles of Health Visiting: A Re-examination*. CPHVA, London.

UKPHA (2009) *Health Visiting Matters: Re-establishing Health Visiting* UKPHA, London. Available from: http://www.ukpha.org.uk/media/14945/health%20visiting%20matters%20final%20report.pdf (accessed 26 February, 2011).

UN (1948) *United Nations Universal Declaration on Human Rights*, United Nations, New York. Available from: http://www.un.org/en/documents/udhr/index.shtml#a25 (accessed 6 March, 2011).

UN (1966) *United Nations International Covenant on Economic, Social and Cultural Rights*, United Nations, New York. Available from: http://www.un-documents.net/icescr.htm (accessed 6 March, 2011).

UN (2000) *United Nations Millennium Declaration* United Nations, New York. Available from: http://www.un.org/millennium/ (accessed 28 February, 2011).

UNICEF (1989) *The United Nations Convention on the Rights of the Child*. United Nations International Children's Emergency Fund. Available from: http://www2.ohchr.org/english/law/crc.htm (accessed: 16 January, 2011).

UNICEF (2009) *The State of the World's Children 2009 Report*. United Nations International Children's Emergency Fund. Available from: http://www.unicef.org/sowc09/ (accessed 2 March, 2011).

UNICEF (2010) *Progress For Children: Achieving the MDGs with Equity*, United Nations International Children's Emergency Fund. Available from: http://www.unicef.org/publications/files/Progress_for_Children-No.9_EN_081710.pdf (accessed 2 March, 2011).

Unite (2009) *Press Release – Fall in Health Visitor Numbers is 'A National Scandal', Nursing Commission Told*. Available from: http://www.unitetheunion.org/news__events/latest_news/health_visitor_crisis_is_a_na.aspx (accessed 1 March, 2011).

Unite/CPHVA (2007) *Record Keeping and the Law*. Unite/CPHVA, London.

Unite/CPHVA (2008) *Omnibus Survey*. Unite/Community Practitioners and Health Visitors Association, London.

Unite/CPHVA (2009a) *Regulatory Issues and the Future Legal Status of the Health Visitor Title and Profession*. Unite/Community Practitioners' and Health Visitors' Association, London.

Unite/CPHVA (2009b) *What Size Caseload Should a Health Visitor Have?* Unite/CPHVA, London.

United Kingdom Public Health Association (UKPHA) (2009) *Health Visiting Matters: Re-establishing Health Visiting*. Available from: www.ukpha.org.uk (accessed 10 March, 2011).

UNOCINI (2008) *Guidance*. Understanding the Needs of Children in Northern Ireland. Available from: http://www.welbni.org/index.cfm/go/publications/key/6832628E-09E1-D43F-4F0E0109B9D314BD:1 (accessed 10 March, 2011).

Van der Kolk, B.A. (1984) *Post-Traumatic Stress Disorders: Psychological and Biological Sequelae*. American Psychiatric Press, Washington D.C.

Verweij, M. & Dawson, A. (2009) The meaning of 'public' in 'public health'. In: *Ethics, Prevention, and Public Health* (eds A. Dawson & M. Verweij), Oxford University Press, Oxford.

Wakefield, A.J., Murch, S.H., Anthony, A. *et al.* (1998) Ileal-lymhoid-nodular hyerplasia, non-specific colitis, and pervasive developmental disorder in children. *Lancet*, **351**, 737-641.

Wasoff, F. & Hill, M. (2002) Family Policy in Scotland. *Social Policy and Society*, **1**(3), 171-182.

Watson, M., Kendrick, D., Coupland, C., Woods, A., Futers, D. & Robinson, J. (2004) Providing child safety equipment to prevent injuries: randomised controlled trial. *British Medical Journal*, doi:10.1136/bmj.38309.664444.8F.

Watt, G. (2002) The inverse care law today. *The Lancet*, **360**(9328), 252-254.

Weaver, B.R. (1977) Conceptual basis for nursing intervention with human systems: communities and societies. In: *Distributive Nursing Practice: a Systems Approach to Community Health* (eds J.E. Hall. & B.R. Weaver), J.B. Lippincott Co., Philadelphia.

Weed, L.L. (1969) *Medical Records, Medical Education and Patient Care*. Press of Case Western Reserve University, Ohio.

Weiner, R. (1975) *The Rape and Plunder of the Shankhill*. Notarms Press, Belfast.

Welsh Assembly Government (undated) *Flying Start Health Visiting Core Programme – Play, Learn, Grow*. Available from: http://www.wales.nhs.uk/site-splus/866/opendoc/140318/&47125823-1143-E756-5C54492FA3987A90 (accessed 10 March, 2011).

Wenger, E. (1998) *Communities of Practice, Learning, Meaning and Identity*. Cambridge University Press, Cambridge.

Wenger E. (2006) *Communities of Practice*. Available from: http://www.ewenger.com/theory/index.htm (pp. 1-5; accessed 4 August, 2010).

While, A., Forbes, A., Ullman, R. & Murgatroyd, B. (2005) *The Contribution of Nurses, Midwives and Health Visitors to Child Health and Child Health Services: a Scoping Review*. NCCSDO, London.

White, R., Carr, P. & Lowe, N. (2002) *The Children Act in Practice*, 3rd edn. Butterworths, London.

Whitehead, M. & Dahlgren, G. (2006) *Concepts and Principles for Tackling Social Inequities in Health: Levelling Up Part 1*, World Health Organisation, Regional Office, Copenhagen. Available from: http://www.enothe.eu/cop/docs/concepts_and_principles.pdf (accessed 6 March, 2011).

Whitlock, E.P., O'Connor, E.A., Williams, S.B., Beil, T.L. and Lutz, K.W. (2008) *Effectiveness of Weight Management Programs in Children and Adolescents*. Agency for Healthcare Research and Quality, Rockville, MD USA.

Whitlock, E.P., O'Connor, E.A., Williams, S.B., Beil, T.L. and Lutz, K.W. (2010) Effectiveness of weight management interventions: a targeted systematic review for the USPSTF. *Paediatrics*, **125**(2):e396-418. Epub 2010, 18 Jan.

Wiggins, M., Rosata, M., Ausaterberry, H., Sawtell, M. & Olicwe, S. (2005) *Supporting Teenagers Who Are Pregnant or Parents: Sure Start Plus National Evaluation: Final Report*. Social Science Research Unit, Institute of Education, University of London, London. Available from: www.ioe.ac.uk/ssru/reports/ssplusevaluationfinalreport.pdf (accessed 10 March, 2011).

Wilson, P. (2002) How to find the good and avoid the bad or ugly: a short guide to tools for rating quality of health information on the internet. *British Medical Journal*, **324**, 9 March, 598-602.

Wilson, P., Thompson, L., Puckering, C., *et al.* (2010) Parent–child relationships: are health visitors' judgements reliable? *Community Practitioner*, **83**(5), 22-25.

Wohl, A.S. (1986) *Endangered Lives: Public Health in Victorian England*. Dent, London.

Woodgate, R.L., Heaman, M.I., Chalmers, K.I. & Brown, J. (2007) Issues related to delivering an early childhood home visiting program. *American Journal of Maternal and Child Health Nursing*, **32**(2), 95-101.

World Health Organization (WHO) (1946) *Constitution of the World Health Organization*, New York, 22 July 1946, World Health Organization, Geneva.

World Health Organization/UNICEF (1978) *Declaration of Alma Ata*. WHO, Geneva. Available from: www.who.int/NPH/docs/declaration_almaata.pdf (accessed 10 October, 2010).

World Health Organization (1986) *Ottawa Charter for Health Promotion*. World Health Organization, Geneva.

World Health Organization (2008) *Primary Health Care: Now More than Ever*. WHO, Geneva.

World Health Organization (2011) *Social Determinants of Health: Key Concepts*. Commission on Social Determinants of Health, World Health Organization, Geneva. Available from: http://www.who.int/social_determinants/thecommission/finalreport/key_concepts/en/index.html (accessed 7 March, 2011).

World Health Organization (WHO) & International Society for Prevention of Child Abuse and Neglect (2006) *Preventing Child Maltreatment: A Guide to Taking Action and Generating Evidence*. World Health Organization and International Society for Prevention of Child Abuse and Neglect, Geneva. Available from: http://whqlibdoc.who.int/publications/2006/9241594365_eng.pdf (accessed 20 March, 2011).

Worth, A. & Hogg, R. (2000) A qualitative evaluation of the effectiveness of health visiting practice. *British Journal of Community Nursing*, **221**(5), 224-228.

Wright, C.M., Jeffrey, S.K., Ross, M.K., Wallis, L. & Wood, R. (2009) Targeting health visitors: lessons from Starting Well. *Archives of Disease in Childhood*, **94**(1), 23-27.

Wright, L.M. & Leahy, M. (1994) *Nurses and Families: A Guide to Family Assessment and Intervention*. FA Davis, Philadelphia.

Young, M. & Willmott, P. (2007 (1957)) *Family and Kinship in East London*. Penguin Modern Classics, London.

Young Foundation (2010) *How Can Neighbourhoods Be Understood and Defined?* The Young Foundation, London.

Young Foundation (2011) *Community Action Toolkit*. Available from: www.youngfoundation.org/community-action-tool-kit (accessed 13 March, 2011).

Index

access to services, 95, 100-101, 106, 127, 131, 230
Alma Ata Declaration, 86
assessment
    health needs, 101, 103, 106-110
    Joint Strategic Needs, 5, 75, 101-102
    vulnerable children, 186-190
Association of Public Health
        Observatories, 4, 110, 221, 242
    Public Health Observatories, 5, 219
audit, 20, 26, 39, 101, 137, 143, 206, 209, 223, 232

Bandura, 134, 228
Big Society, 5, 93
Breastfeeding, 63, 68, 74, 110, 149, 207, 221, 242

CAF, see also Common Assessment
        Framework
caseload, 95, 134, 171, 175, 187-188, 196, 222
census information, 108, 221
child
    abuse, 173-179
        health impact, 177-178
        incidence 182-185
        neglect, 176-177
            Graded Care Profile, 190
        prevalence, 182-185
        significant harm, 179-182
            threshold criteria, 180
        working together, 190-197
    behaviour, 128-129, 233-235
    definition, 165-167
    safety, 148, 152
    vulnerable assessment, 186-190
Child and Maternal Health Observatory, 108, 221, 242
child-centred, 122-123, 170
Child Development Programme, 130-131
    evaluation, 131

child health
    programme assessment, 129
childhood
    definition, 167-168
Children Act, 166, 168, 172, 174-175, 179, 181-182, 186, 190, 193
children in need, 185-189
children's centres, 5, 15, 75, 93, 102, 134, 140, 152
citizen participation, 112
client/health visitor relationship, 146-149, 168, 193
clients' views, 40-46
Common Assessment Framework, 126, 152, 188-190
Communities of Practice, 6, 10, 35-37, 41
community
    definition, 86-88
    development, 67, 86, 95, 109, 111, 141, 145, 152
    impact on health, 89-94
    knowing your community, 101-104
    participation, 112-113
    social climate, 90-92
    theory, 88
    working with communities, 94-101
Community Health Partnerships, 2
Community Mothers' Programme, 131-132, 142
Community Practitioners' and Health
        Visitors' Association, 2, 70, 168, 222, 232
community-based interventions, 85, 112
community-level interventions, 85
confidentiality, 192-193, 224
CPHVA, see also Community
        Practitioners' and Health
        Visitors' Association

data, see also information sources
Data Protection Act, 189, 192
data sources, 40-41, 108, 221

Health Visiting: A Rediscovery, Third Edition. Edited by Karen A. Luker, Jean Orr
and Gretl A. McHugh.
© 2012 Blackwell Publishing Ltd. Published 2012 by Blackwell Publishing Ltd.

deprivation, 62, 76, 93, 110
determinants of health, 4, 72-74, 85,
    92-93, 109, 229
    Dahlgren & Whitehead: Main
        Determinants of Health, 72, 92
domestic abuse, 67-68, 181-182, 204

early home visiting programmes, 130-132
empowerment, 57, 109, 111
environmental influences, 3, 54, 60,
    72-73, 90, 134, 166, 187
evaluation
    care planning, 214-215
        process, 216-217
    concepts, 210-214
    current emphasis, 205-206
    definitions, 209-210
    evaluation research, 217-227
        structure evaluation, 221
        process evaluation, 222-224
        outcome evaluation, 224-227
    example
        weight management, 211-214
    goal attainment, 214-217, 224-227
    record keeping, 231-235
evaluation research, 217-227
evidence
    debate, 44-46
    health visiting, 14-15, 227-231
    sources of, 45, 51, 108-109, 206-207,
        221, 240
evidence based medicine, 16-22
    concepts, 20
    debates, 18-21
    definition, 21-22
evidence based practice,
    barriers, 24-25
    concept, 25-26
    debates, 11-12, 21-35, 44-46
    practice, 16-18
    redefining, 25-26
    translation, 11-12

family
    models of intervention, 121-126
        child-centred, 122-123
        family-centred, 123
        ecological, 122-125, 134, 143
        application, 125-126
        evidence, 128-145, 150
    support, 120, 145-147-149
    public health, 149-150
Family Nurse Partnership, 7, 61, 75, 121,
    124, 127, 130, 132-136
    background, 132-133
    characteristics of programme, 134, 144
    evaluation, 134-136

Flying Start - Wales, 136-137, 143-144
    background, 136-137
    characteristics of programme, 137
    evaluation, 137
Framework for the Assessment of
        Children in Need and their
        Families, 186-188

General Practice consortia, 2
genogram, 123-124, 160-161
GCP see also Graded Care Profile
GP consortia, see also General Practice
        consortia
Graded Care Profile, 7, 190
Guidelines, 6, 18-19, 27-34, 206-207,
    221, 239
    National Institute for Health and
        Clinical Excellence, 19, 50, 108,
        206, 221
    Scottish Intercollegiate Guidelines
        Network, 19, 50, 221

health
    definition, 56-58
    determinants of health, 4, 73-74,
        92-93, 109, 229
    inequalities, 6, 53-54, 60-61, 62, 64-78
    influences, 93-94
    profiles, 109-110
    surveillance, 16, 70, 96-98, 117-118, 127,
        131, 183
health care, 3, 5, 33, 40, 63
Health Equity Audit, 101
Health Impact Assessment, 101, 108
Health Improvement, 57-61, 65, 67, 76-77,
    97, 111, 133, 142, 145
health needs assessment, 101, 103,
    106-110
health promotion, 5, 11, 20, 57-59, 66, 83,
    127-128, 211-213, 222-223,
    228-229
    child-health programmes, 142-145
    models, 110-113
health visiting
    role, 3, 11-16, 94-101, 126-127, 228-231
    public health, 3-6, 20-21, 27-28, 52-61,
        70-71, 85-86, 94-99, 122,
        126-128, 149-50
    prevention, 66, 123, 127-128, 216,
        228-229
    principles of practice, 66-71
    practice, 11-12, 54-59, 65-71, 94-101, 111
        effectiveness, 98, 136, 141, 164, 171,
            196-197, 207-213, 217, 219,
            227-230
        ethical principles, 65
    communities, 94-101

health visiting (*cont'd*)
  standards of proficiency, 70-71, 96-97,
    172-173, 208-209
  competencies, 96-99
health visiting service, 3, 11, 75-76, 94,
    99-100, 124, 186, 196, 211
  access, 95, 100-101, 106, 127, 131, 230
  challenges, 149-153
  community interactions, 99-100
  implementation plans, 5, 54, 99-100,
    101-102, 222, 235-236
  universal, 3, 73, 99-100, 125, 127-130,
    168
  universal partnership 99-100
  universal plus, 99-100
health visitors
  caseload, 95, 134, 171, 175, 187-188,
    196, 222
  leadership, 3, 6, 70-71, 112-113, 117, 163,
    165, 188-189, 195-196, 208
  partnership, 3-4, 23, 58-59, 62, 78,
    95-97, 106-107, 112, 127-128, 145,
    148-150, 166, 169, 193, 228
  role, 3, 11-16, 94-101, 126-127, 228-231
Healthy Child Programme, 3, 54, 60-61,
    77-78, 100, 126, 128, 230
home visit, 12-13, 15, 123, 125, 128-132, 134,
    136-138, 140, 142-143, 146,
    148-152, 162, 207, 230, 232, 234

immunisation, 78, 129, 131, 141-142, 192,
    206-207, 210, 219, 223, 230
inequalities in health, 6, 53-54, 60-61,
    62, 64-78
  Marmot review, 4, 6, 53-54, 73-75, 106,
    108-109, 120, 123, 127-128, 168,
    215, 229
information sharing, 192-193
information sources, 107-110, 219-221, 240
  collection, 31-32, 103-108
interventions
  focussed programmes, 128-132, 137-139,
    180-181
  health visiting, 145-146, 207-208
  threshold for, 180-181, 204
  weight management, 213

Joint Strategic Needs Assessment, 5, 75,
    101-102

knowledge
  clients, 40-44
  communication, 13-16
  define, 10-11
  generation, 27-28, 46
  managing, 4, 27-35, 46
  reflective practice, 6, 36-40, 45, 195

  type, 10
Korner report, 223

leadership, 3, 6, 70-71, 98-99, 112-113, 117,
    163, 165, 188-189, 195-196, 208
libertarian paternalism, 76-77
lifecourse, 54, 73-74
local authority, 2-3, 68, 75, 78, 106, 136,
    179, 186

Marmot review, 4, 6, 53-54, 73-75, 106,
    108-109, 120, 123, 127-128, 168,
    215, 229
models
  child-centred, 122-123, 170
  ecological, 60, 122-125, 134, 143
  family-centred, 122-123, 127, 152
  health promotion, 110-113

National Health Service, 1, 2, 6, 75, 78, 95,
    128-130, 193, 205-206, 208
  Careers Framework, 98-99
  Connecting for Health, 6
  NHS Commissioning Board, 2
  Plan, 2
National Institute for Health and Clinical
    Excellence, 19, 50, 108, 206, 221
needs, 104-106
  Bradshaw's taxonomy, 106
  comparative, 105-106
  expressed, 105
  felt, 105
  Maslow's hierarchy, 190
  normative, 105
neighbourhood, 12, 87-93, 101-102, 107,
    119, 124, 128, 168, 215, 221
NHS, *see also* National Health Service
NICE, *see also* National Institute for
    Health and Clinical Excellence
Nursing Midwifery Council, 2, 9, 19, 65,
    70-71, 95, 99, 164, 223-224
  Code of Conduct, 64-65, 173, 193
  Standards of Proficiency, 70-71, 96-99,
    172-173, 208-209

obesity, 4, 74, 178, 213, 216, 221, 229
Office for National Statistics, 219, 221
outcome evaluation, 224-227

Patient Related Outcomes Measures, 210,
    219, 221
partnership, 3-4, 23, 58-59, 62, 78,
    95-97, 106-107, 112, 127-128, 145,
    148-150, 166, 169, 193, 228
PCTs, *see also* Primary Care Trusts
primary care, 27, 30, 32-33, 75, 86, 94,
    128, 133, 206, 221

Primary Care Trusts, 2, 30, 101, 123, 133, 136, 142, 145
principles of health visiting, 66-70, 77-78, 84-85, 95-97, 127
principles of public health, 77, 228
problem-orientated recording, 232-235
  example
    behaviour management, 233-235
problems
  actual, 215-216,
  potential, 14-15, 215-216, 226, 233
  problem-solving, 35, 214, 216-217, 232
process evaluation, 150, 219, 222-224
PROMS, see also Patient Related
    Outcome Measures
public
  definition, 55-56
Public Health
  definition, 58-61
  England, 2-4, 75
  family-centred role, 126-128, 152
  human rights, 62-65
  ideological perspective, 58-61, 77
  policy, 3-4, 52
  skills, 96-99
  vision, 3-5
  Wales, 2
Public Health Skills Framework, 96-97, 99
public health walk, 102-103, 118

record keeping, 223, 21-235, 242
  audit, 223-224, 232
  problem-orientated recording, 232-235
    example, behaviour management,
    233-235
reflective practice, 6, 10, 36-40, 45, 195
  definition, 37-39

safeguarding children, 163-197
  Common Assessment Framework, 126,
    152, 188-190
  definition, 168-172
  policy, 166-172, 188-189
  working together, 190-197
    information sharing, 192-193
    confidentiality, 192-193
Scottish Intercollegiate Guidelines
    Network, 19, 50, 221
self-care, 3, 205, 227
skill-mix, 99, 118, 127, 132, 150, 205, 222
SIGN, see also Scottish Intercollegiate
    Guidelines Network
significant harm, 7, 169-170, 179-182, 187,
    189, 193, 204

SMART approach, 210, 214-215, 233,
    235, 241
smoking cessation, 4, 74, 30, 74, 94,
    110,142, 149, 150, 221
SOAP recording, 232-235, 242
social capital, 91-93, 111, 153
social climate, 90-91
social networking sites, 6, 41-44, 177
social worker, 99, 106, 121-122, 165, 175,
    179, 187, 231
Starting Well, 124. 137-139. 144. 151
structure evaluation, 219, 222
supervision, 164-165, 180-181, 193-197
Sure Start, 53-54, 61, 76, 95, 134, 140-145,
    151-152, 209
  Children-s Centres, 54, 95, 134, 140,
    144-145, 152

teenage pregnancy, 4, 110, 133
Triple P Programme, 137, 139-140, 144

UNICEF, 53, 163, 170
United Nations Convention on the Rights
    of the Child, 53, 62-64, 163, 166,
    169-171
universal partnership, 99-100
universal plus, 99-100
universal service, 3, 73, 99-100, 125,
    127-130, 168
universalism
  progressive, 127-128, 144, 168, 215
  proportionate, 73, 128, 153, 168,
    215

vulnerable children, 171-173, 180-183,
    186-190
  assessment, 186-190
    Common Assessment Framework,
    126, 152, 188-190
    Framework for the Assessment of
    Children in Need and Their
    Families, 186-188
    Graded Care Profile, 190

windshield survey, 101-102
working together, 190-197
working with communities, 5, 85, 91,
    94-110, 112
workload, 176, 190, 219-220
World Health Organisation
  Alma Ata, 86
  health definition, 56-57
  maltreatment of children, 170
  sources of statistics, 109